KU-497-268

Eat **Well** Live **Long**

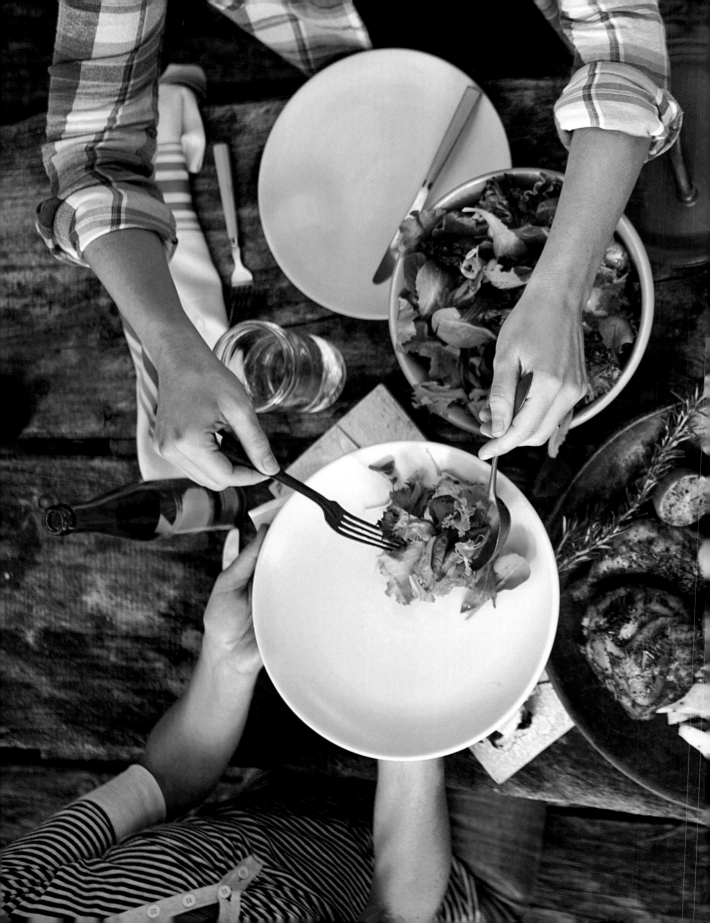

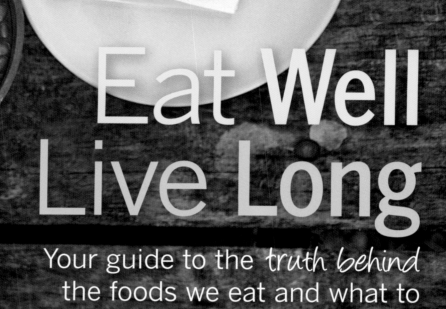

Eat Well
Live Long

Your guide to the *truth behind* the foods we eat and what to choose for *optimum health*

Reader's
Digest

Contents

While the creators of this work have made every effort to be as accurate and up to date as possible, food science and medical knowledge are constantly changing. Readers are advised to consult a qualified nutritionist or medical specialist for individual advice. The writers, researchers, editors and publishers of this work cannot be held liable for any errors and omissions, or actions that may be taken as a consequence of information contained within this work.

Food matters!

Was there ever an age in the modern world when food was so readily available and such a source of interest? We should all be so healthy, so what has gone wrong? Finding out will put you on the path to life-long wellbeing.

Supermarket choice is overwhelming. Restaurants surround us. Food can be bought at pharmacies, petrol stations, bookstores, cinemas, department stores, fitness centres – almost everywhere that people congregate. Cooking programs, glossy magazines, TV advertising and luscious-looking cookbooks bombard us with images of beautiful meals and extravagant feasts. At the same time, doctors, diet gurus and government advisers issue dire health warnings about most of the food we eat. It's all so confusing and contradictory.

That is why this book is so important at this time. It is a clear, fresh and frequently surprising guide to the increasingly complex world of everyday food – the meals, snacks and drinks that most of us consume. It cuts through the clamour of competing interests with one simple message – good, nutritious food is worth seeking out. Why? Because it's delicious, fresh and made from natural or near-natural ingredients, which will promote your good health and that of your family. It will help you live longer. It will make you feel well, help keep you active, combat excess weight and may also protect you against diseases of older age such as dementia.

What our bodies don't need

Finding such food should not be a difficult task. Once upon a time, dairy products or meat were fresh from source; fruit and vegetables came from nearby orchards and farms. But today when so much of what we eat has been sprayed, processed, frozen or manipulated in some other way, there is a clear need for expert, unbiased information about what's good for us and what is not – which *Eat Well, Live Long* supplies.

To make this book and achieve that goal, Reader's Digest assembled a team of leading international nutritionists and food writers, who understand precisely what goes into modern food products and also how such ingredients influence our health. Now that three quarters of all foods sold across the world are processed rather than fresh, these are vital facts we need to know.

While 'processing' can be as minimal as washing leaves or peeling a fruit, it may also strip out nutrients from foods such as grains, while adding any number of preservatives, flavourings, colours, sugar, salt, emulsifiers, gelling agents, thickeners and more. The more highly processed a food, the less likely it is to contain wholesome, natural ingredients. The added extras disguise the fact that popular fast foods – burgers, chicken nuggets, frozen pizza and pasta dishes – are often made out of 'cheap parts or remnants of animal foods,' as a 2013 article in the respected medical journal *The Lancet* explained.

We buy these foods for convenience and also because their sugar, salt and fat appeal to our taste buds; humans are programmed to enjoy – some say even crave – them. In many households today across the Western world, few fresh foods are eaten; ready meals and fast foods are the everyday norm. It is a seemingly unstoppable trend that is driving obesity and global epidemics of diabetes, cancers, stroke and heart disease, as an increasing number of population studies have revealed. Why? Because fast foods and processed snacks typically supply fattening kilojoules but little fibre and few of the vitamins, minerals and other important nutrients that contribute to our wellbeing.

Make the right choices

Fighting back against the commercial juggernaut is the most important thing you can do for your own health and the health of your family. *Eat Well, Live Long* provides the tools and knowledge to do just that. In Parts 1 to 3, you'll find out how food and drink have been industrialised over the last 50 years and the five food enemies of good health that are best avoided. Most importantly you'll discover the five key 'friends' – that not only taste wonderful but also strengthen our bodies and protect against disease. These include luscious fruits, crunchy wholegrain cereals, delectable olive oil, lean protein, water and a little wine. This is not a book devoid of treats. A little of what you fancy – take dark chocolate, for instance – can do you good.

Part 4, 'Easy steps to transform your diet' is packed with tips and strategies to help you shop, cook quick and easy nutritious daily meals, accommodate special diets and control your weight. Then, to help you make the soundest everyday choices – for flavour and good nutrition – Part 5, 'Your live-long food guide' reveals the best (and worst) meats, fish, dairy foods, fresh produce, pasta, grains, snacks, drinks and even restaurant meals and takeaways.

Eat Well, Live Long is a timely book. It is a modern paradox that scientific research has taught us so much more than our grandparents knew about nutrition and health, but most of us are not actually healthier. How did that happen? Surely multinational food companies would want to work with government health experts to ensure that what we eat and drink keeps us well? So why do they encourage the creation of an ever vaster range of tempting sweet and fatty foods and why do they market them so aggressively – encouraging us to consume?

Obesity adds $190 billion to the USA's annual health bill, says *Forbes* magazine. It's costing Australia $120 billion, according to the Herald-Lateral Economics Index of Australia's Wellbeing, and accounts for up to eight per cent of all European health spending. It is ruining lives from childhood onwards – and few dispute that poor nutrition is to blame. This book is the antidote; it will steer you to good health, acknowledging a truth the writer George Orwell identified decades ago:

'Changes of diet are more important than changes of dynasty or even of religion ... Yet, it is curious how seldom the all-importance of food is recognised.'

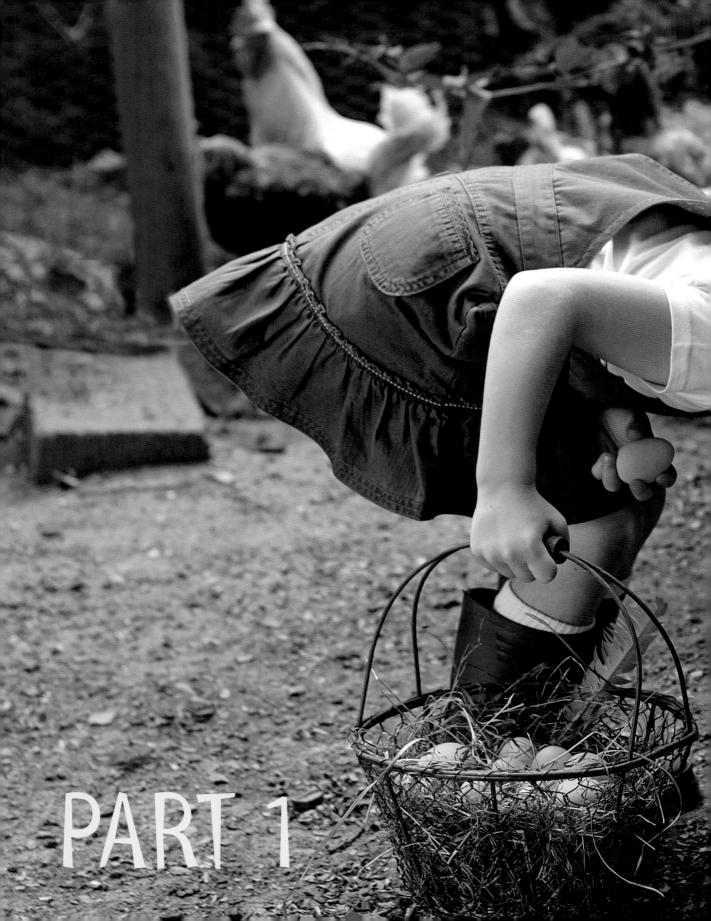

PART 1

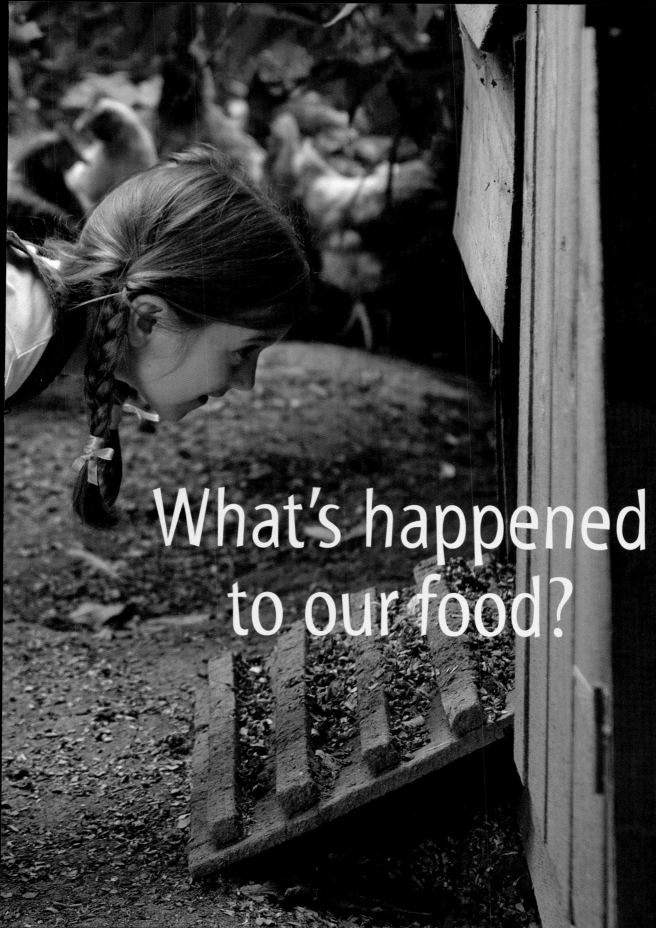

What's happened to our food?

Food, glorious food!

What we eat can be a delight, but food's core role is much more important than that; food is our essential fuel, keeping us well and strong. As you'll discover, the choices we make have never been more crucial for our health.

We live in a world of food abundance. We're not just physically surrounded by the stuff – groaning supermarket shelves, ubiquitous fast-food outlets. We also face a constant barrage of food ads and cooking programs, stimulating appetites and imaginations. Hungry or not, there's almost always a tasty snack to tempt us to eat. It's foodie heaven.

Or is it? If abundance and availability were all that mattered, we should be healthier than ever, but more and more life-threatening diseases today are linked to obesity and to poor diet. In recent decades, choosing what to eat has become increasingly complex.

Once, all dairy products were fresh from source; fruit and vegetables were seasonal and came from nearby orchards and farms. Now, much of our fresh produce is transported across the country; modern preservation and refrigeration techniques mean that food can be stored longer and travel thousands of kilometres before it reaches us.

➡ Once upon a time, fruit and vegetables came from nearby orchards and farms.

Unhealthy 'healthy' foods

So yes, we can enjoy strawberries year round. But the downside is that much non-seasonal produce has been sprayed, processed or manipulated in some other way before it gets anywhere near a shop. A long-distance apple may look red and shiny but seldom tastes as crisp and sweet or contains as many good nutrients as one just picked from your garden.

Then there are 'healthy' foods, such as breakfast cereals. Advertisers suggest they are bursting with fruit and grains and goodness. But when Choice, Australia's consumer organisation, analysed 195 popular cereals in 2012, it found many of them were unhealthily high in salt and sugar. Of the 41 brands aimed at children, 30 were more than 15 per cent

sugar and four were in the top ten of saltiest cereals. Four favourite children's brands contained a whopping 40 per cent sugar or more.

Modern processing and mass production has transformed every aspect of everyday eating, filling supermarket shelves with products that were unknown in our grandparents' time. Attractive packaging and advertising persuade us that this or that food product is what we should take home and eat. But all too often, seductively delicious products contain unhealthy levels of salt, sugar or fats, and few good nutrients.

Faced with the persuasive power of the modern mega-food industry, how do we, as customers, choose food that doesn't just look good but genuinely tastes good and, above all, is good for us? Understanding just what it is you're eating is a 21st-century survival skill.

Why it matters

Because yes, it is a matter of survival. Food is at the heart of good health but, as you'll discover in Part 2, far from sustaining us, some foods and drinks contribute directly to diseases that could shorten our lifespan. Heart disease and many cancers are linked to obesity. And all the evidence suggests that poor dietary choices are primarily to blame for the recent dramatic rise in obesity levels.

Increasingly, too many of us eat processed foods rather than fresh and, although stringent measures have also been introduced in most countries to ensure that foods are safe for consumption, astonishingly, 'safe' doesn't necessarily translate to 'healthy' or 'nutritious'. Too often food products (think anything from chicken nuggets to vegetarian burgers) have become mere industrial widgets manufactured by methods and from a standard of ingredients dictated by profit rather than health considerations. They won't make you ill because they're mouldy or contaminated but, as the 2004 film *Super Size Me* illustrated so well, just 30 days of fast food can have drastic effects on physical and mental wellbeing.

Processing is not the only issue. It's becoming clearer that the intensive, factory-style conditions in which some livestock are raised are not the best for us. Study after study shows that animals which feed or graze in a natural habitat produce not just tastier but more nutritious meat. Higher-welfare beef has up to 700 per cent more beta-carotene than beef from intensively reared cattle, reports Compassion in World Farming. Free-range

▶ Free-range eggs have 100% more vitamin E and 280% more beta-carotene than eggs from caged or battery hens.

eggs, for instance, have up to 100 per cent more vitamin E and 280 per cent more beta-carotene than eggs from caged or battery hens. Similarly, locally grown fruit and vegetables are likely to have lower levels of pesticide and a higher vitamin content than produce transported across the world.

Fighting back

The good news is that you can enjoy good-quality, nutritious, healthy and tasty food at affordable prices, and this book explains how. In Part 3, Five Food Friends, you'll discover which delicious foods fuel your body and also boost immunity, fight disease, build strong bones, nourish your brain and promote longevity. Here and in Part 4 and Part 5, you'll also find out:

- How to resist marketing hype and identify the healthiest and tastiest foods (good food usually tastes best).
- Which potentially harmful foods and drinks to resist or restrict.
- Which 'food friends' will actively keep you well.
- How to enhance your daily meals, ensuring they're packed with essential nutrients.
- The best and worst points of dozens of everyday products, what to buy, what to cook – a complete everyday guide to meats, fresh produce, dairy foods, snacks, drinks, restaurant food and takeaways.

In the larger picture, *Eat Well, Live Long* embraces and champions the new cultural food revolution that is steadily gathering momentum. Consumer power can be remarkably effective. If more and more people across the Western world demand better food, the industry that sells to us must respond. The best supermarkets and food manufacturers are already beginning to take heed. Read on … and join the revolution!

1 We're getting fatter
– but who's to blame?

We're told that it's our responsibility to eat sensibly and get enough exercise. If we're fat, the message often goes, it must be due to our shaky ability to exert self-control when it comes to food. But is that fair?

Twenty-eight per cent of Australians are obese, according to figures compiled between 2011–12, up from 11 per cent in 1989. The same figures reveal that 63 per cent of Australians are now either overweight or obese, up from 44 per cent in 1989. Elsewhere, British obesity levels have – staggeringly – quadrupled in the past 25 years and a third of all Americans are now classified as obese. Medical experts say the situation is reaching epidemic proportions with potentially disastrous consequences for health, while recent studies show that the problem is spreading fast to the Middle East and Asia in countries that have adopted Western-style diets. So is self-control, or rather the lack of it, really the culprit behind all those expanding waistlines? Have so many of us lost our collective willpower? Or are other factors at work here?

Why we love high-energy foods

Simple lack of willpower is not a fair explanation, says David A. Kessler, former commissioner of the US Food and Drug Administration (FDA). He believes that food companies 'addict' us to their processed products with irresistible combinations of fats, sugar and salt, that hoodwink many of us into eating more than we should.

The temptation is compelling because humans are 'evolutionarily prepared to respond to fats and sugars,' explains Marc A. Lindberg, a professor of psychology at Marshall University in Huntington, West Virginia, who has studied the US obesity phenomenon for 30 years. We crave these foods because they promote survival. When humans hunted and scavenged for food, high-kilojoule animal fats were their essential source of energy. Sugars, from fruits and occasionally honey, were rare and highly prized. Much later, 'In a quirk of fate, humans discovered how to take fats and sugars and add them to all sorts of foods to increase production of such foods in homes and restaurants – that's what is responsible for the increases in BMI.'

Perhaps the best example of a food that contains both fat and sugar, one you don't need to be hungry to eat, is ice cream. As Lindberg wonders, given the choice after a big meal, do you want a second helping of the chicken – or the chocolate ice cream? Exactly. The food industry knows this, says Lindberg. It's their business to sell in bulk and make sure we come back for more. Fast foods are engineered specifically to be 'addictive'; manufacturers know that people will buy their fatty, sugary, crispy, gooey products because they tap into an evolutionary human response.

Making us feel pleasure

'Addictive' may not be an overstatement, as something else also happens when we tuck into chips or a creamy cake. Humans are endowed with neural circuitry known as the 'brain reward system', which reinforces certain types of behaviour by making us feel pleasure. Many researchers believe that food can make it light up like a pinball machine in an arcade. In fact, studies suggest that the effect of food on the brain could be similar to that of addictive recreational drugs.

Playing a key role in the brain's reward system is a chemical called dopamine. Properly called a neurotransmitter, dopamine affects brain processes that control emotional response, especially the ability to experience pleasure and pain, among other functions. In effect, it triggers your brain to seek rewards, as the release of dopamine makes you feel good. Drugs such as cocaine increase dopamine levels, setting in motion an addictive cycle. Scientists are now discovering that high-sugar and high-fat foods may also overload the brain with dopamine.

In one study, published in the journal *Obesity* in 2011, researchers at the US Department of Energy's Brookhaven National Laboratory found that the mere sight or smell of favourite foods prompted a surge in dopamine levels in overweight people with compulsive eating disorders. A 2010 study in animals suggests that the same mechanism that promotes drug addiction may be a factor in compulsive eating behaviours and obesity.

ICE CREAM

sales boomed worldwide from US$59 billion in 2007 to US$85 billion in 2012. Food giants Nestlé and Unilever control most of this high-kilojoule market.

➡️ You don't need to be hungry to eat ice cream.

Earlier studies involving people of a normal weight found dopamine releases were linked to hunger and a desire for food.

Rewiring the brain?

It was Kessler's own lifelong struggle with obesity that prompted him to research the problem, talking to food industry experts, scientists and behaviour specialists. He also invested hours of his time observing people eating at fast-food joints and restaurants across America. Finally, he concluded why it was so hard for him to control his eating. He deduced that foods that contain fat, sugar and salt do more than stimulate the brain's reward centre. Over time, consuming them actually rewires the brain to the point where the mere smell or sight of such foods activates the reward centre, creating the urge to indulge. So you eat and in response, says Kessler, the brain releases opioids. The result is a pathway in the brain that activates each time you're reminded of those fatty and sugary foods, triggering the urge to eat, whether you're hungry or not. And food companies will do their utmost to make sure that you never forget how delectable their foods taste.

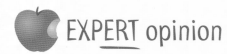

EXPERT opinion

Food advertising makes us eat more

'Food marketing has become more intensive and ubiquitous. It is part of a food environment that has changed in developed countries, where cheap, high-fat, high-sugar foods are widely available. Food marketing can over-stimulate a normal response to foods, with serious potential health consequences. … when we consider the effect of food marketing on children, the argument for protection is even stronger.'

Jane Landon *National Heart Forum*

Awareness is everything

No one is likely to ban the production or promotion of tasty, fattening foods. But making us more aware of them should help. While head of the FDA between 1990 and 1997, Kessler pressed hard for greater accuracy in food labelling. Elsewhere, including Europe, South America and Asia, similar initiatives have been and are still being launched.

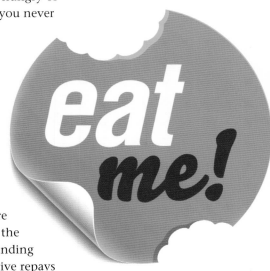

Being aware of the 'Big Food' industry's power to seduce you is a vital first step. Knowing that you're being encouraged to eat unhealthy food is half the battle, reading labels is essential and understanding what your body really needs to grow and thrive repays all the effort. With knowledge comes the power to make better choices. The following pages give you every reason to resist the food marketers' siren call.

2 Faster, cheaper ... better?
Some truths about processed foods

Eating to survive was the goal of our ancestors; now something different is happening. A manufacturing process geared to mass sales and big profits ensures food is plentiful but often transforms and distorts its original, natural form.

In earlier days of food processing, innovation was driven by the need to preserve food for leaner times and to make it available to more people. More recently, in a world of huge global food manufacturers, added imperatives are to churn out ever more products, to encourage greater consumption and boost profits.

The race to produce began in earnest after the Second World War. Farmers began to use industrially produced fertilisers and pesticides, in the USA especially, where subsidies to grow soy and corn encouraged overproduction. The food industry was to find ingenious ways to create a wealth of cheaper fats, sugars and other ingredients from soy and grains.

Crops fuel a food boom

Corn and soybean oils, for instance, were 'hydrogenated', changing their structure to make them more versatile. But the process also created trans fats, now known to be dangerous (*see* page 38) because they increase the risk of serious disorders such as heart attack and stroke. The new processed plant oils were originally thought to be healthier than animal fats and advertisers played on their agricultural origins to give them and other grain products a 'natural' image.

Soy was processed to make animal feed and various food additives; today

Did YOU know ?

The birth of the tin can

Warfare in the early 1800s prompted the invention of airtight food preservation. When starvation was decimating Napoleon's troops, Nicholas Appert invented a way to seal partially cooked foods in corked bottles, which were then boiled. In 1810, Peter Durand patented a similar method in Britain using tin cans. By 1812, when Britain was at war with the USA, a canned food factory had opened in London and was soon shipping 18,000kg of food a year to the Royal Navy.

processed soy can be found in countless meat-replacement products such as 'veggie burgers' and many other foods. 'In fact', writes American good-food advocate and author Michael Pollan in *The Omnivore's Dilemma*, 'you would be hard-pressed to find a late-model processed food that isn't made from corn or soybeans.'

And a controversial sweetener

Versatile, plentiful and relatively cheap, these new ingredients have proved a boon to the food industry – but potentially disastrous for human health. Sugar, originally derived from sugar cane, was once a luxury reserved for the rich. When Europeans colonised the West Indies and parts of South America, production increased but it wasn't until the 19th and 20th centuries, when sugar was extracted from sugar beet and other sources, that its use became widespread.

A new, cheaper, US grain-based source of sweetness was to prove particularly successful. In the 1970s, high-fructose corn syrup (HFCS), was developed. Today it is present in thousands of foods and drinks and has been increasingly linked to health problems (*see* page 46), although its defenders claim that its chemical structure is identical to other forms of sugar.

The truth is that now most of us consume far too many sweet foods and drinks. With sweetness of some kind added to everything from sauces and pizzas to 'healthy' flavoured waters, it's almost inescapable. Yet sugar in almost all its forms provides little more than empty kilojoules. Taken to excess it causes weight gain but offers no nutritional benefits. You'll discover more on this food 'foe' in Part 2.

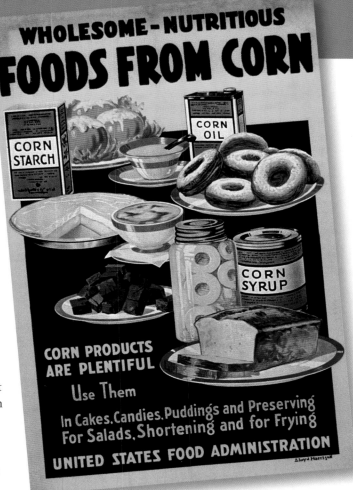

CORN FOODS
enjoyed a healthy, 'natural' image for decades, as a result of their agricultural origins.

Cereal production – behind the scenes

As already revealed, sugar is one of the main ingredients in many common breakfast cereals. But that's not all that happens in the making of this 'healthy' start to the day. The milling process strips away much of the natural goodness of the grain, then what is left of the wheat, corn, rice or oats is often blended with water into a soupy sort of porridge that goes through an extruder machine. Under high heat and pressure, the mixture is forced out of a little hole, which turns it into its designated shape. For other cereals, grains fed into the extruder expand to become 'puffed' cereals. After extrusion, the cereal is sprayed with sugar and oils to help it stay crunchy in milk.

Stripped of its goodness

Milling the grain removes the fibrous husks, which contain the nutritionally valuable bounty of fibre, B vitamins, phytochemicals and some minerals. The heat and pressure during extrusion further destroy the water-soluble B vitamins. Although synthetic vitamins, and sometimes fibre, are often added back into the cereals, the sugar content is often still dangerously high, though many manufacturers have – under government pressure – reduced salt levels in recent years.

But all cereals are not equally bad. Look carefully at your cereal box label. Go for wholegrain cereals, such as breakfast oats, with the minimum of added sugar and salt, and plenty of fibre, which will keep you feeling full. For more information on healthy breakfasts, *see* page 158.

Did YOU know ?

The birth of flaked cereal

Cereals owe their healthy image to a couple of US Seventh Day Adventists-cum-health-fanatics, the brothers Kellogg. Will Keith Kellogg and his brother John Harvey Kellogg ran the sanitorium in Battle Creek, Michigan, USA. House rules for the guests were strict and, by today's standards, not much fun: think yogurt enemas, meal-time 'digestion marches', a no-alcohol policy and a vegetarian diet.

Along the way, the brothers figured out how to process cooked grain into crispy flakes. They launched a wheat flakes cereal in 1894; corn flakes followed in 1898. Here's the irony: the brothers went their separate ways when Will, less health-conscious than his abstemious brother, wanted to add sugar to the flakes to make them tastier. John Harvey refused – ahead of his time, he adamantly believed sugar was unhealthy. So Will formed the Battle Creek Toasted Corn Flake Company in 1906. The brothers fought it out in court over the next 20 years, but never spoke again.

➡ The sugar content of cereals is often still excessively high.

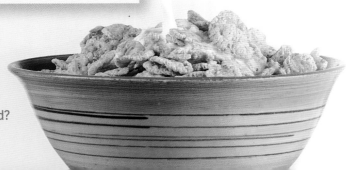

Those added extras

Additives are an integral part of food preserving and processing. And much as we may worry about what is in our food today, it's undoubtedly safer than when there were few, if any, legal constraints.

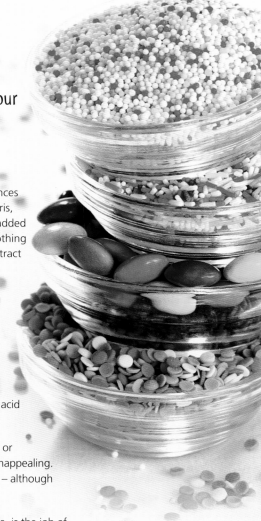

In the past many unscrupulous food providers added substances with little regard for health. For instance, bakers sometimes used plaster of Paris, pipe clay or even sawdust to increase the weight of loaves of bread. Brewers added strychnine to 'improve' the taste of beer – and to save money on hops. But nothing was as terrifying as the way sweets were made – the bright colours used to attract children were often due to poisonous lead, mercury or copper salts.

These days, in Australia and elsewhere, additives are tested for safety and regulated. But the ingredient labels on some food products can make you feel you need a chemistry degree just to work out what you're eating. Food additives that pass safety tests are assigned international code numbers and approved for use. Here are three key roles that some additives play:

▶▶ Antioxidants: When fats and oils combine with oxygen, they can become rancid, so foods made with oils or fats usually also contain antioxidant ingredients to delay spoilage. One of the most common antioxidants is ascorbic acid (vitamin C), which prevents the interaction.

▶▶ Food colours: Chemicals used to colour foods may come from natural or synthetic sources; without them, many processed foods would look decidedly unappealing. It is illegal to use colourings to mask or disguise foods that are inferior in quality – although some infringements might be difficult to trace and prove.

▶▶ Preservatives: Keeping food safe from spoilage, extending its shelf-life, is the job of three different kinds of preservatives. Antimicrobials keep the lid on mould, bacteria and yeast growth. Antioxidants, as noted above, prevent fats turning rancid. The third type of preservative targets enzymes in food such as phenolase, which causes cut apples or potatoes to go brown. Citric acid or ascorbic acid (vitamin C) might be used to inhibit phenolase and keep the browning at bay.

But then there's also the added salt, which is a preservative, but is often included to boost taste. Health experts recommend consuming no more than 6g of salt (2.4g of sodium) per day for adults and much less for children. Take a look at most soups, breads and even biscuits and cereals and note the salt or sodium levels. You'd be surprised at how much 'hidden' salt you'll find, even in foods that don't seem salty. *See also* Part 2, chapter 3. Despite modern regulations, the use of additives in foods remains controversial. And perhaps the major question is simply why do manufacturers add so many of these ingredients? To read more about those that are causing controversy, *see* page 64.

3 Food on tap

Eating habits are changing. More and more of us are grazing – snacking, eating on the run and patronising fast-food restaurants – instead of preparing and cooking most of our main meals at home. It's not a healthy trend.

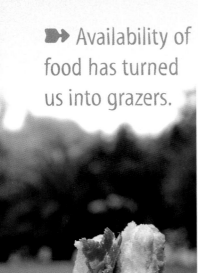

➡ Availability of food has turned us into grazers.

The industrial food revolution that has swept across the world in recent decades has packaged edibles into wonderfully convenient meals and mouthfuls. For many people in industrialised countries, cooking is now a thing of the past, if indeed they ever learnt the skill at all. For them, preparing a meal now means putting something in the microwave, as ready meals with a range of price tags tempt us to reheat manufacturers' concoctions quickly ('fast' is part of their attraction) rather than toil over a hot stove.

Availability has also turned us into grazers – snacking at home, at our desks and as we walk or travel. Fast food is the norm for many workers; in one survey, employees were more likely to go out for a burger than to eat in their workplace canteen or even the local food outlet.

Fast-food childhoods

Beyond Europe and the USA, a growing preference for Western food over one's traditional diet is having an impact on health. One 2012 US study of eating habits among Chinese people in Singapore has linked fast-food intake to a higher risk of diabetes and heart disease. In a 2010 study in Saudi Arabia, researchers noted 'an alarming increase' in the number of overweight and obese teenagers in Jeddah as a result of changing to a Western diet.

One study of Australian children aged 11 to 16 found that over half of the boys and more than one-third of the girls drank soft drinks every day, and up to 20 per cent of the children ate fast food every single week. Globally more than 42 million children under the age of five are overweight or obese – and the World Health Organization blames foods high in sugar and fat. Fast food, in particular, often comes in larger portions, and the food is high in energy and low in nutrients.

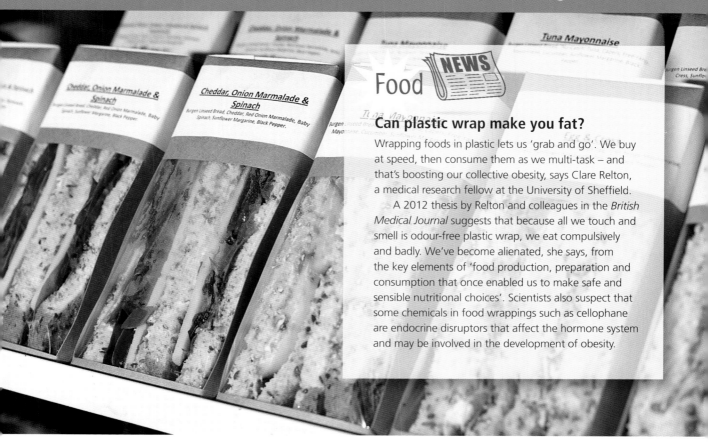

Food NEWS

Can plastic wrap make you fat?

Wrapping foods in plastic lets us 'grab and go'. We buy at speed, then consume them as we multi-task – and that's boosting our collective obesity, says Clare Relton, a medical research fellow at the University of Sheffield.

A 2012 thesis by Relton and colleagues in the *British Medical Journal* suggests that because all we touch and smell is odour-free plastic wrap, we eat compulsively and badly. We've become alienated, she says, from the key elements of 'food production, preparation and consumption that once enabled us to make safe and sensible nutritional choices'. Scientists also suspect that some chemicals in food wrappings such as cellophane are endocrine disruptors that affect the hormone system and may be involved in the development of obesity.

Temptation 24/7

In towns and cities, the invitation to eat appealing (if unhealthy) food is smack in our faces, 24/7. The eat-me-now aroma wafts over every main street, tempting us with fatty, salty, sugary treats. The two top fast-food chains account for most of the money we spend on fast food, but there are hundreds of other outlets vying to cash in on our appetite for a quick bite.

Fast food is now ubiquitous. You can pick up sausage rolls, meat pies, chips, sweets and fizzy drinks with your petrol. Take-away foods are often sold in 'meal deals' that actually encourage you to buy a fizzy drink and packet of chips along with the sandwich at lunchtime. Shops and stalls in railway stations sell fast food of all varieties from early morning onwards. Vending machines everywhere – even at swimming pools and in sports centres, which you might expect to promote healthy foods – dispense anything from sweet drinks and chocolate bars to the very latest hot pizza and freshly fried chips. Cheap, sugary, salty, fatty unhealthy food is virtually inescapable.

SNACKING has become increasingly popular across the world in recent years, according to Euromonitor International, with Brazil, China and India fast becoming the most prolific snackers.

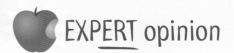

EXPERT opinion

Campaign for better food

'What I say to parents is this: take a look at what you and your kids are eating. Look at the ingredients list and the nutrition information. You may not like what you see, and you may even get anxious. But think: who is to blame? What are the food companies doing, putting this stuff in your food, and spending billions of dollars promoting it to you and the kids – that will turn your anxiety into anger.

'But there's no point being angry and doing nothing. So find out more, join other parents, complain to the supermarkets and start campaigning. Get active!'

Dr Tim Lobstein *International Obesity Task Force*

Why are we doing this to ourselves?

The simple answer is probably because we can. Without giving it a second thought, it is remarkably easy to eat badly and consume many more kilojoules than is good for our health. We eat largely in response to the stimuli around us, says Brian Wansink, Director of the Cornell Good and Brand Lab at Cornell University in Ithaca, New York, USA.

Most of the time we're surrounded by fatty, salty, sugary foods concocted to appeal to our most basic instincts. Fats gave early humans the energy reserves needed to weather food shortages, the sodium in salt helped them to retain water and avoid dehydration, and sugar allowed them to tell the difference between sweet edible berries and bitter poisonous ones, he explains. So, combinations of these ingredients still have the power to hook us.

Making fast food even more irresistible is the fact that manufacturers often price products cheaply and make them supremely easy to obtain. And because it often costs an outlet very little to 'supersize' a fast-food meal, we are encouraged to buy the bigger portion because of its perceived value – boosting our kilojoule intake and the food outlet's profits.

Eating healthily on the run

This is not to say that healthy alternatives aren't often sold alongside the unhealthy ones – of course they are. Burger places now sell meal-sized salads, for example, and most sandwich shops offer vegetarian choices, wholemeal bread and low-kilojoule options. But when you're dashing about on the run, you're likely to be under the kind of stress that makes wise choices harder to make, says Mara Mather, a professor at the University of Southern California, USA, who researches stress and the decision-making process.

'Our research suggests that under stress, the rewarding aspects of an outcome [as in eating a juicy burger] get more attention than the potential negative consequences [as in overloading on salt, fat and

➡ Ask your children – 'What would Batman eat?'

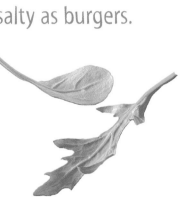

kilojoules].' says Mather. 'Even if you do make the apparently healthy choice, you must beware: if you're not careful, add-ons and dressings can make salads nearly as fatty and salty as burgers.'

Nutrition experts will tell you that the best place to eat is at the family dining table, with a wholesome home-cooked meal set before you. But for much of the time, for many people, that's simply not feasible. You may have to work, pick up the kids, drop them at whatever their activities happen to be, and by the time you get home, cooking dinner – much less sitting together as a family to eat it – is an unrealistic proposition for at least one and often more nights of the week. But that's actually no reason why you shouldn't try to make healthier choices. Here are a few ideas:

- **Mind your portions:** If you must have fast food, choose the smallest possible portion to satisfy your craving, *never* the supersize one – however much of a bargain it appears to be. You'll save more than 800kJ. Or better still share a small portion with friends.

➡️ If you do make the apparently healthy choice, beware: add-ons and dressings can make salads nearly as fatty and salty as burgers.

- **Choose the most choice:** Opt for fast-food sandwich outlets where you're in charge of choosing the bread (pick 100 per cent wholegrain), the dressing (a little olive oil, mustard, balsamic vinegar or lemon juice), and where you can add vegetable fillings. Choose healthier meats such as chicken breast (roasted, not fried) or turkey and other lean options.
- **Salad on the side, please:** Always order a side salad when you can, and opt for the low-kilojoule dressing. It will help fill you up and give you an extra portion of essential vegetables.
- **Visit your grocer:** If you're taking your children on an outing, stop at the supermarket first for bottled water, cut-up vegetables, hummus, yogurt and low-fat cheese – even sushi and salads. Your family might appreciate the al fresco picnic, even if you have to eat in the car.
- **Ask them: WBE? – 'What would Batman eat?'** This simple question encourages children to make healthier fast-food choices, say researchers from Cornell University in America and Utrecht University in the Netherlands. When researchers posed the WBE question, offering children the choice between apple slices or crisps, 45 per cent chose the apple slices. Substitute with your child's favourite superhero if Batman doesn't do the trick.

4 Back to basics

If decades of food industrialisation have amply contributed to obesity and higher levels of sickness, a growing army of good-food campaigners and organisations are now trying to reverse the trend.

Influential television chefs, such as Jamie Oliver, who has taken his fresh, healthy food message into schools in the UK and the USA, or Hugh Fearnley-Whittingstall, who has campaigned for locally farmed produce, sustainable fishing and animal welfare, have been making their mark. The number of farmers' markets in Australia and New Zealand has tripled in the past decade as more people prefer to buy produce that has been grown close to home.

The benefits are clear. As the Harvard School of Public Health points out, most of the fruit and vegetable varieties you'll find in supermarkets were chosen primarily for their yield – how much can be harvested per acre, their growth rate and ability to withstand long-distance transport. These are not qualities that are principally designed to benefit our health, nor are they any guarantee of good taste. Farmers producing for local markets are more likely to prioritise good nutrition and taste, choosing their varieties accordingly.

Taste is the driving force behind another campaign that is gathering momentum across the world. Carlo Petrini founded the Slow Food movement in Italy in 1989 to promote traditional foods and counter the influence of the newly arrived McDonald's chain in his home town. He believes that our taste buds are being numbed by the onslaught of fast and processed foods and wants people to rediscover the delights of fresh, natural, locally grown foods.

Slow Food is encouraging chefs to use local and sustainably produced foods and is helping to revive delicious, traditional local foods.

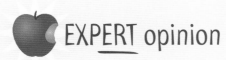

EXPERT opinion

Organic is affordable

'There are many ways that people can buy organic on a budget. Buying seasonally, locally and directly from growers can save people considerable amounts of money on their food bills. We believe it is possible for most of us to shop and cook organically on a budget and without compromising on quality. It might require some creativity and life-style changes, but these changes have the potential to leave both people and the planet healthier and happier.'

Josh Stride *Soil Association*

Making our voices heard

Thanks to the increasing muscle of real-food campaigners – and vocal consumer demand – more local and organic produce is being sold in mainstream businesses, including Pret A Manger and McDonald's, reports Josh Stride, press officer for the UK's Soil Association, which promotes organic food and farming. There are also more online retailers selling organic produce, and box schemes offering customers a selection of seasonal fresh fruit and vegetables have become popular.

But the global food industry is a huge force to turn around. As the recession bites, there is increasing evidence that 'comfort' food, those tempting fats and sugars, are once more threatening to take hold, especially among those on lower incomes.

'Can't afford to go out for a meal? Never mind, you can still spoil yourself,' is the seductive message with many of the 'treats' we are sold. But it's not what we or our bodies need. With *Eat Well, Live Long* as your personal nutritional guide, you'll discover why your food choices matter so much for your health. The changes you make could be life-saving – and the bonus? Enjoying the delicious taste of really good-quality food.

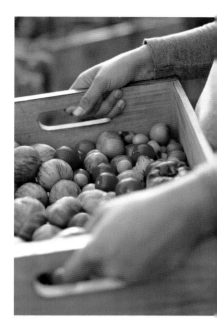

The eat-well message

Seeking out the best-quality food you can afford is a must for good health.
Powerful commercial forces ensure that alluring foodstuffs are more available than ever. But that is no guarantee that products will provide the nutrients your body needs, for strength, energy and to fight disease. It's never been more important to shop wisely and resist the food lobby, its advertisers and marketers. This book shows you how.

➡ **Buy the freshest** whenever you can. Locally grown fresh fruit and vegetables conserve most of their nutrients and lose less in transport.

➡ **Choose meat from grass-fed** livestock and free-range poultry. Studies show they contain higher levels of vitamins and healthy fats than meat from animals that are intensively reared.

➡ **Understand your appetite triggers.** Stress, boredom and the alluring aroma of fast food can all tempt us to snack on whatever is available at the time.

➡ **Avoid highly processed foods.** Fast food or a ready meal are seldom healthy options. Check ingredients, avoid long lists of chemicals and, whenever possible, cook at home.

Food and you

Eating is a physical necessity but our attitudes to food and the choices we make can vary considerably from individual to individual. To assess the role food plays in your life, answer the questions below as honestly as you can.

1 Are you a foodie?

A I like most foods and look forward to meals.
B I don't think much about food and sometimes skip meals if I'm busy.
C I love food. I like to eat the best-quality food I can – it tastes so much better.
D I enjoy eating but worry about my weight so I'm always kilojoule-counting.

2 How do you shop?

A I tend to grab what I need on the way home and do a bit more at weekends if I'm having people round.
B I do a weekly shop at the supermarket and try to buy the best-quality food I can.
C I usually shop around the supermarkets to get the cheapest deals.
D I use a lot of independent shops – butchers, greengrocers or farmers' markets. I enjoy seeking out good, local foods.

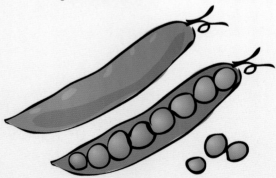

3 Would you call yourself a cook?

A Yes, I love cooking and I often make extra and freeze it for days when I won't have time.
B I cook once or twice during the week and often at the weekend – I'm happy to eat a ready meal or takeaway a couple of nights a week.
C I seldom cook – I like eating out and there are also plenty of good takeaways around to choose from.
D I don't cook much but I do prepare simple meals from fresh ingredients most days.

4 What do you eat for breakfast?

A Just a cup of tea or coffee – I'm never hungry first thing in the morning.
B It has to be something quick – a bowl of cereal with milk, a slice of buttered toast, or sometimes a croissant.
C Porridge or wholegrain cereal with fruit and yogurt.
D A bacon or fried-egg sandwich most days but I do enjoy a full fry-up when I have time.

5 What meat do you prefer in your sandwiches or rolls?

A Chicken.
B Beef.
C Ham.
D Bacon, with lettuce and tomato.

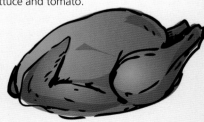

6 Do you eat wholegrain foods – bread, brown rice or pasta?

A Almost every day – I always buy wholegrain bread and pasta.

B Not very often – they're expensive and I prefer white bread and rice.

C I'll have a wholemeal sandwich sometimes, but my local takeaways don't do brown rice or wholemeal pizza.

D About 4–5 times a week, usually wholemeal bread.

7 How about fruit and vegetables?

A I don't really like vegetables.

B I have an apple or orange most days.

C I eat vegetables with my main meal and often snack on fruit during the day.

D I have some most days. I often snack on fruit or eat it for dessert and I enjoy cooking with vegetables.

8 Which dessert would you choose?

A Sticky toffee pudding with ice cream.

B Chopped fresh fruit with plain yogurt.

C Apple pie with cream.

D Fruit-flavoured yogurt or fromage frais

9 How often do you eat fried food?

A Every day.

B Rarely, unless you count stir fries.

C Two or three times a week.

D Never.

10 What kind of fat or oil do you usually cook with?

A Olive or canola oil.

B Butter or lard.

C Whatever vegetable oil is on offer in the supermarket.

D I don't cook.

11 How often do you eat fish or seafood?

A Never – the smell puts me off.

B Fish is expensive, but I like to try something different once a week.

C I have fish and chips once a week.

D If you include canned sardines and canned salmon, I eat fish two or three times week.

12 What do you usually drink?

A Fizzy soft drinks.

B A cordial or juice drink.

C Real fruit juice.

D Water.

13 How often do you eat a takeaway or fast food?

A Less than once a month.

B About once a week.

C Three or four times a week.

D Every day – sometimes more than once.

14 What's your favourite takeaway?

A Pizza – I like the standard margarita (tomatoes and cheese) best.

B Chinese – crispy sweet and sour pork is my favourite.

C Burger and chips, or chicken nuggets.

D My local curry house does a fantastic lamb curry – I like it with mixed vegetables, rice and naan bread.

15 When you need a quick snack, what are you most likely to choose?

A Chocolate biscuits or crisps.

B Cheese and biscuits.

C A piece of fresh fruit or yogurt.

D Dried fruit or unsalted nuts, or sometimes a small piece of dark chocolate.

Your answers matter

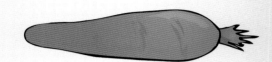

1 A=3, B=1, C=4, D=2

A Many of us do. But not all food is equal; this book outlines the best choices.

B Make sure that what you do eat is nutritious and includes foods from each group (*see* page 120).

C That's great but balance is still important. Take care not to eat too much fat, sugar or salt.

D Try limiting portion sizes, and eating just a little from each food group. *See also* Part 4, Effective weight control, page 210.

2 A=2, B=3, C=1, D=4

A A busy life can lead to poor nutrition. For your health's sake, do buy a variety of foods and include as much fresh produce as possible.

B Do check labels, too – high price does not always equal good nutrition. And you might find better quality local produce elsewhere.

C Nothing is wrong with a good deal. But remember that some fresh foods lose nutrients with age.

D You know what you're looking for. You may find further tips in Part 4, Shop for quality, page 132.

3 A=4, B=3, C=1, D=2

A Admirable! Especially if you cook balanced meals.

B Home cooking is always preferable to ready meals or takeaways; try preparing more quick, easy dishes.

C You may never really know what's in your food. But Part 5, Restaurant foods & takeaways, page 300 will help you make healthier choices.

D Not a bad idea, if you're eating foods from each group. *See* Part 3, Are you missing out?, page 120.

4 A=1, B=2, C=4, D=1

A Try to get the breakfast habit or at least keep a healthy snack handy to satisfy mid-morning hunger.

B 'Quick' can be healthy if you choose a wholegrain cereal that keeps you feeling full. Toast/croissants are quickly digested so you soon feel hungry again.

C An excellent combination, supplying fibre to keep mid-morning hunger at bay and plenty of vitamins.

D Eating lots of fried food is inadvisable; it can lead to weight gain, and bacon is high in salt and nitrates. *See also* Part 4, chapter 4, Breakfast review.

5 A=4, B=3, C=2, D=1

A White meat is the best choice. Recent studies show that eating processed meat regularly may be linked with a raised risk of heart disease and some cancers.

B Red meat may be linked to increased cancer risk. Best not to eat more than 500g a week.

C Ham, however fresh, is a processed meat so best to eat sparingly and prefer chicken, fish or egg fillings.

D Good to include salad in your sandwich, but bacon is a fatty, salty processed meat, which medical research suggests you should not eat every day.

6 A=4, B=1, C=1, D=3

A Whether it's because you prefer the taste or know the science, this is an excellent choice.

B Consider eating wholegrain products at least once a day – for the healthy fibre and nutrients they supply.

C Look around your supermarket; most sell wholemeal pizzas that just need heating up.

D Try to eat whole grains every day. The fibre helps lower cholesterol and protects against heart disease, diabetes and cancer, particularly bowel cancer. For more about fibre *see* page 92.

7 A=1, B=2, C=3, D=4

A You're missing out on so many healthy nutrients – vitamins, minerals and protective phytonutrients.

B Health experts talk of 'seven a day' or more, so try to include vegetables in soups and main meals.

C Don't forget how versatile vegetables are, too. You can snack on them or use them to make soups or juices or to bulk out and flavour numerous dishes.

D Good, and to benefit from all the different nutrients in fresh fruit and vegetables, choose a rainbow of colours and try experimenting with new flavours.

8 A=1, B=4, C=2, D=2

A Delicious – but strictly as a treat. It supplies few good nutrients but racks up about 2000kJ; that's more than 25% of a woman's daily kilojoule count.

B Excellent for vitamins, minerals and taste. Choose luscious fruits and enjoy with creamy plain yogurt – the small amount of fat helps you to feel fuller.

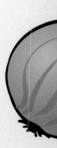

C Nice as an occasional treat. There's some fibre in apples but they lose vitamin C in cooking, and the pastry, sugar and cream add lots of extra kilojoules.

D Fruit-flavoured yogurts or fromage frais may not be as 'healthy' as their image – check sugar content.

9 A=1, B=3, C=2, D=4

A It's worth cutting back. Research has consistently linked fried foods to increased risk of heart disease, blood pressure and obesity.

B Stir-fries cooked with vegetables and minimal oil are pretty healthy but don't let the oil burn as it might produce some unhealthy trans fats.

C It's healthier to eat less. Marinate meat and grill it, bake potatoes, and boil or poach eggs.

D Excellent, and easy enough at home but surely tricky when you eat out? 'Occasionally' is allowed.

10 A=4, B=1, C=2, D=1

A This is the best choice as olive and canola oils contain more healthy monounsaturated fats.

B Both butter and lard are high in unhealthy saturated fats. To mimic a buttery taste, try a soft margarine that is a mix of plant oil and skimmed milk.

C Choose olive or canola oils if possible. Cheaper sunflower oil is high in less healthy omega-6 fats.

D Check ingredient labels and avoid trans and saturated fats. *See also* Part 2, Bad fats, page 34 and Part 3, Good fats, page 98.

11 A=1, B=3, C=2, D=4

A That's a shame as fish adds protein, vitamins and minerals, for far fewer kilojoules than meat.

B Don't forget oily fish, such as fresh mackerel, which is cheap but rich in healthy omega-3 fatty acids.

C Tasty, but too much fried food is not advisable, and the chips and batter are laden with unhealthy fats.

D That's good but whenever you buy canned fish, do look for the salt or sodium levels as some are very high. *See also* Part 5, Fish and seafood, page 240.

12 A=1, B=2, C=3, D=4

A Fizzy drinks don't really quench thirst and can be packed with sugar, prompting weight gain.

B Check the sugar content of both these drinks.

C Real fruit juice is also high in sugar but rich in vitamins. Try diluting it a little if you drink it regularly.

D The best choice as a thirst-quencher and to keep your body and brain well-hydrated.

13 A=4, B=3, C=2, D=1

A It makes a nice change once a month or so.

B Check the ingredients and choose wisely.

C Too often for good health. Mass-appeal fast food/takeaways tend to have lots of fat, sugar and salt.

D You need to know what's in your food. When did you last ask a takeaway outlet about its ingredients?

14 A=3, B=1, C=1, D=3

A The baked dough and tomatoes are healthy enough but avoid fatty, cured meats and too much cheese.

B Many delicious soups and steamed dishes to enjoy here, but avoid too much 'crispy' (deep-fried) food.

C Healthy burgers have become quite trendy, so go for quality, but beware of most chicken nuggets.

D To avoid too much fat, opt for plain rice and non-fried vegetable-based dishes. *See also* Part 5, Restaurant food & takeaways, page 300.

15 A=1, B=2, C=4, D=4

A Snacks should fill a gap but neither biscuits nor crisps are a good choice. Both cause a blood glucose surge for a quick burst of energy that won't last.

B Cheese is digested more slowly, maintaining energy and blood glucose levels for longer.

C & D Fresh or dried fruit, nuts, yogurt and even a small piece of dark chocolate are all good options that should help sustain you until the next meal. *See* Part 4, Healthy snacks, page 168 for more ideas.

Total scores:

Over 50 Bravo! You clearly love good food. Read on to get the latest news on food and health.

40 to 49 Most of your food choices are very good; a few tweaks could make your diet excellent.

26 to 39 You're getting many things right, but you'd benefit from paying more attention to what you eat.

15 to 25 Making a few key changes now will help you to avoid future health and weight problems.

PART 2

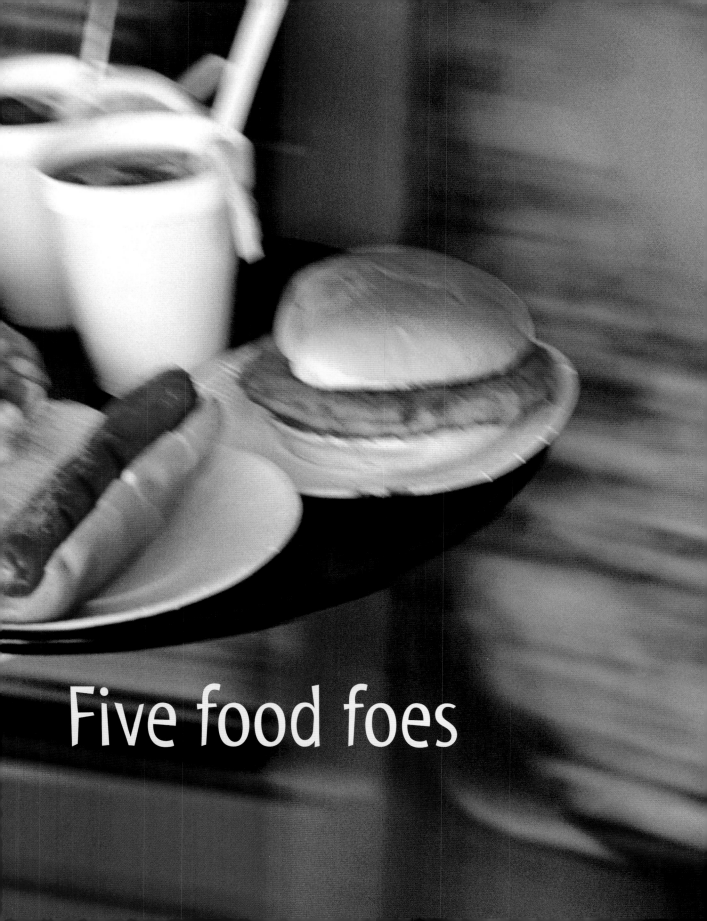

Five food foes

Getting off the bad-food rollercoaster

If you don't like the shape you see in the mirror, or if you often feel tired or easily catch colds – the Five Food Foes described in the following pages could be conspiring against you.

Do you find that the weight piles on all too easily and keeps piling on year by year? If so, you're far from alone. The simplistic view is, that if you're overweight, you must be eating too much and taking too little exercise. The truth is more complex than that.

Much of what we eat today – fast foods, biscuits, chips, fizzy drinks – supplies lots of kilojoules without satisfying hunger. Energy soon flags, together with mood, so we eat some more. It doesn't end there; the fatty, sugary or salt-laden foods so available in our modern world may actually alter body chemistry in ways that make weight gain and other ills more likely.

Those physical changes are not always as visible as excess kilograms; people can be a 'healthy' weight and still be poorly nourished. A diet that consists mainly of snacks and fast foods undermines the body's immune system.

Most worryingly, eating like this year after year can encourage the onset of serious, debilitating and life-threatening diseases including cancers, heart disease, diabetes, osteoporosis, arthritis and dementia.

Enemies of good health

As the world's obesity crisis worsens, the damaging role played by the Five Food Foes is gradually being revealed.

➡ **Bad fats** People have worried for years about the animal fats in meat, cream and butter and their potential for clogging our arteries and causing heart disease. But it took a century for the world to recognise that trans fats, found in certain processed hard margarines and oils, are even worse for our health. Some governments have banned them altogether. You'll discover what sorts of foods contain them and why it's best to steer clear of fast fried-food outlets unless you know that the oil used for cooking is trans-fat free.

➡ **Dangerous sugars** In one form or another, sugars turn up in everything from pizzas to low-fat sauces and yogurts, in most cases adding nothing but empty kilojoules. Learn how to track them down under their many pseudonyms. And find out why cutting back on added sugar and eating naturally sweet foods instead can boost health and also help hold back the years.

Worldwide, more than **500 MILLION** adults are obese.

Ultra-refined foods Many of us eat these most of the time. They're the biscuits, pies, ready meals, processed meats and cereal products that line supermarket shelves and make their manufacturers a fortune. But, as global experts have made clear, a constant diet of high-fat, high-sugar, low-fibre fast foods is a major driver for serious, life-threatening ills.

An excess of additives These days, you need a chemistry degree to identify all the preservatives, flavourings, colourings, bulking agents and more that go into everyday products. Are they strictly necessary? What are they all for? And could some of them be affecting our health? You'll learn some label-reading skills to help you identify the ones that are causing controversy.

Evil spirits The fifth foe is alcohol when drunk to excess. Encouraged by powerful marketing forces, it's the richer nations who are indulging, young and old alike. The Australian Bureau of Statistics reports that over 30 per cent of males and 10 per cent of females in the 55–64 age group consume alcohol in quantities that pose a health risk over their lifetime. The better news is that drinking wine in moderation and following a few simple rules can boost heart health.

Fighting back

You don't have to ban fatty, salty and sugary foods completely. But if they form a large part of your diet, cutting back on them will improve your health. Food should nourish rather than harm us, and there's a whole world of great tastes to discover and enjoy. As we learn to appreciate the natural flavours of good food, processed convenience products start to lose their appeal.

Too many fatty, sugary and salty foods may alter your body chemistry and make you ill.

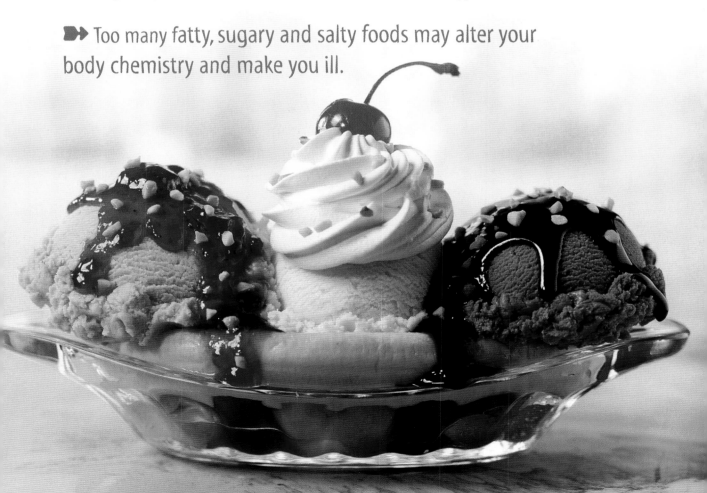

1 Bad fats

Some common fats are so bad for us that certain governments now ban them. Others should be eaten occasionally rather than every day. Here are the facts.

If you've followed food news over the years, you may have found media coverage of fats confusing. Like in a challenging 'whodunit', it's been hard to spot the villain as advice ricochets from 'this fat will kill you' to 'this fat will save your life' to 'this fat, which we used to think was bad for you, is actually quite healthy and it's OK to eat a little more of it'.

It was back in the 1950s when US doctors first branded saturated fat the ultimate baddie, linking high levels of animal fats in food to the nation's clogged arteries and surging levels of heart disease. By the 1970s, this became dogma and the food industry weighed in with a powerful and hugely profitable new low-fat, no-fat revolution. Soon supermarkets were packed with low-fat alternatives for everything from cheese to soups.

Yet close examination of low-fat foods revealed that some had more kilojoules than their full-fat counterparts because they contained more sugar. What's more, after 20 years of low-fat living, people weren't getting any healthier; levels of heart disease and obesity were still rising. In a further plotline twist, animal fats came back into vogue as people who wanted to lose weight embraced the low-carb, meaty high-protein diets of rebel doctor Robert Atkins and his successors. Heart doctors were, understandably, shocked and dismayed.

What we now know

The decades-long confusion is not surprising but a clearer picture has gradually emerged. We know that fat is not, in fact, a single entity but made up of many different fat types, some of which are much better for us than others. Although the jury is still out on a few more obscure fats, most of the rogues and angels have been revealed.

What is also clear and important to understand is that some fat in the diet is essential for the development and maintenance of our bodies and brains. But because fat is densely packed with

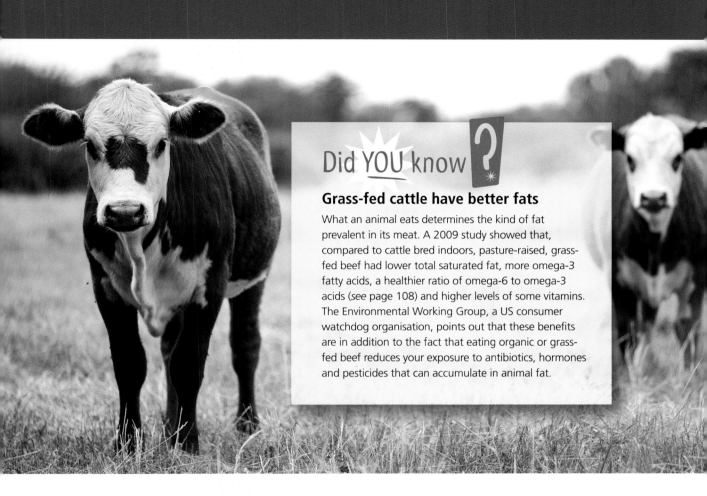

Did YOU know ?

Grass-fed cattle have better fats

What an animal eats determines the kind of fat prevalent in its meat. A 2009 study showed that, compared to cattle bred indoors, pasture-raised, grass-fed beef had lower total saturated fat, more omega-3 fatty acids, a healthier ratio of omega-6 to omega-3 acids (*see* page 108) and higher levels of some vitamins. The Environmental Working Group, a US consumer watchdog organisation, points out that these benefits are in addition to the fact that eating organic or grass-fed beef reduces your exposure to antibiotics, hormones and pesticides that can accumulate in animal fat.

kilojoules, health problems arise when we eat too much of it, especially the wrong kind. The main types of dietary fat to look out for are these:

✗ **Saturated fat**
✗ **Trans fat (hydrogenated vegetable oils)**
✓ **Polyunsaturated fat**
✓ **Monounsaturated fat**
✓ **Omega-3 fats**

In this section we put the first two under the microscope – saturated fat, the original culprit, found in animal and dairy products, and the newer 20th-century villain, trans fats that are produced in the manufacture of certain hard margarines and hydrogenated oils. You'll discover why you should limit the former and banish the latter. In Part 3, Five Food Friends, you will read much more about the polyunsaturated and monounsaturated fats, omega-3 and omega-6 fatty acids, their virtues and the role they all play in a good, healthy diet.

6 SOURCES OF SATURATED FAT

- Fatty cuts of meat
- High-fat cheese
- Cream and whole-fat milk
- Butter
- Dairy ice cream and ice-cream products
- Palm and coconut oil

Did YOU know ?

Some fat is essential

A totally fat-free diet would quite literally kill us. Here are four of the vital jobs that dietary fat performs:

- Fat fuels energy, and once stored in the body, helps to regulate body temperature.
- Fat cushions and protects vital organs and is essential in the membrane structure of the body's cells.
- The body needs fat to absorb the fat-soluble vitamins A, D, E and K, plus other fat-soluble nutrients.
- Fat plays a role in regulating hormones and chemicals that help control basic processes such as metabolism.

When all fat was good

From prehistoric times up until just a century or two ago, all fat was desirable because it was generally difficult to get enough of it. Experts in early human nutrition have shown that the animals hunted by Stone Age hunter-gatherers were lean and sinewy, and the make-up of their meat was very different from the meat of today. Only about seven per cent of the kilojoules in meat from an ancient antelope came from fat, and almost all of that would be unsaturated. Game meats such as venison are the modern-day equivalents. More typical of red meat today is beef from grain-fed cattle bred indoors, in which five times the kilojoules – 35 per cent – come from fat, much of it saturated fat.

So for most of human evolution fat was scarce, an energy-dense treat when available and something to be feasted on when times were good. Then, in the 20th century, far-reaching innovations in science, food production and processing dramatically altered the availability and affordability of fat. Suddenly it was everywhere and in everything from meats to margarines, biscuits, crisps and doughnuts. The problem was that we humans were not prepared for the change. Our evolutionary history still guides our food preferences and we remain predisposed to crave the flavour and 'mouth-feel' of fat.

Saturated fat ... and the 'junk' enzyme

The fat that makes meat, cream and butter taste so good is saturated fat; the term 'saturated' refers to its chemical structure, which is saturated with hydrogen. These fats – often from animal sources – are widely used because they're stable, have a long shelf life and a high melting point.

Eating too much saturated fat – more than the 20g to 30g a day nutritionists suggest – may cause weight gain and has been linked to heart disease, stroke and diabetes. This is because saturated fats raise cholesterol and contribute to a phenomenon known as inflammation – which upsets certain functions in the body. In one recent US study, researchers discovered that saturated

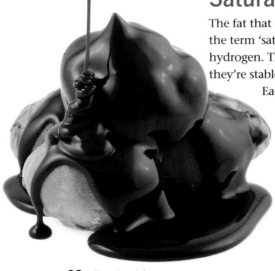

➨ The fat that makes chocolate and butter taste so good is called saturated fat.

fat can 'turn on' a kind of enzyme, called Jun N-terminal kinase (JNK). This so-called 'junk' enzyme interferes with the way that body cells communicate with each other. One of the processes that can go awry when JNK is triggered is the proper functioning of insulin. This crucial hormone enables your body to extract energy from food and controls glucose levels in the blood; it 'unlocks' cells to allow glucose (sugar) to enter them and perform its energy-promoting action. A diet heavily laced with saturated and trans fats can make cells resistant to insulin.

This sets the stage for inflammation, which subtly alters your internal chemistry so it starts to work against your body, rather than for it. Eventually, inflammation leads down the road to what health experts call 'metabolic syndrome', a precursor to type 2 diabetes, and other inflammatory conditions including heart disease, arthritis and kidney disease, to name just a few.

Triggering digestive problems

In another piece of the inflammation puzzle, scientists have linked an excessive intake of saturated fat to colitis, a painful swelling of the large intestine that causes diarrhoea and other digestive woes. In 2012, researchers from the University of Chicago showed that when mice were fed on a diet high in saturated fat (from milk), it encouraged the growth of a harmful, gut-dwelling species of bacteria.

✓ 6 WAYS TO EAT LESS SATURATED FAT

- Trim visible fat off meat before you cook or eat it.
- Avoid meats with a marbled, fatty appearance.
- Remove skin from poultry before cooking.
- Roast potatoes in a little canola or olive oil.
- Choose a lower-fat pizza topped with vegetables, fish or prawns instead of salami or extra cheese.
- Eat fewer or avoid full-fat dairy products; drink low-fat rather than whole milk, for instance.

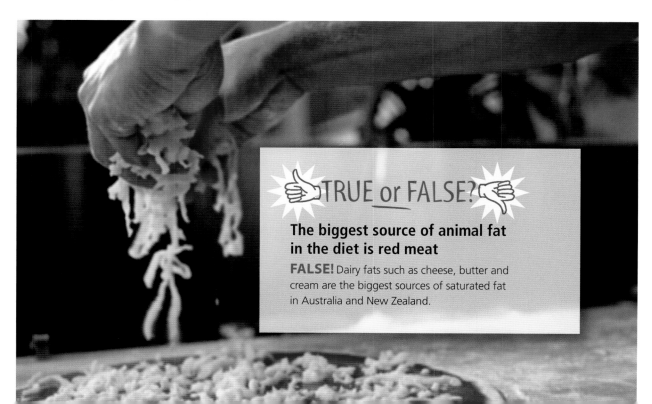

👍 TRUE or FALSE? 👎

The biggest source of animal fat in the diet is red meat

FALSE! Dairy fats such as cheese, butter and cream are the biggest sources of saturated fat in Australia and New Zealand.

Did YOU know ?

The healthy saturated fat limit

How much saturated fat is too much? Current health guidelines suggest that a maximum of 10 per cent of total daily energy should come from saturated fat. Fat has 39kJ a gram, so for women consuming 8000kJ a day, a 10 per cent maximum would be about 21g of saturated fat, and just under 26g for men on 10,000kJ a day. Many of us consume much more.

The researchers say that a booming population of the bad bacteria can attack the immune system, triggering gut inflammation leading to colitis, irritable bowel syndrome and other intestinal inflammations. Reducing saturated fat may be key to preventing these ills.

Limit, rather than exclude

In the health story so far, all saturated fat is dubbed 'bad' but this does not give the whole picture. For this type of fat is made up of several kinds of fatty acid, found in both animal and non-animal sources. Scientists are discovering that some of these are better, and some worse, for our health than others. Take stearic acid, for example, which is found in dark chocolate and in animal fat. Studies have shown that stearic acid does not raise harmful LDL cholesterol levels in the way that other saturated fats do. On the other hand, two commonly consumed saturated fats – palmitic and myristic acid – probably are harmful. They are found in palm kernel oil and countless processed foods, as well as animal fats such as butter. Some studies suggest they promote inflammation, hardening of the arteries and heart disease.

The problem for even the best-informed consumer is that saturated fat is usually made up of both 'bad' and 'OK' kinds of fatty acids. So what do we do? Since it's almost impossible to cut out saturated fat altogether, the answer is to limit the amount we consume every day. For most people a little as part of a healthy balanced diet is nothing to worry about. Which is good news for those who love tasty food.

Trans fats – dubbed 'Frankenfats'

When it comes to food, nutrition writers don't usually like to paint anything edible as being completely unhealthy. 'Everything in moderation' is the motto. But with trans fats – or 'Frankenfats', as some have called them – normal rules may not apply.

Research into the link between trans fats and heart disease began back in the 1950s. But at that time, as heart disease was reaching epidemic proportions in the USA, the American Heart Association (AHA) had started to focus on the need to reduce saturated fat in the diet. The nation's love affair with fast-food burgers, chips, fried fish, chicken sandwiches and the

Crisco – the original hydrogenated fat

The process of hydrogenation of fats was invented in Germany by chemist Wilhelm Normann in 1901, but it was in the USA that it first made an impact on the food supply. In 1911, Procter & Gamble launched Crisco, the first synthetic, solid fat to be marketed commercially for baking and frying. Sales of hard margarines and shortenings received a massive boost during World War II when butter was in short supply. Being cheaper than butter, they remained popular with thrifty housewives in the 1950s.

like had begun – a love that big business encouraged people across the world to share. At first, fast-food chains such as McDonald's fried their foods in beef fat, but as warnings about saturated fat gradually condensed into health campaigns, pressure would mount to abandon the practice. The hydrogenated fat business was about to get a major boost.

In 1984, most outlets switched to using partially hydrogenated oils for frying; the notion was that these plant-based, albeit lab-transformed, fats would be healthier. In fact, by the mid-1980s, some studies were already indicating that the unnatural trans fatty acids produced during hydrogenation were potentially harmful. Further research confirmed this in the 1990s and today trans fats are of great concern to health experts.

Chemically altered, 'twisted' fats

Although a small amount of trans fat occurs naturally in the saturated fat of cow's milk, the trans fats that have been hitting the health headlines are all synthetic. These are corn or soy oils that have been chemically altered by the process called hydrogenation. In this process the oil is heated to a very high temperature and hydrogen is pumped through it. This changes the way that the hydrogen atoms bind to the carbon atoms in the oil, turning the liquid vegetable oils into solid fats.

For food manufacturers, solid fats have distinct advantages over liquid oils. They are easier to handle and don't become rancid so quickly, so foods made with hydrogenated or partially hydrogenated vegetable oils have a longer shelf life. With these benefits, it's hardly surprising that this seemingly user-friendly fat found its way into practically every corner of the food-processing industry. It became an ingredient in a huge variety of processed foods from biscuits and baked goods to breakfast cereals and ice cream. The problem, as scientists discovered, was that it turned out to be less friendly to the health of the consumer.

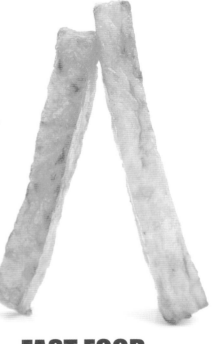

FAST FOOD
outlets began using partially hydrogenated oils (trans fats) for frying in the 1980s; many still do.

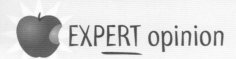

EXPERT opinion

Danger of trans fats

'Trans fats are literally toxins (as declared by the World Health Organization in 2009). Ideally, they should form no part of anyone's diet, because there is no safe level of consumption.'

Dr Alex Richardson *Senior Research Fellow, University of Oxford, UK*

To understand what's so bad about trans fats, it helps to compare them directly to the healthiest types – the essential, polyunsaturated fats omega-3 and omega-6. These fats are essential to the normal structure of body cell membranes, says Dr Alex Richardson, a senior research fellow at Oxford University. They keep the cell membranes fluid and flexible, which is necessary for normal 'cell signalling'. This scientific term is pretty much shorthand for the intricate, inner communication process that keeps all our body systems functioning properly.

By contrast, trans fats are 'twisted' versions of the natural polyunsaturated fats and act in a very different way. 'The twisted trans fat molecules pack closely together in cell membranes,' explains Dr Richardson. 'That stiffens them and makes them less flexible, which interferes with normal cell signalling.' As a result, eating trans fats increases the risk of a multitude of serious health problems, including:

- **Higher cholesterol and increased risk of heart attack and stroke**
- **Insulin resistance and type 2 diabetes**
- **Obesity**
- **Infertility**

EATING THE WRONG FOODS on a regular, long-term basis can encourage the onset of serious, debilitating and life-threatening diseases.

Emerging research also suggests that a high level of trans fats may affect brain development and harm mental health. The brain is particularly susceptible because it is largely made up of fat – 60 per cent of your brain is fatty tissue. When this tissue takes up the 'twisted' molecules in trans fats, it tries to use them as it would good fats. The result? According to new studies, people who eat a lot of trans fats may also be at increased risk of:

- **Depression**
- **Aggression**
- **Irritability**
- **Manic behaviour**
- **Dementia**

Should trans fats be banned?

Governments and health organisations across the world are beginning to regulate trans fats. Many countries have now removed trans fats from margarines – though some experts worry about the saturated fats in the palm and palm kernel oils which have replaced them.

Certain countries were swifter than others to react and regulate. In 2003, Denmark became the first country to introduce a partial ban on hydrogenated oils by limiting amounts in foods to just 2 per cent. Over the next two decades, this move is expected to

➡ When you cook, use liquid vegetable oil instead of solid shortening.

reduce deaths from heart disease in Denmark by 50 per cent. Other countries which limit trans fats include Switzerland, Iceland, Sweden and Austria. Argentina and Brazil are also reducing levels of trans fats in foods. Canada has been considering trans-fat legislation for years, but to date, only British Columbia enforces trans-fats limits.

In Australia the federal government supports a trans-fat reduction policy, but the country's current labelling laws don't require the listing of trans fats. In 2003, the American Food and Drug Administration mandated that labels should list the amounts of trans fats contained in food products. Since then New York City, Seattle and the state of California have introduced trans fat limits.

Is voluntary action enough?

Without formal legislation, we rely on voluntary action from the food industry to remove dangerous trans fats from products. Some supermarkets and food companies, such as McDonald's, have indeed taken appropriate action to eliminate trans fats from their own products. Elsewhere, you have to ask or check food labels. If a food label indicates 'hydrogenated' or 'partially hydrogenated fats', the product may contain an undesirable level of trans fats.

Food and Behaviour (FAB) Research, a Scotland-based scientific group, is highly critical of the reliance on voluntary action, claiming that far from being effective, it will ensure that parts of the food industry continue to use trans fats. The government's policy, says FAB, 'fails to protect the public, and particularly the most vulnerable members of our society'.

☑ TO AVOID TRANS FATS

- Do not buy or eat products listing hydrogenated or partially hydrogenated fat or oil on the label.
- Skip fried foods when you eat out unless you're assured they're not fried in partially hydrogenated oil.
- Cook with vegetable oil instead of solid shortening.
- Avoid cakes, pastries and biscuits unless you're sure that they are trans fat-free.

2 Dangerous sugars

Everyone loves a sweet treat but sugar, in its myriad forms, is now an ingredient in thousands of drinks, snacks and also savoury foods. For our health, it's a worrying trend.

No one is going to mistake sugar for a health food. But you might be wondering why it has been generating so much heated controversy. At least one health expert has called sugar a toxin that ought to be regulated like alcohol. Some feel the fault lies with specific types of sugar, such as fructose. Others say that singling out any one sugar is a distraction from the central issue: that eating too many kilojoules in general, particularly the 'empty' kilojoules in sweet foods and fizzy drinks, threatens our health in deadly ways. They also draw attention to the sugar added to a host of unexpected processed foods – the 'empty' kilojoules that many of us don't realise are there.

Did YOU know ?

Fizzy drink menace

If you had to lay responsibility for the world's obesity crisis at the door of just one villain, the most likely suspect is sugar-sweetened beverages (SSBs). One recent study estimated that a 15 per cent decrease in sugar-sweetened beverage consumption in Australia would mean over 100,000 fewer people with obesity.

A simple source of energy?

Sugar is a simple form of carbohydrate. Carbohydrates ('carbs' for short) are the sugars, starches and fibres found in fruits, vegetables, grains and milk products. Your body converts the starches and sugars in food to glucose, which fuels your brain, central nervous system and red blood cells. Any excess glucose is stored as glycogen in your liver and muscles, or is converted to body fat. If you eat too many simple carbs, you're likely to gain weight.

This was revealed all too clearly as the dietary habits of Western populations changed in the last decades of the 20th century. Over this period, the proportion of fat in the average diet actually decreased, and

➡️ Fizzy drinks are full of unnecessary 'empty' kilojoules.

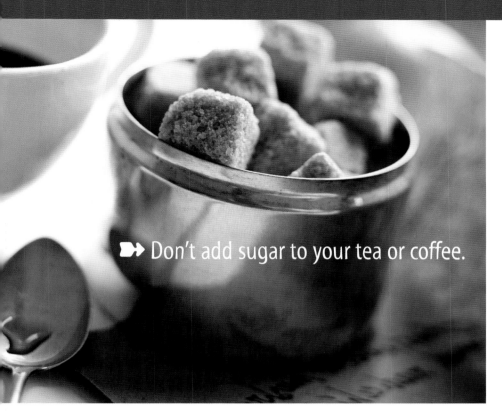

➠ Don't add sugar to your tea or coffee.

✓ SLASH YOUR SUGAR INTAKE

- Just say no to sugary fizzy drinks. In their place, enjoy fizzy water – on its own or with a slice or squeeze of lemon or lime, or with a splash of real fruit juice.
- If you add sugar to tea, coffee or cereal, wean yourself off it. Use a little less every day and within just a few weeks, you'll find you don't miss it at all.
- Read labels carefully and avoid food products that list any kind of sugar among the first few ingredients.
- When you buy canned fruit read the label to make sure it is in its own juice, not in sugar syrup.
- When you feel that you need something sweet, reach for a piece of real fruit or even a small square of dark, bittersweet chocolate.
- Choose wholegrain breakfast cereals and avoid those coated with sugar or honey.

yet obesity levels more than doubled. In the same period, the proportion of carbohydrates increased. This suggests that the dramatic increase in a nation's weight gain might have less to do with the consumption of fat and now more to do with the consumption of sugar.

'Added sugar' versus 'natural sugar'

The 'food foes' highlighted in this chapter are the sugars added to foods – not those that are contained in whole fruit and vegetables, dairy foods or grains. When you eat natural, unprocessed foods, you also get vitamins, minerals, fibre and phytochemicals, which help your body to digest those sugars and convert them to energy, supporting your health and vitality.

On the other hand, the sugars added to sweets, fizzy drinks, cakes and pastries add nothing that benefits your health. Sugary products are more likely to contribute to dental problems and often take the place of more nutritious foods that would otherwise be in your diet. For example, studies show that the more fizzy drinks a person consumes, the less milk he or she drinks. Milk, of course, is packed with calcium, protein and vitamins, while fizzy drinks are a nutritional black hole.

You might ask: how much added sugar is too much? That question doesn't have an easy answer. Different countries have quite different recommendations (*see* page 46). Australia and New Zealand have no official limit but in the UK, depending on age, size and activity levels, the NHS suggests a daily maximum of 70g of added sugars for men and 50g for women. As one rounded teaspoon of sugar equals 5g, this means no more than 14 teaspoons for men per day and 10 teaspoons for women. Does that seem a lot? In fact, it's remarkably easy to consume: just one regular 330ml can of cola packs 35g (7 teaspoons) of sugar.

The calculation below shows how grams of added sugar can translate into excess weight if you're eating too much and not burning off the energy in physical activity. Converted to kilojoules, this is what the female's maximum daily 50g adds up to:

1g of sugar = 16kJ

↓

16 x 50g (added sugar) = 800kJ each day

↓

800kJ per day x 365 days = 305,000kJ per year

↓

305,000kJ over one year = almost 9.5kg of added weight

The American Heart Association is more conservative than the UK and suggests that women should have no more than 6 teaspoons of added sugar a day (about 500kJ), while men should limit themselves to 9 teaspoons. For women, that's about the same amount of sugar as in a 50g chocolate bar and less than in two average scoops of ice cream.

Hidden sugars

Packed with sweetness

You expect to find sugar in chocolate and confectionery. The surprise is how much some savoury and even supposedly 'healthy' products contain, as the illustrated examples show. Some of the sweetness may be natural sugar from fruit or vegetables, but much is added sugar; food labels seldom distinguish between the two.

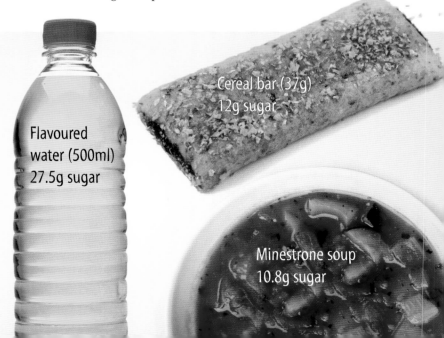

Flavoured water (500ml) 27.5g sugar

Cereal bar (37g) 12g sugar

Minestrone soup 10.8g sugar

The 'toxic' side of sugar

The omnipresence of sugar has got many of us hooked. Are you an addict? The answer for most people is probably 'yes'. To some extent, a liking for sugar is built into our human make-up. For much of our history, sugar, like fat, was hard to come by. It was only readily available during harvest time. People would gorge on sweet, ripe fruit, not unlike bears and other mammals fattening up for winter hibernation, or store it to help them through the long, cold days ahead.

These days sugar is available in quantities that have never been known before. Our innate taste for it and the allure of many foods that contain it encourage consumption – with consequent adverse effects on health.

Added sugar, particularly when consumed in drinks, is not a satiating source of energy - it does not help us to feel full, so it is easy to overeat. As well, it is harmful to teeth.

Its ageing effect

One controversial researcher, Dr Robert Lustig, suggests that sugar also speeds up the ageing process. 'The same "browning reaction" that occurs when you slather spare ribs with barbecue sauce occurs in all your cells when exposed to sugar.' This process, he asserts, leads to the kind of cellular damage that can shorten your life.

Perhaps the most controversial part of Dr Lustig's argument is his belief that sugar should be regulated like alcohol. He's not alone – in the USA, Michael Bloomberg, the mayor of New York, has caused a stir by fighting for a so-called 'Big Gulp' ban on sweet fizzy drinks larger than 480ml from restaurants, cinemas and other venues, which the beverage

KNOW YOUR SUGARS
as sweetness comes in many different guises. If any of the following items are listed on a food label, then the product contains sugar. Since ingredients are listed by weight on labels, if you see sugars among the first few ingredients, you know that the product contains a substantial amount of sugar.

- Brown sugar
- Cane juice
- Cane syrup
- Confectioner's sugar
- Corn sweetener and corn syrup
- Dextrose
- Fructose
- Fruit juice concentrates
- Glucose
- Granulated white sugar
- High-fructose corn syrup
- Honey
- Hydrolysed starch

➡ Check food labels Look for 'Carbohydrates – sugars'. More than 15g of total sugars per 100g is high; 5g of total sugars or less per 100g is low. Total sugars will include both natural and added sugars, although it's usually impossible to tell how much there is of each.

Creamy korma sauce 10g sugar per portion

Red kidney beans in chilli sauce 9.2g sugar per portion

Children's fromage frais (50g) 6.1g sugar

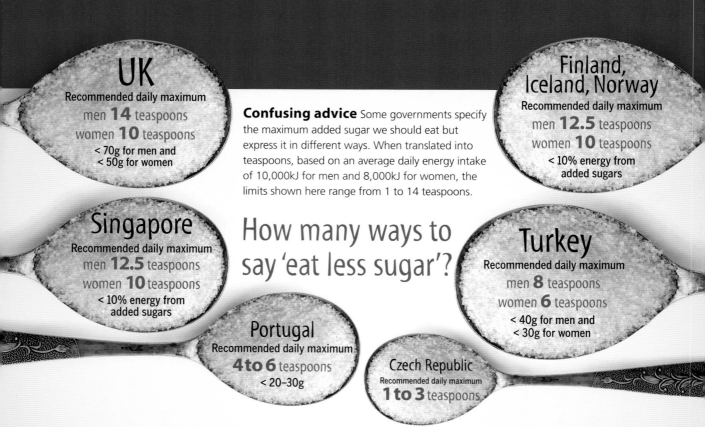

UK
Recommended daily maximum
men **14** teaspoons
women **10** teaspoons
< 70g for men and
< 50g for women

Confusing advice Some governments specify the maximum added sugar we should eat but express it in different ways. When translated into teaspoons, based on an average daily energy intake of 10,000kJ for men and 8,000kJ for women, the limits shown here range from 1 to 14 teaspoons.

Finland, Iceland, Norway
Recommended daily maximum
men **12.5** teaspoons
women **10** teaspoons
< 10% energy from
added sugars

Singapore
Recommended daily maximum
men **12.5** teaspoons
women **10** teaspoons
< 10% energy from
added sugars

How many ways to say 'eat less sugar'?

Turkey
Recommended daily maximum
men **8** teaspoons
women **6** teaspoons
< 40g for men and
< 30g for women

Portugal
Recommended daily maximum
4 to 6 teaspoons
< 20–30g

Czech Republic
Recommended daily maximum
1 to 3 teaspoons

Denmark and Sweden suggest a daily maximum of added sugars equivalent to 9 teaspoons, but only for children and people on energy-restricted diets, while for obese people and diabetics, France recommends a daily maximum equivalent to 12.5 teaspoons sugar for men and 10 teaspoons for women. Other countries, including Australia and New Zealand, have advice that is general, such as 'limit sugar consumption', 'avoid excessive consumption of sugars, sweet foods and drinks', 'reduce intake of kilojoules from added sugar' or 'reduce intake of sugar-sweetened beverages'. Thailand simply says 'avoid sweet foods', while Greece suggests 'limit sweet desserts to one every other day'.

industry is resisting. Meanwhile, in France a tax on sweetened drinks came into force in 2012. Hungary had introduced a tax on 'junk foods' including sweetened drinks the previous year. Other European countries are debating similar measures, including the UK where doctors have led the call for a tax on sweet fizzy drinks.

Is corn syrup the worst sugar?

Evidence is mounting that one form of sugar may be more dangerous than others: high-fructose corn syrup (HFCS). The sweetener is produced from corn. HFCS is much less expensive to produce than sucrose, the traditional sugar derived from sugar cane and sugar beet, so manufacturers, especially in the USA, prefer to use it in processed foods and beverages. Chemically, sucrose and HFCS are different, and some experts believe they behave differently in the body. Sucrose, familiar to us all as table sugar, is made up of fructose and glucose units joined together in equal amounts: when you consume sucrose, your body has to split the two units so they can be absorbed.

In contrast, HFCS is usually made up of 55 per cent fructose and 42 per cent glucose (plus oligosaccharides). Crucially the units are not joined together, so once consumed, the fructose and glucose are readily available and immediately absorbed. One study from Princeton University in the USA showed that rats with access to HFCS gained much more weight than rats with access to table sugar, even when they ate the same amount in kilojoules.

In 2010, researchers at the University of Colorado in the USA wrote that 'excess fructose intake should be considered an environmental toxin with major health implications'. In 2011, results of a US study published in the journal *Metabolism* suggested that drinking high-fructose corn syrup beverages raised both blood pressure and blood glucose levels higher than did sucrose-sweetened beverages. Research published in *The Journals of Gerontology* in 2010 has also linked excessive fructose intake to dementia. HFCS producers have challenged the findings and are contesting the claims.

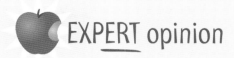

EXPERT opinion

Corn syrup warning

'Some people have claimed that high-fructose corn syrup is no different than other sweeteners when it comes to weight gain and obesity, but our results make clear that this just isn't true, at least under the conditions of our tests ... When rats are drinking high-fructose corn syrup at levels well below those in soda pop, they're becoming obese – every single one, across the board. Even when rats are fed a high-fat diet, you don't see this – they don't all gain extra weight.'

Bart Hoebel PhD *former Professor of Psychology, Princeton University, USA*

A clear message

All the evidence suggests that we should consume fewer foods and drinks that contain added sugars – and avoid excessive intakes of HFCS under any of its many names. Start cutting down as soon as you can. Gradually reduce the amount of sugar you add to tea and coffee, for example, or cut it out completely – you'll soon get used to the taste. Try diluting fruit juices to reduce their sugar content.

As your sugar intake decreases, your body will thank you; sweet treats send blood glucose see-sawing, with consequent energy and mood fluctuations. Fruits, fresh or dried, are a much more nutritious source of sweetness, offering vitamins, minerals and fibre, too. Eat naturally to fuel your body with essential nutrients – and see how much healthier you feel as a result.

✅ **AGAVE SYRUP** – a sweetener produced from a succulent Mexican plant is about 30 per cent sweeter than sugar or honey and has a very low glycaemic index (GI) so is absorbed more slowly by the body.

3 Super-refined ...
but far from cultivated foods

Research shows that the closer food is to its natural fresh state, the more nutritious and healthier it tends to be. But to make food as plentiful and convenient as it now is, a huge global industry is at work, transforming produce into a seductive and often low-cost commodity.

We talk about processed or 'refined' foods, but what are they? In fact, practically all the foods you buy in the supermarket are in some way or another processed or refined. So much happens to our food from the moment a crop is harvested or an animal is slaughtered to the point where it arrives on our plates. Processing ranges from the simplest and most basic actions, such as washing vegetables, to transforming foods via chemical additives and machine processes.

To preserve and protect

At the minimal-intervention end of the scale are actions that don't substantially change a food's composition or its nutritional value. Apart from washing, these would include peeling (although for many fruit and vegetables peeling and chopping accelerates the loss of vitamins). Expert freezing, drying and even fermenting are processes that may preserve many of a food's nutrients. Juicing (when the whole fruit is used with few additives) is also considered a minimal process. But it does alter the

➡ Processing and packaging foods ...

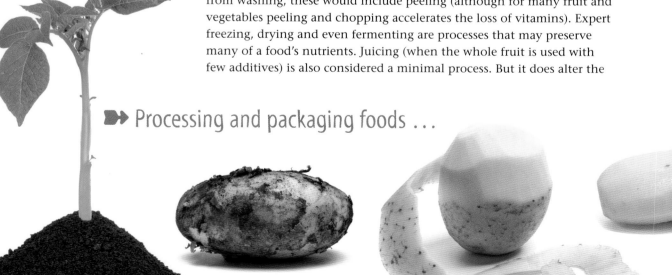

structure and food value of a fruit by removing pulp, which contains fibre and nutrients. Moving further along the processing continuum, some perishable packaged foods may have preservatives added to prevent the growth of pathogens – harmful bacteria or mould – and to prolong shelf life. Other foods are exposed to heat, or even radiation, to kill pathogens. Milk, for example, is heat pasteurised to kill potentially harmful bacteria.

The best preservation techniques retain the nutrients in the food, or most of them. Foods that are properly frozen and canned, for instance, will have good levels of natural nutrients and can play a valuable part in a healthy diet.

Transforming natural foods

All manner of natural ingredients are processed and treated to render them longer-lasting and easier to use in fast or packaged food production. Altered by various means are grain and oil seeds that are milled, refined, crushed and/or exposed to chemicals. These techniques can drastically change the nature of the original raw materials, up to and including processes that turn them into substances such as partially hydrogenated oil and high-fructose corn syrup – ingredients which are now believed to contribute to various health problems.

When natural ingredients are processed, they often lose their goodness because manufacturing can refine the nutrients right out of them, stripping grains, for instance, of bran, fibre, vitamins, minerals and phytochemicals to make them easier to package, store, sell and serve. As in the case of hydrogenated vegetable oil, there can be unforeseen consequences. The low-cost fat has a longer shelf life and is industrially convenient. But it also contains a high level of trans fats, which health experts say can trigger inflammation in the body. Inflammation can exacerbate everything from arthritis, carpal tunnel syndrome and diverticulosis to fibromyalgia and irritable bowel syndrome (*see also* Bad fats, page 38).

STRIPPED BARE of their vitamins, minerals, fibre and phytochemicals during manufacturing, many processed foods are left high in 'empty kilojoules'.

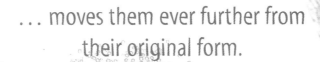

... moves them ever further from their original form.

A further potentially unhealthy aspect associated with super-refined foods is the manufacturers' tendency to make their products more instantly appealing to consumers by adding the flavours and textures that so many have come to crave (crispy, meaty, gooey, creamy, sweet) via the addition of fats, sugars, salt, artificial colourings, flavourings and preservatives (*see also* Chapter 4, page 64). This, of course, only encourages us all to eat more of certain nutritionally inferior foods.

Fortified with synthetic vitamins and minerals

Sometimes, addition in the form of fortification is a 'good thing'. Take salt, for example, to which the mineral iodine has been added. Iodine deficiency is the world's leading preventable cause of mental disability. It is also responsible for swelling of the thyroid gland in the condition known as goitre. The World Health Organization (WHO) is encouraging iodisation of salt across the globe. In some countries milk is fortified with vitamin D, which health experts suggest northern dwelling people may need more of, especially in winter when the sunshine needed to synthesise the vitamin is scarce. B vitamins and iron are often added to grain products.

The irony is that in the manufacture of foods such as cereals or bread, the makers often fortify the products with the very nutrients that were removed originally when the raw ingredients were processed. The manufacturers then claim nutritional benefits for their fortified foods, which may include highly sweetened breakfast cereals and snacks. But nutrition research by experts at the Johns Hopkins Bloomberg School of Public Health in Baltimore, Maryland, USA, suggests that the synthetic vitamins used may not offer the same nutritional benefits as vitamins that occur naturally. Part of the reason may be that vitamin supplements contain only the known vitamins, and not the myriad other natural substances in food that work together as a 'team' to benefit our health. Without all the members of the team, in the right proportions, it is not surprising that the effect is not the same.

In an article in the journal *Medical Hypotheses* naturopath Dr Robert Thiel explains it this way. Most synthetic vitamins 'are processed with petroleum

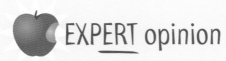

EXPERT opinion

Natural vs fortified foods

'There are no quick and easy magic-bullet solutions to good health that can be found in a dietary supplement or fortified-food product … I am a firm believer that we should get our nutrients mostly from real foods and not from synthetic sources. For me there is still too much left unknown about these substances to assume that they are automatically the same, or safe or healthy for consumption.'

Allison Righter MSPH RD *Johns Hopkins Bloomberg School of Public Health, USA*

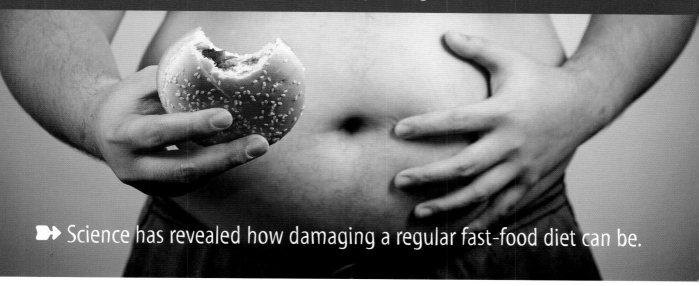

largely, say experts, as a result of unhealthy eating.

➠ Science has revealed how damaging a regular fast-food diet can be.

derivatives or hydrogenated sugars' and are chemically and structurally different from vitamins obtained from natural sources. As a result, their action on the body is likely to differ from the effect of natural vitamins.

Compelling reasons to choose better

There are many incentives to reach for convenient, often cheaper, fast food. You're busy perhaps and time is limited. As you look at the burger, chips and cola, you know you're not making the healthiest lunch choice, but how bad for you can a meal like this be just once in a while?

In 2007, a German study, known as the Hamburg Burger Trial, tried to find out. The researchers fed 24 healthy volunteers one of three meals: a regular burger-chips-fizzy drink meal; a vegetarian burger with the same drink and chips; or a vegetarian burger with a salad, yogurt and orange juice. The volunteers were tested at 2 hours then 4 hours after eating to see if their blood vessels responded differently to the different meals: 'stiffer' blood vessels would indicate an immediate negative impact on heart health. In fact, the groups showed no measurable differences, arguably proving that a highly refined, fast-food meal now and then won't kill you.

Don't get the fast-food habit

The problem with fast food is not the occasional burger and fries. The trouble starts when such foods are eaten more often. On that topic, the science has revealed just how damaging fast foods can be when they are consumed frequently and become a regular part of the diet.

EATING OUT OF BOREDOM

rather than actual hunger increased the odds of being super-morbidly obese by 35 per cent in one US study.

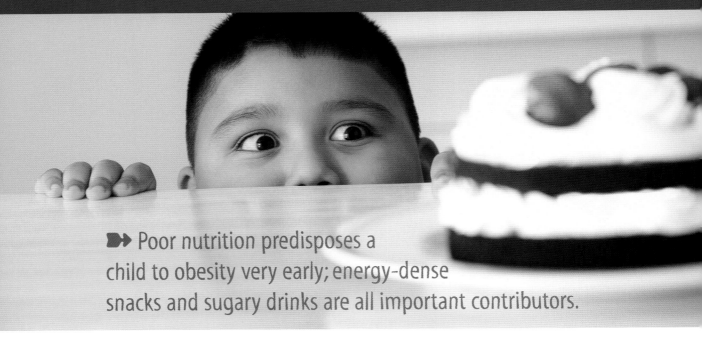

➤➤ Poor nutrition predisposes a child to obesity very early; energy-dense snacks and sugary drinks are all important contributors.

The link between fast foods and obesity is becoming ever clearer. In a study in 2012, researchers from the University of Texas, USA, were investigating the effects of behaviour on obesity. They gave their questionnaire to 270 obese people, all of whom were scheduled for bariatric surgery to help them reduce their weight. What the researchers discovered was that, on average, the people in the study ate fast foods nearly three times a week.

Furthermore, when they graded the people into three groups of worsening obesity – 'obese', 'morbidly obese' and 'super-morbidly obese' – they found that the risk of becoming 'super-morbidly obese' increased by 40 per cent with every additional refined, fast-food meal eaten per week.

Children and fast food

The effect of fast food on children is of particular concern to health experts. While poor diet and inactivity are often blamed in equal measure for obesity in adults, some believe that eating chips, burgers and high-kilojoule snacks has a much greater role to play in the worldwide obesity epidemic among the very young.

According to the World Health Organization, more than 42 million children under the age of five are now overweight, many of them in developing countries, putting them at risk of future heart disease and early type 2 diabetes, a disease once only seen in adults. This has enormous potential implications for life expectancy.

MEN WHO EAT TAKEAWAYS

twice a week or more are 31 per cent more likely than average to be moderately obese, and women with similar takeaway habits are 25 per cent more likely, according to a 2009 Australian study.

'It is said this will be the first generation where a significant number of parents will outlive their children,' says the EarlyBird Diabetes Trust, a UK research program. 'We need to find out why.'

The Trust's researchers followed a group of 300 normal, healthy children, monitoring their health and lifestyle for 12 years from 2000. In 2010 they announced, controversially, that it wasn't lack of exercise that produced fat children. Their studies showed clearly that a child's weight gain came first, often in the very earliest years of life. Their data reveals how poor nutrition predisposes a child to obesity and that 'portion size, energy-dense snacks and sugary drinks are all important contributors'. Other key findings from this long-term study include:

- Most excess weight is gained before a child ever starts school.
- All children today are at risk, regardless of family income or postcode.
- Parents are often unaware and unconcerned about obesity. Parents can be oblivious to their children's weight, says the Trust. 'Overweight is now perceived as the norm.'

The Trust's research and other studies that link fast-food consumption to adult health problems point in the same direction. We're not designed to consume overly processed foods. Eating fresh, natural produce, home-cooked rather than industrially manufactured, is likely to have a much more positive impact on future health.

Breaking bread

Modern bread is a perfect example of a staple that can lose a lot of its natural nutrition during refining and processing. The nutritional value of a loaf can vary hugely according to what goes in it and how it is made.

More than 50 years ago, the UK was at the forefront of a new production method that is now widely used also in Australia, New Zealand and India, and has spread to 28 countries worldwide. Scientists at the laboratories of the British Baking Industries Research Association, based at Chorleywood, had set out to create faster-baking, softer, cheaper, whiter loaves that sliced more uniformly and stayed fresher

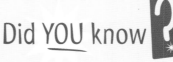

Did YOU know

Grain goodness

The health benefits of eating whole grains – from wheat, oats and other crops – in bread, muffins, biscuits, pasta, breakfast cereals and more include:

- Protection against diabetes: Harvard University researchers found that a diet high in cereal fibre is linked to a lower risk of developing type 2 diabetes, a finding supported by a number of other large, well-conducted studies.
- A reduced risk of heart disease: a 2007 analysis of seven major studies showed that people who eat 2.5 servings of wholegrain foods a day (compared to those who ate less than 2 servings a week) have a 21 per cent lower risk of developing heart disease.

for longer. In 1961, they worked out that adding solid fat, extra yeast and various chemicals to the dough, then mixing it at super-high speeds, dramatically reduced the rising and baking time required, and yielded the soft white loaves they were after. As a bonus their process, known as the Chorleywood Bread Process, enabled bakers to use home-grown British wheat, which previously had been too low in protein for bread-making.

Commercially, the Chorleywood process was a huge success, enabling bread to be made more quickly and cheaply. But from a health perspective, it transformed a vital staple food for the worse. Nutritionally speaking, bread made by this process is inferior to its browner, grainier predecessor.

According to Andrew Whitley, founder of the Village Bakery and author of *Bread Matters*, the quality of the wheat used presents another problem: 'The best traditional varieties of wheat have twice the iron and zinc of modern hybrids, and a recent French study revealed that the mineral content of French wheat is 30 to 40 per cent below that of older varieties.'

Added extras – for looks and shelf-life

Next, there's the milling of that wheat. Most industrial bakers use white flour milled by a fast rolling method in which the grain is exposed to very high temperatures (over 400°C). The process slashes some vitamin and mineral content by up to 86 per cent compared to wholemeal flour. Then there are the 'extras' either used by the millers or added in the baking process to achieve a light, white uniform loaf. These include flour treatment agents which help the bread to rise more, making it appear a larger loaf. Chlorine dioxide gas is used in milling to make flour whiter. Hard fats promote volume, softness and shelf-life. Emulsifiers help the dough to hold more gas (volume again) and also slow the rate at which the bread goes stale, an effect more generally promoted by adding

HIDDEN SALT Most of us expect to find salt in obviously salty foods such as chips and dips, but salt is also present, sometimes in high levels, in foods that are not obviously salty. Bread is a good example. A 2011 survey conducted by CASH (Consensus Action on Salt and Health) in the UK looked at 300 breads and found many had a high salt content, so be sure to check the nutritional analysis on the packet.

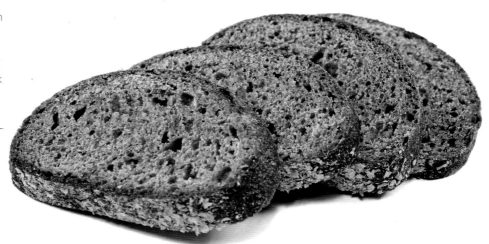

Key differences

Average white bread V. Wholemeal bread (100g = 4 slices)

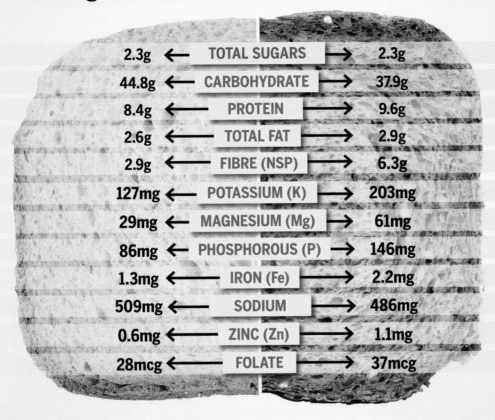

Average white bread		Wholemeal bread
2.3g	TOTAL SUGARS	2.3g
44.8g	CARBOHYDRATE	37.9g
8.4g	PROTEIN	9.6g
2.6g	TOTAL FAT	2.9g
2.9g	FIBRE (NSP)	6.3g
127mg	POTASSIUM (K)	203mg
29mg	MAGNESIUM (Mg)	61mg
86mg	PHOSPHOROUS (P)	146mg
1.3mg	IRON (Fe)	2.2mg
509mg	SODIUM	486mg
0.6mg	ZINC (Zn)	1.1mg
28mcg	FOLATE	37mcg

preservatives. This is a long way from the four ingredients needed to make bread: flour, water, yeast (for rising) and salt.

Finally, there is the sheer speed of the Chorleywood Bread Process. Andrew Whitley believes this may be the biggest problem of all because the dough isn't fermented long enough to allow beneficial natural bacteria to destroy harmful elements in the dough and make key nutrients available to the body. According to Whitley, modern bread-baking techniques could be one reason why digestive woes such as coeliac disease are becoming more common. He recommends radical action: 'From wheat to finished loaf, industrial baking needs to be reconstructed from first principles.'

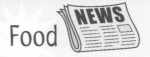

Food NEWS

Is it beef or horse meat?

In 2013, DNA testing in the UK and Europe revealed that some ready meals labelled as beef contained horse meat. Although not a threat to human health, the fact that a food product contained unlisted surprise ingredients shocked consumers and retailers alike. The discovery highlighted the long and complicated road that many ingredients now travel before being put into products and reaching the shops. Meats from more than one country are routinely mixed together during processing. This is not apparent as labelling reflects where a product is made, not the source of its ingredients. Consumers have called for tougher laws.

Convenience foods

'Why cook?' you might ask yourself, as you push your trolley through the aisles of your brightly lit, well-stocked supermarket at the end of a busy day. You'll be seduced by images of 'special' slow-cooked beef lasagne, chicken curry, Greek moussaka or a meat or fish pie, staring at you from the fridges, tempting you to take them home.

'Luxury' may not equal 'healthy'

Perhaps surprisingly, sales of 'ready meals' in industrialised countries have continued to grow despite the recession of recent years. In Europe the UK has been leading this trend with more than 40 per cent of total sales; France and Germany account for around 20 per cent each. It seems that as consumers reined in spending on eating out, food manufacturers and retailers found they could sell us more 'premium' ready meals as an affordable treat.

But as you contemplate whether to splurge on that ready meal for the family instead of cooking from scratch, it might be worth remembering that money may not be the only thing you're splurging on, especially if you opt for the 'luxury' version.

In a 2012 study run by Glasgow University, Scottish researchers visited several supermarkets to purchase and compare a range of the meals. Here's what they discovered:

● One beef lasagne contained more than 77 per cent of an adult's daily maximum saturated fat intake – twice the fat contained in the same store's basic beef lasagne; its saturated fat content was 36 per cent of the recommended daily limit.

● One supermarket brand of 'finest' cottage pie contained 39 per cent of the recommended saturated fat limit, while a 'value' version had less than half that (18 per cent) and also half the amount of salt.

● Another store's 'extra special' macaroni cheese weighed in with a whopping 118 per cent of the daily saturated fat limit; the bargain version contained 48 per cent.

Of the 67 products tested, almost half did not have enough kilojoules to constitute a proper meal, while 10, including

Saturated fat in the 'luxury' beef lasagne was more than 77% of an adult's daily maximum intake.

By contrast, the basic beef lasagne contained 36% of an adult's daily maximum saturated fat intake.

Did YOU know?

Bacon, beware!

Not only is bacon a processed meat, which experts now believe is linked to an increased risk of cancer, heart disease and type 2 diabetes, it's also a huge contributor of salt in Western diets. Just two rashers can contain more than half your daily salt maximum, which is 6g, and some even more, although certain suppliers are now taking action to reduce salt levels. Since Consensus Action on Salt and Health, a scientific group concerned with the serious effects of salt on health, issued its report in 2012, at least one major supermarket chain is reported to be launching lower-salt bacon products.

➤➤ **Just two rashers of bacon can contain more than half your daily salt maximum, which is 6g.**

premium products, had more than 3,000kJ. Researchers were astonished by the nutritional disparities. 'Generating simple standards for ready meals would cost little, upset few and would help consumers,' said Mike Lean, chair of human nutrition at Glasgow University. 'The need for food manufacturers to consider nutrition should be pretty obvious by now.'

That price is not always the best indicator of good nutrition is also evident from another study, this one conducted by a UK shopping website in 2012. A high-priced fruit and nut muesli in one store had almost three times the sugar of its bargain counterpart. 'Basic' cookies in another store turned out to have a third less fat and 25 per cent less sugar than its 'luxury' cookies that were three times the price. And there were similar findings for pizzas, quiches, pies and pasties – in all cases, the budget store brands had less fat, sugar and fewer kilojoules than the higher-priced alternatives.

Pleasurable as food browsing is, being a savvy shopper means turning over the colourful packaging and paying close attention to the nutritional information in the small print, and understanding what it means. The possible advent of front-of-pack labelling (*see* Part 4, Shopping for quality, page 145) may make all this clearer and might persuade manufacturers to rethink the ingredients they use.

Processed meat and you

Curing meat is an ancient preservation technique dating back to Roman times. Back then, the procedure involved little more than salt, smoke, vinegar and oil. The expensive and delicious modern descendants include Italy's prosciutto di Parma, Spain's jamón serrano and France's Bayonne ham.

When you indulge in such delicacies, you're likely to savour a small amount – because of the price, and also because a little goes a long way. But it's eating processed meats – bacon, sausages, hot dogs or luncheon meats – frequently and in quantity that appears to pose the greatest danger. Given what science now knows about the health impact of cured, smoked and salted meats, you'll be doing yourself and your family a favour if you relegate them to the 'every now and then' spot reserved for gastronomic indulgences like gourmet ham.

One 2010 study from the Harvard School of Public Health, USA, found that people who regularly ate processed meats had a 42 per cent higher risk of heart disease and a 19 per cent higher risk of type 2 diabetes. The World Cancer Research Fund reviewed thousands of clinical studies and its guidance in a 2012 report was clear: 'We advise people worried about cancer risk to avoid processed meat whenever possible.'

PINK SLIME is how Americans describe beef that is mechanically recovered and processed from low-grade trimmings First approved for pet food, it is now widely used as a filler in US meat products.

Red for danger, or something more?

Why is processed meat so bad for us? First, because most of it starts as red meat, which has also been linked to higher rates of cancer and heart disease. But it seems that something else is going on. In a 2012 study published in the *British Journal of Cancer*, researchers who examined 1,171 cases of people diagnosed with bladder cancer learned that people who ate the most processed meat had the highest risk of developing the disease – 41 per cent higher than people who didn't eat the stuff. And those who frequently ate 'white' processed meat, such as turkey and chicken, also had a 28 per cent higher risk of bladder cancer. Other prominent studies have echoed these findings.

Blame it on the chemicals, says one of the study's co-authors, Rashmi Sinha, PhD, deputy chief of Nutritional Epidemiology at the National Cancer Institute in the USA. Processed meats contain several additives that preserve the meat, including nitrate or nitrite, which form compounds that are harmful; studies in animals have found they can cause tumours. And many other additives are used during the processing, smoking or salting of meats that could also promote cancer. Processed meats, says Sinha, are 'associated with a high risk of type 2 diabetes, heart disease, stroke and certain cancers ' – risks that are higher than those for unprocessed red meats.

Re-formed meat

There may be other reasons to question what exactly is in supermarket packets of processed meat. If you've examined labels on some of the cheaper products you may have noticed the words 'reformed' or 'reconstituted' and wondered precisely what that means.

There is a food-processing system called 'mechanically separated meat' (MSM), or 'mechanically recovered meat' (MRM), which removes meat from flesh-bearing bones of pigs and poultry, resulting in a sort of slurry-like meat product. MSM must be separately labelled in the ingredients list

Anatomy of the chicken nugget

Perhaps nothing symbolises the modern food-processing industry more than the chicken nugget. Invented in the 1950s by a professor of food science at Cornell University, USA, nuggets didn't take the world by storm until industrial-scale chicken farming and food processing could supply demand. In the 1980s, chicken nuggets were launched by McDonald's as the 'healthy option' (compared to beef), so perhaps it's not surprising that many of us thought they really were a healthy choice. After all, they contained pure chicken protein, didn't they? Better-quality chicken nuggets may contain breast meat but here's what can lurk behind that crispy exterior:

1. Mechanically deboned poultry meat, minced up with skin and other carcass bits – skin is essential to the texture and taste: one manufacturer reckons about 16 per cent is best.

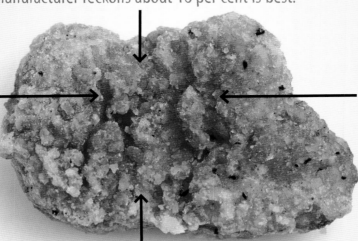

2. Salt, eggwhite, soy products and other fillers and binders, and in some cases additives to make the mixture hold water.

3. The mixture is extruded into nugget shapes, which are dusted with flour, battered and breaded, then deep-fried.

4. Nuggets are frozen, vacuum-packed and sent off to retailers, where they are fried again before being served to customers.

Source: Johns Hopkins Bloomberg School of Public Health.

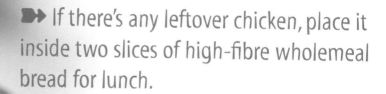

If there's any leftover chicken, place it inside two slices of high-fibre wholemeal bread for lunch.

of a product. Re-formed meat may contain MSM or other surplus parts of meat and the manufacturing process 'glues' them together to resemble normal cuts. These are safe to eat, but we're possibly right to question their quality – and look carefully at other ingredients, which often include other additives, preservatives and added water, compared to freshly carved meats.

The better lunch choice

So what should you have in your lunchtime sandwich? If there's leftover chicken from last night's dinner, carve it up and place it inside two slices of high-fibre, wholemeal bread, with some sliced tomato and lettuce. Buy freshly carved meat from the deli counter and choose sliced packaged meats – not those described as 're-formed'.

Cereal and cereal bars

Most breakfast cereals are pretty far removed from natural grains and laced with more sugar, fat and salt – and far less fibre – than is good for us. What is surprising, however, is that some high-profile cereals specifically marketed as 'healthy' are among those high in sugar and salt, as Australian consumer organisation Choice discovered in 2012. Sugar levels were extremely high in no fewer than 112 of the 195 cereals analysed.

One reason why it's so tricky to choose a healthy option is that few use front-of-pack labelling that the World Health Organization recommends to help us all shop more sensibly (*see* page 145). Further confusion arises because the serving sizes quoted differ from brand to brand, and some manufacturers include milk in the 'per serving' nutritional information, while others don't.

When it comes to cereal bars, matters are even worse. The manufacturers would have you think that these 'grab and go' products are perfectly healthy mini-breakfasts that pack the nutritional 'oomph' you need to give a good start to your day. They may be called 'nutri'-something or the minimal fruit or nuts they contain is often highlighted to make the

SALT LEVELS

were generally down in a 2012 survey of cereals by Choice, as a result of a 2010 agreement between Australian cereal companies. The survey found that of 195 products tested, only 49 met that year's sodium target of 120mg per 100g.

product more convincing. However, when the consumer organisation's researchers examined 28 different cereal bars available on Australian supermarket shelves, this is what they found:

- **High sugar levels** – of the 28 bars examined, 14 were more than 30 per cent sugar. Although in many bars some of the sugar came from fruit, all contained added sugar as well.
- **'Trick' labelling** – by law, manufacturers must list ingredients in order of weight in a particular product. But if a product contains different kinds of sugar, these can be listed separately. This loophole allows manufacturers to list oats, say, higher up the list than the three different kinds of sugar in the product – even though the total sugars may outweigh the oats.
- **Packed with fat** – 11 of the 28 bars were high in saturated fat. Some of the bars (including brands labelled 'no artificial colours, flavours or preservatives') contained synthetic hydrogenated vegetable oil, which may increase the risk of heart disease (*see* page 38).

➦ Be careful with cereal bars, some contain as much as 18g of sugar per bar – that's nearly four teaspoons!

In addition, Choice reported that seven of the bars contained more kilojoules than a Mars Bar. The overriding message for parents was don't assume these products are healthy and read the labels like a hawk: you might think that by putting a cereal bar into your child's lunchbox you're giving them a nutrition boost, but in some cases it's just a crunchy candy bar.

Beware not-so-healthy 'health foods'

These days, food manufacturers know that putting words such as 'healthy', 'natural', 'low-fat' and other such labels on their packaged foods increases their appeal to customers seeking nutritious foods. But as it turns out, not everything labelled 'healthy' actually is. Many are packed with sugar, fat and salt – or come with other extraneous ingredients you don't need. The key advice is this: carefully read nutrition labels on all the food you're buying. Don't be lulled into thinking that healthy-sounding labels guarantee a healthy product. Here are some examples of 'unhealthy' food traps for the unwary.

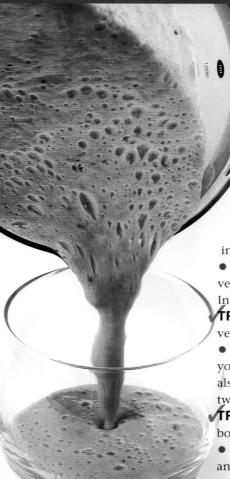

- **Smoothies** – nutritionally speaking these might be an improvement over many fizzy drinks, but that doesn't make them all healthy. Smoothies – which come in many varieties – may contain some crushed fruit and fruit juice, which sounds fine, but fruit juice has none of the important fibre that you get from fresh fruit. And if you sip juicy smoothies slowly over time, the acidic juice can damage your tooth enamel. Some smoothies are very energy-dense and may contain syrups, sugar, and even peanut butter and chocolate.

✓**TRY THIS INSTEAD** When buying a ready-made smoothie, make sure it contains whole fruit, not just juice. Better still, make your own: in a blender whizz together fresh fruit and unsweetened low-fat yogurt.

- **Vegetable crisps** You think you're sneaking in a tasty serving of vegetables by choosing these instead of potato crisps, but you're not. Instead, you're getting lots of kilojoules and fat.

✓**TRY THIS INSTEAD** Air-popped popcorn or a packet of freeze-dried real vegetables – just beware of added fat or salt.

- **Bran muffins** Anything labelled 'bran' sounds as if it must be good for you, because it has plenty of fibre. Not true. Mega-sized bran muffins can also have plenty of fat, sugar and kilojoules, and often contain more than two servings.

✓**TRY THIS INSTEAD** Keep to small bran muffins, or better still, enjoy a bowl of bran cereal with low-fat milk and fresh fruit.

- **Flavoured vitamin and mineral waters** Plain old H_2O has become another hot commodity these days, and added vitamins, minerals or caffeine make it seem as if you're getting something extra for your money. But why pay extra for stuff that you don't need? Some of the enhanced waters on the market are also laced with sugar, so read labels carefully. Similarly, so-called 'natural' flavourings in mineral waters with fewer ingredients contain flavouring and up to 30g of sugar per half litre – that's a whole six teaspoons of sugar.

✓**TRY THIS INSTEAD** Tap water that's been chilled in the fridge with a large slice of lemon in it.

- **Granola** The increasingly popular crunchy, toasted-oat breakfast food, granola is not all bad news. It's often fibre-rich and low on the glycaemic index, so it keeps you feeling full for longer. It may also contain omega-3 and omega-6 fatty acids, B vitamins, iron and folate from the rolled oats, fruits, nuts and seeds. On the down side, many granolas are high in sugar, with more than 12.5g per 100g; high in saturated fat (5g per 100g); and high in total fat (20g per 100g).

➡ Better still, make your own smoothies in a blender.

✓TRY THIS INSTEAD By sprinkling nuts, seeds or fruit over your porridge or muesli, you can get the same taste and nutrition as granola and you'll slash your sugar and fat intake, says Bond. Or make your own granola, by mixing together dried fruit, nuts, a little honey and canola oil and pouring this over rolled oats, then baking it in the oven.

● **Frozen yogurt** You avoid the ice cream in the supermarket frozen foods section, going for frozen yogurt as a leaner, healthier option. But is it? Some versions are packed with sugar, so your best bet is to scrutinise the labels before you buy.

✓TRY THIS INSTEAD Low-fat versions of Greek yogurt, with live active cultures, are a good choice here.

● **Couscous** If you think you're making a healthier carbohydrate choice than white pasta when you eat couscous, think again. Couscous, like pasta, is made from semolina flour and the processed white version contains little fibre or nutrients.

✓TRY THIS INSTEAD Wholemeal couscous, or better still try whole grains such as quinoa or wild rice.

● **Wrap sandwiches** Substituting a thin-looking wrap without butter for a traditional bread sandwich might seem a skinnier option, but it's not. The tortilla wrap alone can sneak in as many as 1,000kJ to 1,500kJ, and that's not counting the filling.

✓TRY THIS INSTEAD A sandwich of wholemeal bread, the grainier the better, spread with a little low-fat mayonnaise then filled with egg, roast turkey or chicken, plus a pile of tomatoes, roasted capsicum and dark green lettuce.

Making the best choices

In all but the freshest foods, some form of processing is evidently unavoidable. And when it helps to keep a food from rotting or, for instance, transforms inedible grains into flour, it is of course to everyone's benefit. Although companies are not legally obliged to reveal all their ingredients, many now do, so understanding food labels is important to help establish good-quality products from something, however well-dressed, that is merely pretending to be good.

Read on to discover more about the many additives that manufacturers use. Some help to preserve a product, others are there for bulk or appearance; relatively few are included for your good health.

'LIGHT' foods
There is no law governing what 'light' means on a food label – 'light' could refer to pale colour or mild flavour, and not be low in kilojoules.

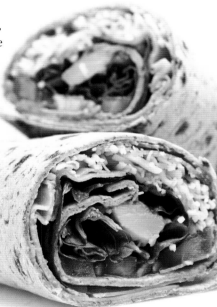

4 An excess of additives?

Pick up any packaged foodstuff today and you'll often find that its nutrition label includes a number of mystifying ingredients from code numbers and emulsifiers to sulphites and nitrites. Do we need them all?

We take it on trust that food ingredients are good for us – after all the industry is properly governed and regulated, isn't it? The answer is yes, and sometimes no, as this chapter explains. And while most of what is added is technically 'safe', the other question is, are all these additional extras strictly necessary or conducive to good health?

The urge to spice

Adding condiments to food is nothing new. In early human society, spices were used mostly to preserve food. Salting food or soaking it in seawater lengthened its life and as a bonus infused it with extra flavour. Gradually, through experimentation, people learned to use spices obtained from the fruit, seeds, bark and roots of plants – many of which have antibacterial or antifungal properties – to do a similar job of preserving and flavouring. As trade developed, spices were among the most valuable commodities. The desire for these exotic flavourings drove much of the seafaring exploration in the Middle Ages.

Today, a vast array of spices is readily available and used imaginatively by amateur cooks and professional chefs. But within food manufacturing, flavour and food preservation are usually achieved in a rather different way.

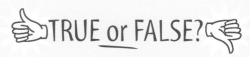

TRUE or FALSE?

Curry's fiery ingredient, the red hot chilli, is native to India

FALSE! When Christopher Columbus sailed to the New World, his discoveries opened up a whole new realm of foods and spices, too. Among them was the pungent chilli which has been grown in Central America since 7500BC. Just as the spices of the East Indies came west along the trade routes, so the chilli was taken via Europe to Asia in the 1500s. South American chillies are now synonymous with much Asian cuisine and India is the largest chilli producer in the world.

Salt – natural but misused?

It is one of the most ancient preservatives – and today the most widely used additive in processed foods. What makes salt so popular in the industry is its capacity for enhancing flavours – in cereals, biscuits, nuts, crisps and much more. Research suggests that at least 75 per cent of our salt intake comes from restaurant and processed foods. Salt adds the edge, encouraging us to eat and drink more. Most of us consume more than the recommended maximum of 5g to 6g daily (2g to 2.4g sodium).

Why does this matter? Research worldwide has linked a high salt intake to high blood pressure, a dangerous risk factor for heart disease and stroke. Health authorities including the World Health Organization say that millions of premature deaths could be avoided if we all cut back and food manufacturers reduced the sodium content of their foods.

How much is too much in processed foods? Ideally, look for foods with less than 120mg sodium and restrict your intake of high-sodium foods. More than 600mg sodium per 100g is 'high'. Low-salt foods have 0.3g (0.1g sodium) or less per 100g. And try not to add extra salt to food; you'll find you soon lose the taste. Instead, use more spices and herbs to flavour dishes.

FOOD ADDITIVES

are officially defined as 'any substance not normally consumed as a food itself' that is used for a 'technological purpose in the manufacture, processing, preparation, treatment, packaging, transport or storage of food'.

From condiments to chemicals

What about other food additives – the vast array of chemicals we see listed on food labels? Some are natural, extracted from those once-exotic spices – such as the colouring curcumin from turmeric – and other plant or animal sources. Most are artificial, either recreating a natural substance or inspired by chemicals occurring somewhere in nature.

Evil additives of the past …

History records that unscrupulous merchants often used ingredients other than spices to add flavour or bulk to food – and boost their profits. Everything from mashed potatoes to plaster of Paris gave bread more heft, while various bitter compounds, including the poison strychnine, were put into beer because they were cheaper than hops. In the late 18th century, toxic lead, copper or mercury salts were often used to colour children's sweets. Tea and coffee might be adulterated with anything from sheep's dung to chemical colours. From the 19th century, governments across the world adopted safety measures. Today volumes of regulations dictate what can or can't go into food and drinks.

In the developed world, at least, governments have put in place standards and regulations that govern the testing, licensing and use of chemical additives. Although there is common ground internationally, these standards vary from country to country. Take butter: in some countries salt and antioxidants are added, plus yellow pigment to keep the colour consistent, while Ireland prohibits any additives other than the traditional salt.

Approved additives are assigned an international code number. This numeric system was developed as a language-free labelling method. Public response has been less positive; partly because people don't understand them, code numbers have aroused suspicions and been blamed for a number of ills.

In fact, most of the additives used world-wide have clear and distinct functions. They can be broadly classified into six main groups.

- **Antioxidants** help to prevent foods from spoiling or going rancid, particularly those prepared with oils or fats, which could include everything from meat pies to mayonnaise. They also help to preserve bakery products, soup mixes and sauces. Common antioxidants include ascorbic acid (synthetic vitamin C, 300) and tocopherols (306).
- **Emulsifiers, stabilisers, gelling agents and thickeners** are the various agents that keep foods from separating, enable foods to gel, and help to add body and thickness. Lecithin (322) and monoglycerides and

➡ Butter from pasture-fed cows is a deeper yellow than that of grain-fed cows because of the carotene present in grass.

diglycerides of fatty acids (471) are among the most common. Pectin (440) is the gelling agent used in jams and jellies.

• **Flavour enhancers** bring out the flavour of foods without imparting any of their own. Monosodium glutamate (MSG) is one of the best-known additives in packaged foods (621). *See also* pages 69–70.

• **Food colours** are used to add colour lost through processing, storage or seasonal variation and to make the food conform better to consumer expectations. But – and this is an important 'but' – it is illegal to use food colours to disguise inferior quality. Common colours include caramel (150a), used in products such as gravy and soft drinks, and curcumin (100), a yellow colouring extracted from the roots of the turmeric plant.

• **Preservatives** limit the growth of micro-organisms, enabling foods to be kept for longer. Sometimes, preservatives are simple compounds such as salt, sugar or vinegar. Common preservatives – sulphur dioxide (220) stops mould and bacteria growth on dried fruit; bacon, ham, corned beef and other cured meats rely on nitrate and nitrite (249 to 252).

• **Sweeteners** used alone or with sugar, make foods taste sweeter. Common artificial sweeteners include aspartame (951), saccharin (954) and sorbitol (420).

The pros and cons

It is no exaggeration to say that the modern food industry could not exist without its stock of food additives. Those in favour point out that without preservatives, for example, many foodstuffs would be far more unsafe than they are and that chemicals in food are used only in minute quantities. Many, such as pectin, have a long history in cooking and are known to be harmless; others, such as ascorbic acid (a synthetic form of vitamin C), are actually good for you. Some are even permitted in organic food products.

Critics argue that the food industry does not use additives only for the benefit of customers but also to increase profits, that there are far more additives (including salt, *see* page 65) than are strictly essential in foods and that minute quantities can build up over the long term, with potentially serious effects for health. Certain additives are also the subject of heated controversy because they are suspected of directly provoking allergies or behavioural problems. As such they have become the subject of further research and a target of good-food campaigners.

MORE THAN 700

substances are used worldwide as food additives. Around 400 of these have been assigned international numbers; food standards regulations in each country control how these can be used.

Can additives worsen behavioural problems?

For more than 35 years, researchers have been trying to establish if there is a connection between certain food additives and children's behaviour, specifically Attention Deficit Hyperactivity Disorder (ADHD).

In 2007, the UK's Food Standards Agency commissioned a study by Southampton University to examine the effects of certain artificial food colours and the preservative sodium benzoate (a combination often found in favourite children's foods). The researchers reported that, while not conclusive, their results did suggest a connection between certain artificial food colours and sodium benzoate and children's behavioural problems. As a result, the British government asked food manufacturers to enact a voluntary ban on certain food colourants.

Another UK research team evaluated children with hyperactivity, and discovered that most of them experienced increased behavioural problems when they consumed tartrazine and sunset yellow. An increased incidence of eczema, asthma and allergies was also reported in children who consumed high levels of these artificial colours.

Yet, the link is far from clear. The evidence to date does not prove that any artificial colourings actually cause ADHD, as a 2012 review of 35 years of research in the journal *Clinical Paediatrics* points out. But it is known that some children with ADHD will improve significantly on a diet free from artificial colourings; this may be due to a more general sensitivity to food chemicals. The authors suggest that parents who believe that certain additives or foods are exacerbating their children's symptoms should ask their doctor if the child could be tested for hypersensitivities. They could then experiment with an elimination diet that excludes the trigger foods.

THE ARTIFICIAL COLOURINGS

that British research suggests may be linked to children's behavioural problems are:

110 (sunset yellow)
104 (quinoline yellow)
122 (carmoisine)
129 (allura red)
102 (tartrazine)
124 (ponceau 4R)

➡ Sixty per cent of children experienced increased behaviour problems after eating foods containing synthetic colours and flavours.

Allergies and food intolerances

It is important to make a clear distinction between food *allergies* and food *intolerances*. An allergy is an immune response to even a tiny amount of a food protein. As most food additives aren't proteins, allergies to them are rare. A true allergy is more likely to be caused by foods such as nuts, peanuts, shellfish, milk, wheat, eggs, soy or sesame seeds.

Food intolerances seem to be quite common, but studies have cast doubt on just how frequently they really occur. For example, up to 20 per cent of parents report their children as 'intolerant' of food additives, says Allergy UK. But research using 'blind' food challenges estimates that actual adverse reactions to additives occur in fewer than one in 100 children.

The bottom line for any food or additive is that anyone can have an allergic or intolerant reaction to anything, but some of us are more sensitive to additives than others. If you suspect an untoward reaction to colourings, aspartame, MSG or any other additive or food, the best advice is to read labels carefully and avoid food products that contain them. To check whether your suspicions of a specific ingredient or food are correct, as a first step, allergy experts recommend that you keep a food diary. Then, seek your doctor's advice.

MSG – good or bad?

It is now more than 40 years since 'Chinese restaurant syndrome' first hit the headlines. The symptoms included numbness in the neck, tingling of the cheeks, palpitations and headache, and its onset was blamed on high levels of monosodium glutamate, MSG for short, in a Chinese meal. The effect on Chinese restaurants was so serious that some started advising patrons that their food was 'MSG-free'. Since then, the substance has been subjected to extensive scientific scrutiny, but with mixed results: some experts remain convinced it is harmful; others exonerate it of any blame.

Monosodium glutamate was created in the early 20th century by a Japanese professor, Kidunae Ikeda, inspired by his wife's delicious seaweed soup. He worked out that the taste was produced by glutamate, a natural substance. He then isolated glutamate as a chemical and stabilised it by adding salt and water, to make monosodium glutamate.

The cheap and simple additive he had discovered enhanced the flavour of savoury foods, and made his fortune. Today, worldwide production of MSG – mostly for the food industry – is estimated to be in excess of 3 million tonnes, with China by far the largest producer and consumer.

MSG remains a source of suspicion among Western consumers, although research has failed to provide supporting scientific evidence.

20%–30%
of children with asthma are sensitive to sulphite preservatives, found in dried fruits, drinks, sauces and many other foods, according to a World Health Organization report.

Can you avoid MSG?

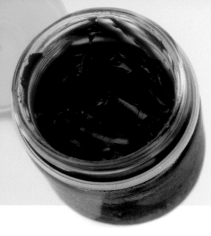

MSG is now widespread in food manufacture. Even if it is not listed in the ingredients of a food product, its active ingredient, glutamate, could still be present under a different name such as 621, glutamic acid, autolysed yeast extract or sodium caseinate. Glutamate occurs naturally in so many foods that it is not possible to avoid it completely. Two popular foods with very high concentrations of naturally occurring glutamate are yeast extract (aka Vegemite) and parmesan cheese. And herein perhaps is a clue: we naturally consume these full-flavoured foods in very small amounts, so the answer, as in so many things, lies in balance and moderation.

It is far more likely that the symptoms are actually associated with intolerance to glutamates in general, and susceptible people should avoid consuming large amounts of high-glutamate foods, including both natural sources and processed foods containing MSG.

Chemicals that mimic 'real' flavours

MSG is by no means the only synthetic flavour enhancer that manufacturers use to tempt our tastebuds. Scientists have isolated the most dominant flavouring components in foods such as strawberries, coffee or lemons. Today legions of 'flavourists' match these 'natural' or cheaper synthetic chemicals to create tastes for use in processed foods and drinks. Some grape drinks, for instance, have absolutely no 'grape' in them, relying on lab-created flavour chemicals for their taste. People with food chemical sensitivity may find that they react to some added flavourings as well as to concentrated sources of natural food chemicals. If you are concerned, check labels and avoid anything that is listed as an added flavouring.

ARTIFICIAL SWEETENERS such as saccharin, aspartame and sucralose may actually contribute to weight gain, rather than helping people to lose weight, say researchers.

The obesity connection

New research from Austria is putting other food additives under the microscope and may help to explain why so many of us put on too much weight so easily. It is early days but scientists at the Innsbruck Medical University believe that the food preservatives sodium sulphite and sodium benzoate could play a role in obesity. According to their work, conducted so far in test tubes and published in the *British Journal of Nutrition* in 2012, the common additives appear to delay the release of a hormone, leptin, which is known to decrease appetite. This suggests that eating foods containing these additives could suppress the body's natural inclination to feel full after eating, encouraging us to eat more.

Artificial sweeteners, such as saccharin, aspartame and sucralose, are also accused of contributing to obesity. Some research has found that, far from helping people to lose weight, they may actually contribute to weight gain. When consumed regularly, one theory suggests, they fail to satisfy the body's urge for energy-rich food, encouraging an endless cycle of cravings for sweet foods, which leads in turn to eating more. A 2009 study in the US journal *Diabetes Care* linked drinking diet drinks daily to a high waistline circumference and a 67 per cent increase in type 2 diabetes.

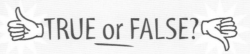

TRUE or FALSE?

Switching to diet cola drinks helps you to lose weight

FALSE! It may seem counter-intuitive to think that a drink with no kilojoules could cause weight gain, but three studies in recent years seem to support this notion.

- A 2011 study published in the *American Journal of Clinical Nutrition* reported that diet soft drinks can increase fat storage in the liver.
- A study presented at the 2011 American Diabetes Association's Scientific Sessions pointed to the possibility that drinking diet soft drinks could expand your waistline.
- A 2009 study published in *Diabetes Care* suggests that drinking diet soft drinks every day could increase the risk of type 2 diabetes by 67 per cent.

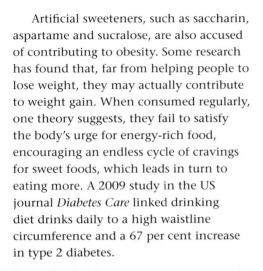

What else about artificial sweeteners?

Back in the mid-20th century there were fears that saccharin and cyclamates might pose a cancer risk for humans. Research has discounted this. But aspartame (951), another artificial sweetener, which is about 200 times sweeter than sugar, has been linked to health problems, including headaches, depression and even cancer. Studies have reported contradictory results, but it is clear that some people are highly sensitive to its effects. If you're one of them, you will want to avoid any products sweetened with it.

Additives and you

Most of us cannot and would not wish to scrutinise the ingredients of everything we eat. But reading the label for additives that might possibly have an adverse effect makes perfect sense in an era when so much is added to manufactured food. If you or someone close to you suffers any sort of reaction shortly after eating a particular processed foodstuff, find the packaging and keep a note of ingredients for future reference. Food manufacturers comply with hygiene and safety regulations but they're not health providers. Consumers should be alert and careful.

5 Evil spirits?

Many people enjoy alcohol. Across the world, a glass of champagne or beer or a colourful cocktail is synonymous with celebrations. We drink when we're happy – and sometimes to dull the pain of sadness. What's the harm in that?

Plenty, as it turns out. Drink in the Western world – rather like food – has seldom been so ubiquitous or so readily available. While some governments have restricted advertising in recent years, films, soaps and general peer pressure perpetuate alcohol's 'happy' image. It remains the Western drug of choice – socially acceptable until we drink to excess or become addicted, when it can have a devastating effect on health and individuals' lives.

How we rank

According to a 2011 report from the World Health Organization (WHO), amongst Australians and New Zealanders over 15 years of age who drink alcohol, per capita consumption of alcohol is 11.89 litres and 11.97 litres of pure alcohol per year, respectively.

But how and what we drink can be as significant as how much. Not everyone's drinking carries the same degree of risk. The report also graded countries for 'hazardous' drinking behaviour on a scale of 1 (low risk) to 5

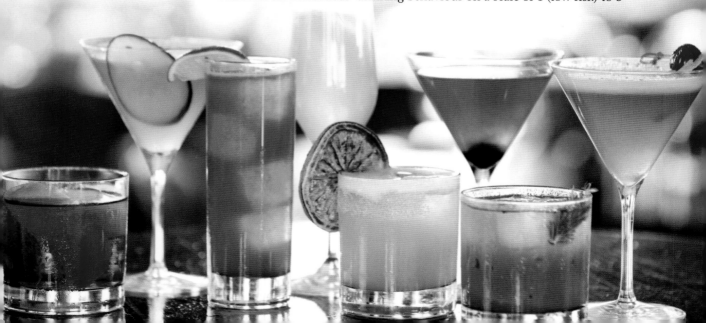

(high risk) and some countries with high consumption scores show surprisingly low scores for risk. France comes in at number 14 for consumption. Yet this nation, where wine is practically its own food group, scores a safe 1 on the hazardous drinking scale, compared to Australia, where around 10 per cent of the population has been classified as drinking at levels posing a high risk to health, or New Zealand where the figure is 19 per cent. (Both Australia and New Zealand scored a 2 on the hazardous drinking scale.)

Did YOU know ?

The rising cost of alcohol misuse

Across the world, alcohol takes its toll on lives and livelihoods. The Australian Institute of Criminology estimated that alcohol costs the Australian community about AU$14 billion when taking into account health costs, violence and loss of work productivity. The figure for New Zealand is about NZ$5 billion.

Risky drinking patterns

The types of drinking behaviour that come with a health warning include drinking outside mealtimes, drinking in public and so-called 'binge drinking', the results of which can be seen in practically every Western city at weekends. Moderate-risk 'level 3' behaviour is seen in the UK, much of Central and Eastern Europe, South America, and perhaps more surprisingly India and parts of Africa and the Far East.

Canadians, Americans, Australians and the Chinese are considered by WHO to be less risky on a score of 2. Moldova, which topped the consumption table, has a 4 for risk behaviour, together with several countries that consume less overall such as Kazakhstan, Mexico, South Africa and Zimbabwe. In many countries where abstention rates are high, those who do drink consume at high levels, which pushes up the risk behaviour score. Russia and Ukraine, 4th and 5th in consumption, display the riskiest drinking habits of all.

Worldwide, it is estimated that alcohol plays a direct part in almost 4 per cent of deaths – that's 2.5 million people each year – mainly through cancer, cardiovascular disease, liver cirrhosis and alcohol-related injuries and accidents. In Russia and neighbouring countries, alcohol is involved in the deaths of 1 in every 5 men.

2.5 MILLION

deaths are caused each year by alcohol misuse – more than those resulting from AIDS or TB – according to a 2011 WHO report.

How alcohol harms

The numbers affected by alcohol are rising. A recent report revealed that around 30 per cent of Australian men and 10 per cent of women drink more than the recommended daily limit, and a quarter of those drink more than twice the limit. In women, drinking increased by almost a third in the decade to 2008, with working women the most likely to exceed safe limits.

Did YOU know ?

'Time, gentlemen, please'

Alcohol consumption may create problems but it can also boost a state's tax revenue. So, throughout history, periods of greater restriction have been interspersed with more liberal times. In Australia and New Zealand, the recent trend has been to extend licensing hours, making alcohol more readily available in shops and licensed premises. But alcohol's relatively low cost – particularly in liquor chain stores – has fed a steep rise in consumption in the last decade.

And which of us are most at risk? Contrary to the general perception that hazardous drinking is the province of the young, it is, surprisingly, the 55 to 74 year-olds whose alcohol-related problems cost most in terms of health care. The so-called baby-boomers are a whopping eight times more likely to need hospital treatment because of alcohol than 16 to 24 year olds.

Drink-related diseases

In one way, perhaps this is not so surprising – this group has, after all, had far more time to spend drinking than the young. But they do seem to be behaving irresponsibly even for baby-boomers. According to Professor Sir Ian Gilmore, a former president of the UK's Royal College of Physicians and an expert on liver disease: 'It is the unwitting chronic middle-aged drinkers who are taking serious risks with their health … People simply do not realise that chronic drinking significantly increases their chances of suffering health problems.' What he is talking about, in the long term, includes:

- **Depression**
- **Liver and kidney disease**
- **Acute and chronic pancreatitis**
- **High blood pressure**
- **Several cancers**
- **Stroke**
- **Heart disease**
- **Overweight**

Alcohol misuse can also be fatal in the short term, and it is here that younger age groups are often most at risk. Sudden death can

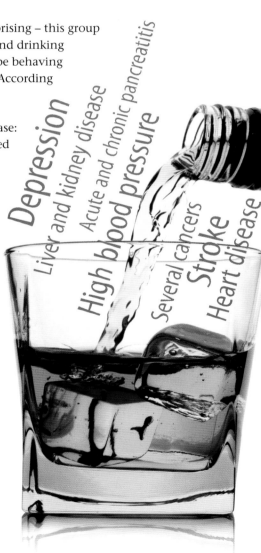

result from acute alcoholic poisoning, and from accidents while people are intoxicated. Drinking can harm an unborn child. And the extra kilojoules in alcohol and the sugar that often comes with it are not good for anyone.

The risk for women

Women need to be particularly cautious because alcohol can increase levels of oestrogen and other hormones linked to hormone-receptor-positive breast cancer. Another reason drinking can increase breast cancer risk is that it can damage cellular DNA.

Compared to teetotallers, women who have three drinks a week have a 15 per cent higher risk of breast cancer than non-drinkers. According to Breastcancer.org, experts estimate that the risk of breast cancer rises by 10 per cent for each additional drink women regularly have each day.

Newer research has drilled down deeper into the cause and effect relationship between alcohol and breast (and potentially other) cancers. Scientists from the Universidad Autónoma del Estado de Morelos in Mexico presented their findings at the Experimental Biology 2012 conference held in San Diego, California.

What they had discovered, explained Dr María de Lourdes Rodríguez-Fragoso, professor of pharmacology and toxicology and the study's co-author, is that when cells work to remove toxic substances such as ethanol (the chemical term for alcohol), it sets in motion a mechanism that produces other toxic substances – including some that are linked to the development of different cancers.

Messing with your brain

Unless you've abstained all your life, you won't need to be told what effect overindulging in alcohol has on your brain. Inhibitions are one of the first things to go, but the fact that you might become a star karaoke singer doesn't compensate in any way for the danger you put yourself in when you drink too heavily.

Some of the other obvious effects include having trouble walking in a straight line, slurred speech, slower reaction times and impaired memory – some people suffer blackouts and cannot recall anything that happened while they were drunk.

ALCOHOL is the second biggest risk factor for cancer after smoking and it is the better off who put themselves most at risk. Of the highest-income people, nearly 90 per cent reported being drinkers, compared to just over 70 per cent of the lowest-income people.

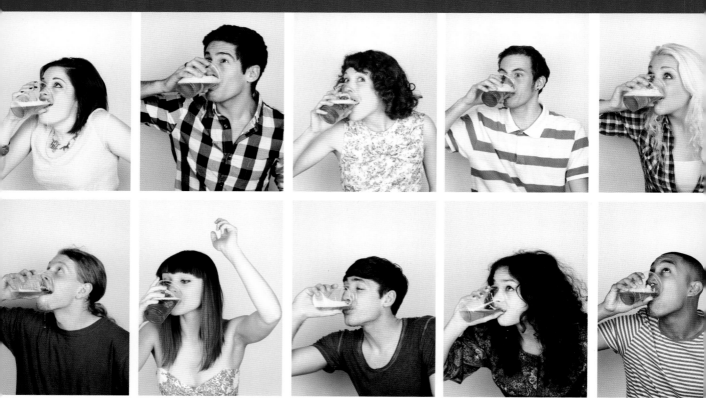

Anyone daft enough to drive becomes a potentially lethal weapon, to themselves and to others; most countries now have a zero-tolerance attitude to drink-driving.

Psychologically, it does you no favours either. Whatever your elation after one or two drinks, alcohol is ultimately a depressant. Which makes it especially ineffective for dulling unhappiness; as most drinkers will admit, it can only make you feel worse.

Long-term effects

Beyond the immediate hangover, alcohol can do longer-lasting damage. Over time, people who repeatedly drink heavily put themselves at risk of brain damage. Advanced imaging techniques, such as MRI scanning, reveal that regular heavy drinking can actually shrink the brain and interfere with its miraculously complex communication system.

This is one reason why health experts are so concerned about teenage drinking, because alcohol can do far more damage to young brains, especially if young people drink to excess. They may drink less frequently or less overall than their elders, but when they do drink they often tend to binge drink. These statistics were revealed in a 2008 poll, commissioned by *The Wall Street Journal*, of more than 17,000 people in 13 EU countries. This found that in France, for example, 25 per cent of people aged over 50 said they drank alcohol at least once a day, compared to just 3 per cent of those aged 14 to 29. But when those young people do drink, they can drink a lot – 43 per cent said that they had five or more drinks before feeling drunk. In Belgium, 56 per cent of young people said they drank five or more drinks before feeling impaired by the effects, compared to 33 per cent of young Americans, 29 per cent of young Germans and 20 per cent of young Swiss.

These figures back up other research that suggests adolescents may be less immediately sensitive to the effects of alcohol than adults – in other words they can drink more before feeling intoxicated – which exposes their brains to greater risk of damage. The teenage brain is so susceptible to harm because it is still developing, and two studies published in 2009, in *Clinical EEG and Neuroscience* and *The Lancet*, show that alcohol abuse could be an even greater cause for concern in this area than marijuana.

TEENAGERS are twice as likely as adults to have tried alcopops, according to a study by the US Alcohol Policies Project.

Tempting the young – the bitter truth about alcopops

They're sweet, they're cheap and they taste a lot like fizzy soft drinks. But there's nothing 'soft' about these alcoholic beverages, the most recent addition to the alcoholic drinks market, now widely sold in supermarkets and other youth-accessible outlets. The alcohol content of alcopops could come from wine, spirits or fermented malt, but the taste comes from the fruit juices and other flavourings that are added.

Either way, they are the alcoholic drinks of choice for underage teens, particularly girls, and no matter what the drinks industry PR says, they seem designed to appeal to young drinkers. Experts have called them a 'gateway' beverage to alcohol abuse by young people. The theory is that by 'hooking' young drinkers on a brand-named alcopop, marketers create loyalty for their 'adult' liquor brands as those drinkers mature.

Because of the colourful packaging and playful advertising that drinks companies use to promote alcopops, many people believe them to contain less alcohol or be in some way lighter than other alcoholic beverages. Not so – a 275ml bottle of alcopop, a 125ml glass of wine or a schooner of strong beer all contain about 1.5 units of alcohol and have the same intoxicating effects.

But because alcopop drinks are so sweet, young people often fail to detect the taste of alcohol at all. In one 2008 study by the consumer group Choice, reported in the *Sydney Morning Herald* in 2012, almost a quarter of young people couldn't taste the alcohol in creamy drinks.

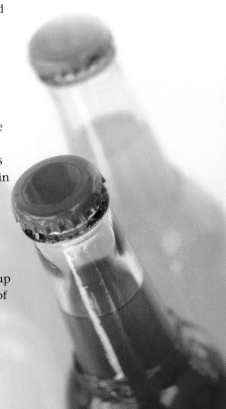

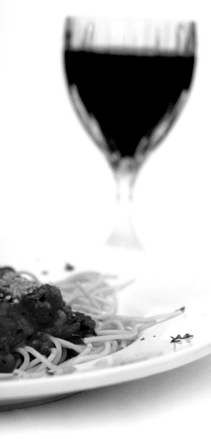

Drinking alcohol with meals is better for you than drinking alcohol on its own.

Sold the dream

As insidious as the drinks themselves is the manufacturers' marketing approach. The sponsorship of music festivals, the use of social media and the product placement in music videos all seem clearly designed to add glamour to the products, attracting young – potentially underage – drinkers. These tactics worry experts such as Mike Daube, the director of Australia's McCusker Centre for Action on Alcohol and Youth, who has described alcopops as 'trainer wheels for drinkers'.

Some countries have gone further than others in restricting advertising in a bid to protect young people. Norway has banned drinks advertising, while of EU countries France and Ireland have the stiffest regulations, including a ban on all television advertising of alcohol and on the sponsorship of sporting events. In Australia and New Zealand, however, moves to restrict sport sponsorship by alcohol companies have met with strong resistance.

Whatever the rules, it's hard to browse a glossy magazine, or sit through the ads before a film at the cinema, or even just watch an evening of TV without encountering some sort of exotic image with alcohol at its heart. In a survey by Alcohol Concern of 2,300 children and young adults, 60 per cent said they favoured stronger regulation of alcohol advertising, and 70 per cent of young women in the survey wanted clearer health guidance on labels.

But aren't there health benefits, too?

So, after all the warnings, what about the media reports that claim that red wine is good for your heart? Or that it can protect against dementia, or even lessen the risk for type 2 diabetes? Is the drinks industry making it up? Where's the truth?

The fact is that many reputable studies show a variety of health benefits associated with drinking alcohol in moderation, as you'll discover in Part 3, Five food friends. The American Heart Association (AHA) agrees that strictly moderate drinking can raise levels of 'good' HDL cholesterol, lower blood pressure, prevent artery damage caused by 'bad' LDL cholesterol and reduce blood clot formation. The key is 'strictly moderate', which Australia's health authorities define as no more than two drinks a day for men and just one for women.

Some people cannot tolerate any alcohol: for people who have suffered any chronic illness drinking can make matters worse and is something that should be discussed with a doctor. In addition, anyone taking medication should ask their doctor whether it is safe to drink alcohol.

Top tips for happy drinking

If you're in good health, a little alcohol may do no harm. Here are a few guidelines that will help to keep your drinking safe and sociable.

- **Keep alcohol for mealtimes** Evidence from France and other wine-producing countries clearly shows that drinking alcohol with meals is best.
- **Space your drinks** Sip slowly, so that you're consuming no more than one or at the most two drinks per hour.
- **Never drink on an empty stomach** When alcohol hits an empty stomach, it is immediately absorbed into the bloodstream before the body has a chance to break it down. Eating before drinking – especially proteins, fats and wholegrain carbohydrates – slows alcohol absorption.
- **Order on the rocks, not neat** Warmer drinks are absorbed faster – and therefore inebriate more quickly – than colder drinks.
- **Watch your mixers** Carbonated mixers such as tonic and soda add extra kilojoules and speed up the absorption of alcohol, so you get tipsier faster.
- **Know your cocktails** Some contain several shots of spirits: be sure to ask what's in an unfamiliar drink, and alternate with non-alcoholic 'mocktails'.

The eat-well message

Some foods contribute so little to good health they are best avoided.
Food enemies include trans fats and any products whose main ingredients are added sugar, fat and salt. Cut down on highly processed foods which have often lost 'healthy' natural nutrients – and gained less desirable ones. Check labels to learn precisely what has been added – often for commercial reasons to extend shelf-life, enhance taste and add bulk.

➤ **Know your fats** As a simple rule, stick to olive and canola oils, enjoy low-fat dairy foods, and avoid products that contain trans fats.

➤ **Look for 'hidden' sugars** It's easy enough to say 'no' to table sugar. Watch out for the sugars that appear in sauces, soups or pizzas.

➤ **Cut back on 'super-refined' foods** Study after study links highly processed foods to obesity and serious health problems – from babyhood onwards. You owe it to yourself and your family.

➤ **Be kind to your body** It simply cannot tolerate a diet of fast food and unnatural additives. Similarly, it makes no sense to take a toxic chemical, such as alcohol, and consume it to excess, thus damaging your physical and mental health.

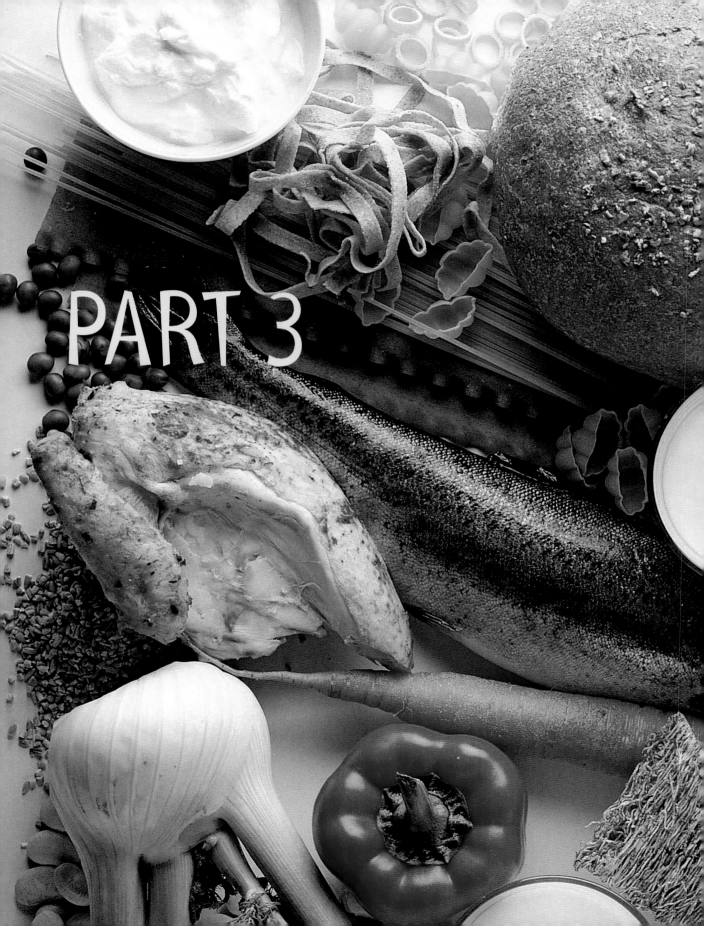

PART 3

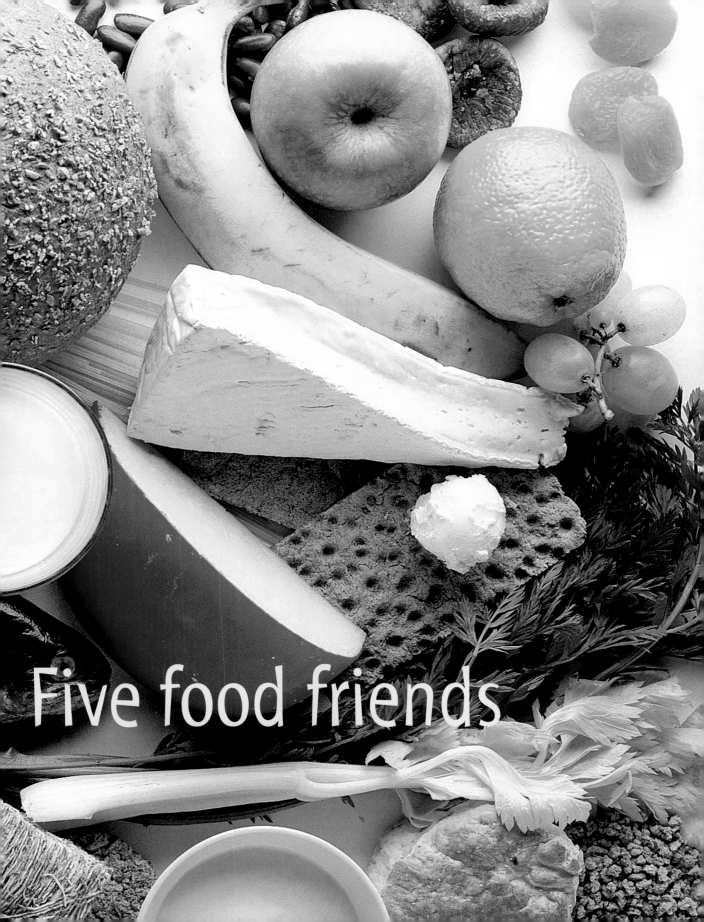

Five food friends

Welcome to the world of the delicious

Good food can excite the senses and offer so much more than a fast-food fix. By eating well we fuel our bodies with the essential nutrients we need to survive and thrive.

Think of fresh bread baking, a meaty casserole cooking or the aroma of freshly brewed coffee. It's not just fast or processed foods that turn us on. There are dozens of irresistible aromas, vibrant and subtle colours and, above all, delicious flavours and textures in the world of natural foods.

The trick lies in getting to know foods that are quite different from those in the previous chapter. For every kilojoule-laden, artery-clogging, blood-glucose boosting, over-processed, ultra-refined food out there, there is an equally tasty counterpart that will feed your body with the energy and power you need to feel healthy and live longer.

So what is the difference? It's simple, really: the foods described in this section are real foods that remain closer to the way nature made them. To put that another way, they are as 'unprocessed' as possible. This doesn't mean you have to raise your own chickens and grow your own potatoes – although more and more people who have the space and inclination are doing just that.

Instead, you'll discover how to navigate the supermarket aisles and explore other food retail options so you can make better, healthier choices for you and your family.

Five friends for life

These are the five types of tasty foods and liquids which, in different ways, do most to nourish your body, safeguard your health and extend your life by reducing your potential for developing serious diseases.

▶▶ **Fresh produce** The colourful world of fruit and vegetables is perhaps our most important ally against disorders ranging from common infections to diabetes and heart disease. All plant foods including legumes, nuts and seeds are packed with vitamins, minerals and other micronutrients that keep us well. You'll also meet some true superfoods that are among the best of the best.

▶▶ **Fibre** It may not sound tasty but there is plenty to enjoy in this group. You'll find out why fibre is so essential for a healthy diet and how you can ensure you get your daily quota; emerging science suggests that this is one of the best things you can do for your body. This really doesn't mean eating bowl upon bowl of bran cereal. Crunchy wholegrain cereals, grains, nuts and legumes, plus some of our tastiest fruits and vegetables are veritable fibre factories that slow the absorption of glucose into your bloodstream and help protect your gut lining against different cancers.

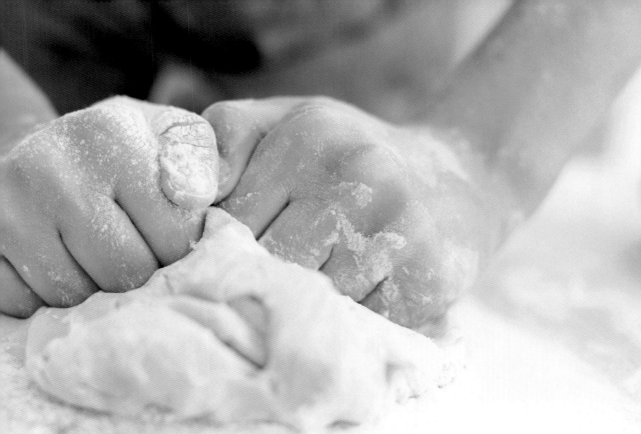

'Good' fats Aren't all fats unhealthy and bad for you? Wrong – some, such as delectable olive oil, are actually good for you. You'll learn why a certain amount of fat is essential and why; contrary to popular belief the best weight-loss diets may not be those that slash your daily fat intake. In fact, some recent science proves that adding certain fats to your diet can actually lower cholesterol levels and reduce the risk of a heart attack or stroke.

Lean protein This vital nutrient provides the building blocks that form our muscles, bones and other tissues, and comes in many tasty forms. Find out which are the best protein sources from meats, fish and other foods and how much protein you need at different stages of your life. If you're going vegetarian or vegan, you'll also discover how to get the right balance of proteins.

Water, water and ... A healthy diet is also about what you drink, and first and foremost among liquids is water. Find out how much of it you really need and whether foods and other liquids count. Does it matter what type of water you drink? Trundle the aisles of any supermarket and you'll find a quite bewildering array of bottled waters – some of them quite pricey. When safe, clean water comes out of the tap, does your body need more expensive options? And how do fruit juices and beverages compare? Finally, why not raise a glass to toast your health? Wine and other alcohol, it seems, can have a place in a healthy diet, and here's why.

Are you missing out?

This section charts the many different nutrients we should try to include in our daily meals for wellbeing and longevity, and how to achieve a healthy balance. You'll find out which vitamins and minerals are essential, what happens if you don't get enough and the best food sources for all of them. Think of this as your quick-reference guide to everything your body needs.

1 Fresh produce
– natural health

The least processed of our foods – fruit and vegetables – also turn out to be exceptional health-boosters. With so many delicious flavours to explore, there is every reason to make sure we eat plenty of them every day.

From the delights of a luscious peach to juicy blueberries, raspberries and strawberries or ripe, red tomatoes, tender asparagus or leafy green spinach, fruit and vegetables provide an abundance of sensational flavours and colours. But flavour is far from the only reason to enjoy the 'seven a day' or more that doctors recommend.

Never before has there been so much evidence that these foods promote good health. Here are three for starters:

- Studies involving hundreds of thousands of people all over the world show that those who eat the most fruit and vegetables have the lowest risk of developing heart disease.
- Eating plenty of fruit and vegetables may lessen the risk of developing cancer, particularly colon and stomach cancer.
- Those whose diets contain lots of fresh produce have a lower risk of developing type 2 diabetes.

So simply eating fresh produce helps protect against three of the major non-infectious diseases in the world today. You could think of it all as almost medicinal. But what medicine ever looked or tasted so good?

The key to their protective powers

What first intrigued scientists was that certain populations whose diet comes mainly from plant sources have relatively low rates of certain major diseases which are widespread in the West. They then began to focus on different plant chemicals to find out how they might act on the body and their healing potential. Some, such as vitamins, are now well known. Most fruit and vegetables are excellent sources of multi-tasking

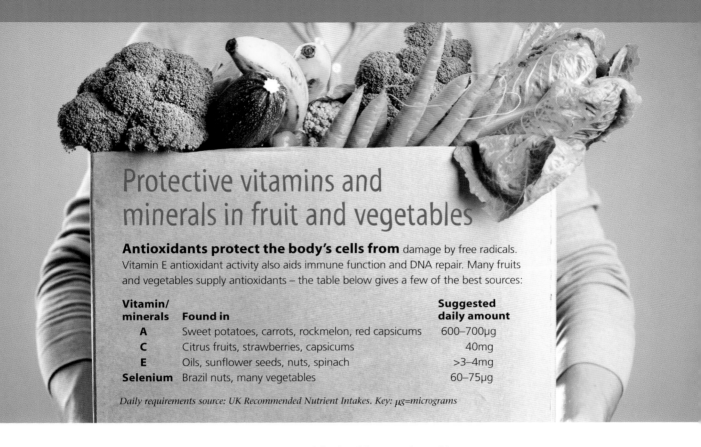

Protective vitamins and minerals in fruit and vegetables

Antioxidants protect the body's cells from damage by free radicals. Vitamin E antioxidant activity also aids immune function and DNA repair. Many fruits and vegetables supply antioxidants – the table below gives a few of the best sources:

Vitamin/minerals	Found in	Suggested daily amount
A	Sweet potatoes, carrots, rockmelon, red capsicums	600–700µg
C	Citrus fruits, strawberries, capsicums	40mg
E	Oils, sunflower seeds, nuts, spinach	>3–4mg
Selenium	Brazil nuts, many vegetables	60–75µg

Daily requirements source: UK Recommended Nutrient Intakes. Key: µg=micrograms

vitamin C, for instance. Vitamin C is essential for building teeth and bones, strengthening blood vessels, healing wounds and creating collagen, the connective tissue that holds cells together and keeps skin smooth.

Fighting free radicals

Vitamin C, together with vitamins A and E, and the mineral selenium are also antioxidants. They help combat an excess of oxygen-derived free radicals – unstable atoms with one or more unpaired electrons. While free radicals fulfill important biological functions, problems arise if our bodies produce too many – often in response to aggravating factors such as smoke, alcohol or over-exposure to ultra-violet light. In a reaction with other molecules called oxidation, free radicals in search of an electron may then oxidise and damage cells, leaving them susceptible to disease.

Scientists believe that is where antioxidants play their vital role, deactivating the oxygen-derived free radicals in various ways before damaging reactions can occur. The table above shows which foods are good antioxidant sources and how much of them we need each day.

LEAFY GREENS are

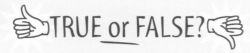

TRUE or FALSE?

Vitamin pills can be just as effective

FALSE! You might think that taking vitamins or other supplements would be as effective as eating fruit and vegetables. You'd be wrong. Most studies using supplements have not yielded the same positive results as eating the plant foods themselves. Scientists don't know why but they suspect that a fruit or a vegetable contains as yet unknown compounds, and that the natural nutrients work together in ways that are beneficial to health. Isolating one element and taking it in pill form doesn't appear to have the same impact.

Flavour, colour and powerful compounds

The slightly bitter taste of cruciferous vegetables, such as brussels sprouts, broccoli and cabbages, has been linked to a variety of plant compounds (phytochemicals) which are believed to protect against cancer. The vibrant colour of many fruits and vegetables is also not a side-show. The so-called anthocyanin pigments are often the very components that give fresh produce many of its health-giving properties. That said, plant foods don't have to be highly coloured to be rich in beneficial phytochemicals; cauliflower, linseeds, nuts and legumes are all packed with these nutrients. A single serving of most vegetables or fruit will contain hundreds of these potentially disease-fighting substances.

In fact, researchers have now identified thousands of phytochemicals and classified them into groups, but only a fraction have been studied closely. Some of the most important ones known so far, together with their sources and possible benefits, are summarised in the table opposite. Their apparent potential for combating major disorders such as cancer and heart disease excites scientists searching for future phytomedicines. However, as yet, study after study suggests that regularly eating lots of whole fruits and vegetables offers the greatest protective benefits.

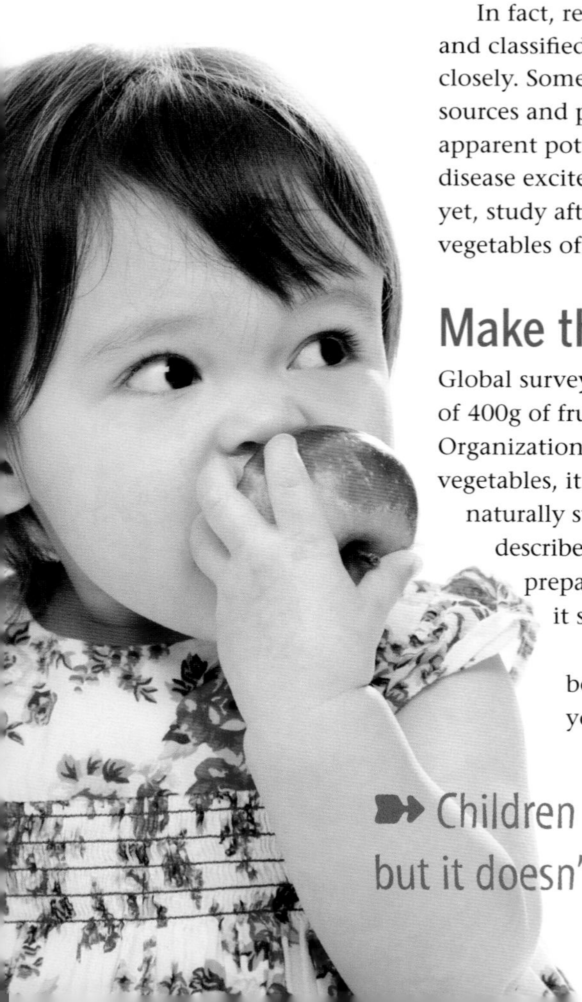

Make the most of fruit

Global surveys show that most of us get far fewer than the daily minimum of 400g of fruit and vegetables recommended by the World Health Organization for lifelong health. While children may object to certain vegetables, it doesn't take much to persuade them to eat fruit because it is naturally sweet and delicious when properly ripe. Fruit could rightly be described as the ultimate convenience food, requiring minimal, if any, preparation. So why do so many of us either fail to buy it or leave it sitting in the fruit bowl until it's ready to be thrown away?

The trick is to make fresh fruit a habit. Work out how it can best fit into your daily diet, and before you know it you'll reach your two serves a day and more. It might start at breakfast,

Children may object to certain vegetables, but it doesn't take much to persuade them to eat fruit.

Healing nutrients: what science is discovering

Class	Fruit & vegetable sources	Potential benefits

Carotenoids
Beta-carotene
Lutein
Zeaxanthin
Lycopene
	• Carrots • Red capsicums
	• Sweet potatoes • Papaya
	• Spinach • Silverbeet
	• Tomatoes, • Kale
	   and processed • Asian greens
	   tomato products
		An important source of vitamin A, carotenoids boost immune system function, protect against free-radical damage and support cellular communication, a function that may help to prevent cancer. Lutein and zeaxanthin may help maintain good vision; lycopene may help protect the prostate

Flavonoids Anthocyanidins	• Berries • Red grapes • Cherries • Sweet potatoes	These antioxidants help protect cells from DNA damage and may also support brain function
Flavanols (catechins, epicatechins, procyanidins)	• Tea • Apples • Cocoa • Grapes • Chocolate	Flavanols help to protect heart health
Flavanones	• Citrus fruits	Both flavanones and flavonols have an antioxidant effect. They neutralise free radicals, helping to protect cells from DNA damage
Flavonols	• Onions • Tea • Apples • Broccoli	
Proanthocyanidins	• Cranberries • Grapes • Cocoa • Wine • Apples • Peanuts • Strawberries • Cinnamon	These chemicals play a protective role in urinary tract and heart health
Isothiocynanates Sulforaphane	• Cruciferous vegetables: cauliflower, broccoli, brussels sprouts, cabbage, kale, spring greens, horseradish, watercress	Sulforaphane may help to detoxify unhealthy compounds in the body and boost cellular antioxidant defences
Phenols Caffeic acid, ferulic acid	• Apples • Citrus fruits • Pears • Some vegetables	Phenols may help maintain cellular antioxidant defences and enhance heart and vision health
Sulphides/Thiols Diallyl sulphide, allyl methyl trisulphide	• Onion family: onions, garlic, leeks, spring onions	These chemicals help to detoxify undesirable compounds in the body and maintain healthy immune function
Dithiolthiones	• Cruciferous vegetables: cauliflower, broccoli, brussels sprouts, cabbage, kale, Asian greens, horseradish	Dithiolthiones help maintain healthy immune function

© Jessica Iannotta, Department of Nutritional Sciences, UMDNJ School of Health Related Professions

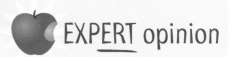

EXPERT opinion

Getting a taste for fruit and veg

What a mother eats during pregnancy can influence her child's tastes, says Julie Mennella, a biopsychologist. Children naturally prefer sweet tastes as this primes them to like their mother's milk but are more sensitive to bitter tastes, so may dislike vegetables. 'We find that the more a mother eats fruits when she's pregnant, the more a child will accept fruit *and* vegetables,' she says.

Julie Mennella PhD *Monnell Center, Philadelphia, USA*

adding bananas or seasonal berries to yogurt or cereal. Or a juicy orange could replace an afternoon cup of tea and biscuit. Or simply take the 10 minutes – it's probably no more – to chop up a selection into a fruit salad, and there's dessert. Where possible, buy fruits in season. Take children on outings to pick ripe berries or to help choose them in farm shops and markets. The more variety you eat, the greater the health benefits.

Superfruits that need no hype

One cup (150g) of blueberries supplies:

9% of your daily fibre

24% of your daily vitamin C

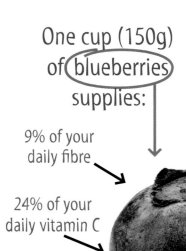

and contains only 250kJ

Every so often little-known fruits will be plucked from obscurity to be acclaimed as bringers of almost miraculous benefits. Think acai berry, pretty mangosteen or goji berry. Are any of them worth adding to your shopping list? Despite all the promotional hype, the scientific evidence is inconclusive. Studies suggest that more readily available fruits have equal or superior powers. Here is the low-down on some true superfruits:

● **Apples** French research reveals that two substances found in apples, boron and a flavonoid called phloridzin, may increase bone density and protect against osteoporosis. Other studies suggest that eating apples may greatly reduce the risk of developing cancers of the lung, colon, liver and breast. Apples also appear to protect against – and reduce the severity of – asthma in children. The pectin in apples may help lower levels of 'bad' LDL cholesterol and help control diabetes by reducing the body's need for insulin.

● **Blueberries** One cup (150g) blueberries supplies 24 per cent of daily vitamin C needs and just under 10 per cent of your fibre needs, as well as vitamin K and the trace mineral manganese. What's more, 150g blueberries contains only 250kJ. Blueberries also contain a diverse group of phytochemicals that help decrease the kind of inflammation that leads to chronic diseases. Research has linked eating them to heart, cognitive and eye health benefits, while test tube and animal studies suggest they might help fight several different cancers. In fact, all berries – raspberries, blackberries, blueberries and strawberries – qualify for superfood status.

● **Citrus fruits** All these fruits are low in kilojoules and packed with helpful nutrients. UK research in 2011 suggested that the flavanones in citrus fruit may protect against stroke and heart disease. Studies also show that a high intake of citrus fruits can reduce the risk of stomach cancer by 28 per cent.

● **Kiwifruit** These are one of the most nutritionally powerful fruits. A single large kiwifruit contains a day's worth of vitamin C, and is one of the few fruits to contain vitamin E. Kiwifruit also offers fibre and potassium. For easy eating, just cut them in half and scoop out the interior with a spoon.

Nut and seed goodness

Both nuts and seeds are delicious to snack on and packed with protective nutrients, too. Most nuts and seeds are a rich source of B vitamins, such as folate, and vitamin E, as well as minerals including potassium, calcium and iron. The fats in nuts and seeds are the best kind; walnuts are particularly high in heart-healthy omega-3 fatty acids. Nuts and seeds are a good source of protein, too, and generally high in fibre; several studies have shown that eating them may help to lower 'bad' LDL cholesterol. But as nuts are also high in energy it is best to eat no more than one serving a day – a small handful of shelled nuts. Seeds have fewer kilojoules and add variety.

Vital vegetables

We've probably all come across people who don't like vegetables; the bitter taste of brussels sprouts or cabbage that indicates their powerful plant chemicals can put children off. The good news is that when vegetables are prepared properly, with flair and imagination, they are delicious – as a main ingredient in meals, for making protein go further, or as accompaniments; they are cheap compared to meat or fish.

Perhaps the biggest favour you can do for your health – and your budget – is to learn how to cook with them so that they can become an important, enjoyable part

EATING FEW

or no fruit and vegetables contributes to 14 per cent of all deaths from stomach cancer, 11 per cent of heart disease deaths and 9 per cent of stroke deaths, the World Health Organization has estimated.

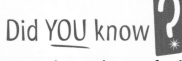

Did YOU know

Frozen is next best to fresh

When fruit or vegetables are flash-frozen straight after harvesting, their nutrient content remains pretty close to that of fresh-picked, so as long as they are well-packaged and stored at the correct temperature. In fact, frozen produce can have more nutrients than fresh produce that has been shipped from afar, stored in less than optimal conditions or left on a shelf for a couple of days. Not all fruit and vegetables freeze successfully – some lose flavour or texture. Peas and corn are two of the best.

VITAMIN

levels in vegetables vary according to their age and colour. Young, tender greens contain more vitamin C than older plants. The darker green outer leaves of lettuce and cabbage contain more vitamin A, calcium and iron than the lighter-coloured inner leaves. The thinner and greener the leaf, the richer it is in nutrients.

Asparagus is rich in the B vitamin folate and is also a good source of potassium.

of your everyday diet. To benefit from all their nutrients you need variety. Here are some vegetable superstars:

- **Alliums (the onion family)** – onions, garlic, leeks, shallots and spring onions all contain vitamin C and several B vitamins, as well as important minerals and antioxidant phytochemicals. They also have natural antibiotic qualities that help to reduce inflammation and infection. Cooks celebrate onions and garlic for the flavour they bring to so many dishes.

- **Broccoli** – and its cruciferous cousins, such as brussels sprouts and cabbage, are loaded with fibre (*see* page 92) and are good sources of vitamin C and beta-carotene, which the body converts to vitamin A. The vegetables may also help protect against cancer. A team of US cancer experts has shown that phytochemicals in broccoli, called isothiocyanates, may be capable of destroying mutant genes, thought to be responsible for up to half of all cancers, while leaving healthy cancer-fighting genes intact.

- **Leafy vegetables** – such as kale and spinach not only supply helpful minerals, vitamins and fibre. The results of a 2010 study suggests that eating 1½ extra servings of leafy vegetables a day can reduce the risk of type 2 diabetes by 14 per cent. Dark green leafy vegetables contain the pigments lutein and zeaxanthin, which research suggests help vision, protecting against cataracts and macular degeneration.

- **Legumes (peas, beans and lentils)** – dried or canned, beans (especially red kidney beans and black beans) pack a powerful combination of nutrients that, among other benefits, encourage healthy sleep and a stable mood. One serving contains as much protein as 60g of chicken or fish. They're also rich in fibre; eating them regularly helps to stabilise blood glucose and helps keep heart disease and other chronic illnesses at bay.

- **Stalks and stems** – think asparagus and celery. Asparagus, a late spring treat, is rich in the B vitamin folate, which helps to prevent birth defects. It is also a good source of the mineral potassium and many micronutrients, as well as the antioxidant rutin which is antibacterial and may help to guard against infection. Celery contains folate, vitamin K and phytochemicals that may help reduce inflammation and fight cancer.

Produce from far and near

Few would dispute that a home-grown tomato or an apple from the garden or a local farm often tastes better than a supermarket fruit that has been flown across the world. But is local more nutritious? The answer is, probably. Many factors determine the nutritional quality of produce, such as how it was grown, how ripe it was when harvested, the way it is handled and stored, and the distance transported.

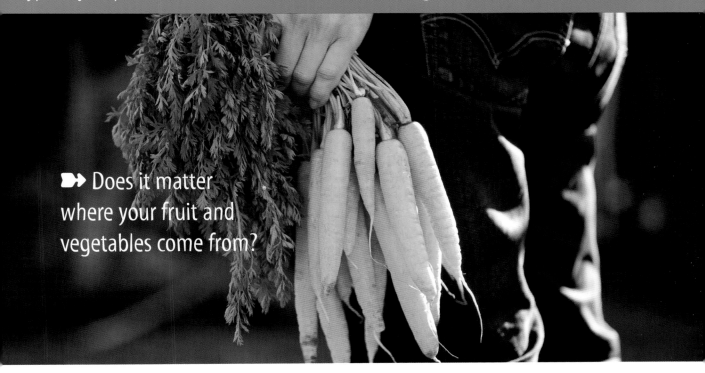

➡➡ Does it matter where your fruit and vegetables come from?

Here are five important facts highlighted by the Harvard School of Public Health in the USA:

- Most varieties of supermarket fruit and vegetables are grown because they produce a good yield and can withstand long-distance transport, rather than for taste or nutrient levels. This also limits our choices.
- So-called climacteric fruits, including apples, melons and peaches, can ripen after harvesting so are often picked early for long-distance transportation. As a result their nutrient levels may be lower than those of fruits picked when they are ripe, according to some studies.
- Transporting fruit and vegetables – especially at speed on roads bumpy enough to cause bruising – can further deplete nutrients.
- Cutting, chopping or slicing long-distance produce to create a 'prepared' product can make it more susceptible to microbial spoilage, alter its chemical make-up and cause it to lose nutrients.
- Storing fresh produce can also affect its texture, appearance and flavour.

The reality is that many of us enjoy fruits and vegetables that cannot grow locally or are out of season but available thanks to modern preservation, storage and transportation techniques. However, as the points above illustrate, there is every incentive to buy local, seasonal produce when we can – for freshness, nutritional quality and superior taste.

For top tips and more advice about choosing, buying and serving fruit and vegetables, see Part 5, pages 248–263.

2 Fibre – far more than roughage

There's so much more to fibre than people once thought. New research is beginning to uncover the complexities that underlie the power of this humble substance, which may help prevent cancer, heart disease, type 2 diabetes and more.

In simple terms, dietary fibre is the edible bits of plants, such as cellulose and bran, that resist digestion and absorption in the gut. Most of us know that this substance, also known as 'roughage', is important for keeping constipation and other chronic digestive complaints at bay.

It is usually described as having two main components:

● **Insoluble fibre** – found in wholegrain cereals, bran, brown rice, nuts, seeds, vegetables and root vegetable skins. As it moves through the gut largely unchanged, insoluble fibre absorbs up to 15 times its own weight in water. This helps to bulk up stools and to speed the passage of waste out of your system to prevent constipation and maintain gut health.

● **Soluble fibre** – found in wholegrain cereals, fruit, legumes and other vegetables. Soluble fibre dissolves in water to form a gel-like substance that makes you feel full. By slowing the digestive process, dietary fibre helps to regulate blood glucose and insulin levels, reducing the risk of developing type 2 diabetes. It also helps to lower 'bad' LDL cholesterol levels, by binding to excess cholesterol in the gut and by moderating its effects.

Disease-fighting powers

Scientists are now discovering that 'soluble' or 'insoluble' is not the whole story. What fibre-rich foods do for us is more complex and far-reaching than once thought. Certain beneficial effects appear to be due to the way that various components of different fibre-foods interact with the trillions of 'good', life-supporting bacteria that live in our gut. Such interactions are thought, for instance, to bolster the immune system, helping our bodies to fight disease, and may even improve mood and memory, as Professor Gregory Freund from the University of Illinois, USA, explained in a 2012 article in the journal *Metabolism*.

What researchers have also discovered is the important role fibre plays in feeding our gut bacteria, giving them a base of support. The best way we can help, they say, is by eating lots of different fibre-rich foods. Just like their human host, it seems our gut microbes need a varied diet that includes a range of fibre components in order to thrive – and when they thrive, so do we. Here are some other findings.

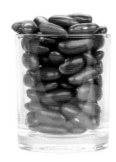

Combating cancer

Researchers have uncovered links between fibre-rich diets and a lower risk of bowel cancer and also oral, larynx and breast cancers. Bowel or colon cancer is common, especially in the Western world where more processed foods are eaten. One significant finding to emerge from a 2009 study of 520,000 people in ten European countries was that those who ate the most fibre had a 25 per cent lower risk of bowel cancer than those who ate lower levels of fibre. The findings also suggested that the protective effect of cereal fibre was stronger than that of fibre from fruits, vegetables or legumes.

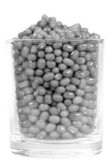

Although scientists have yet to uncover precisely why eating fibre might have a protective effect, what they suspect is:

- When fibre passes through to the large intestine, bacteria there ferment it to produce short-chain fatty acids, which have anti-tumour properties.
- As fibre speeds the transit of waste through the gut, it shortens the time that potentially cancer-causing toxins are in contact with the gut walls.
- Increasing daily fibre intake means you get more antioxidants, which can prevent the cellular damage that leads to cancer.

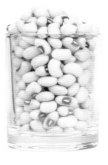

Boosting heart health

Getting plenty of dietary fibre lowers your risk for the whole spectrum of problems collectively known as 'heart disease'. Recent studies have shown that every 10g of additional fibre in your diet can decrease the chances of dying from heart disease by 27 per cent. Here are some of the reasons why:

- High cholesterol levels are implicated in more than half of all heart attacks, so it is vital to keep your cholesterol at healthy levels. Soluble fibre works to decrease both total cholesterol and 'bad' LDL cholesterol levels by increasing the rate of bile elimination – out with the bile, out with the cholesterol.

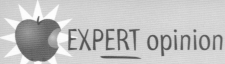

EXPERT opinion

Eating fibre protects against diabetes

Eating 25g fibre a day could reduce your risk of developing diabetes by 25 per cent. For most people in the West, this would mean doubling their intake – the current adult average is around 13g. Insoluble fibre from cereal products appears to be most effective. In one study of 17 obese or overweight people, none of whom suffered from diabetes, fibre-enriched bread significantly improved insulin sensitivity – the body's ability to control blood glucose levels, potentially reducing the risk of diabetes.

German Institute of Human Nutrition Potsdam-Rehbrücke

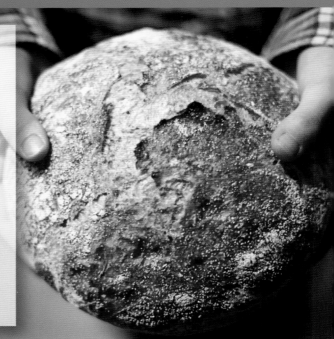

- The short-chain fatty acids produced when fibre ferments in the large intestine during digestion are thought to inhibit the process by which the body makes cholesterol.
- Eating a fibre-rich diet helps to maintain a healthy weight, which is one of the keys to keeping heart disease at bay.
- Dietary fibre has anti-inflammatory effects within the body, which may help to keep plaque stable so it doesn't break free from blood vessel walls to form blockages within the vessels.
- Fibre may help to lower blood pressure and control blood glucose levels.

Protection from diabetes

Once thought of as an adult-onset disease of the affluent West, type 2 diabetes is rapidly becoming a global health scourge of the 21st century. According to the International Diabetes Federation, diabetes affects almost 370 million people worldwide, 60 per cent of them in Asia, and cases in children are rising with childhood obesity. Type 2 diabetes which is directly related to diet and weight is the most common type.

Eating a fibre-rich diet helps in two ways: it stabilises blood glucose levels and it satisfies hunger with fewer kilojoules, thus helping to control weight. A study published in the *New England Journal of Medicine* found that people who ate 50g of fibre a day, both soluble and insoluble, demonstrated better control of blood glucose than those who ate less fibre. Another large study of 42,000 men found that eating fibre from whole grains produced the most significant effect.

Here's how fibre acts. As you digest a carbohydrate food, your body turns it into blood glucose, producing a temporary glucose rise before insulin begins to regulate the process. If the food contains fibre, your body has to work harder to break it down and digest it, which slows the rate at which the food is absorbed and converted to blood glucose. This makes it easier for your body to regulate blood glucose levels and reduces the amount of insulin required to do so.

Soothing digestive problems

Up to 30 per cent of people around the world are affected by various digestive problems, such as irritable bowel syndrome, constipation and diarrhoea. As different as these conditions are, eating more fibre is often helpful. A high-fibre diet effectively clears out waste from the digestive system and may reduce the 'bloated' feeling that many sufferers experience.

Fibre in the fight against obesity

Far wiser than following a low-carbohydrate weight-loss diet is to increase the amount of fibre-rich carbohydrate foods that you eat. People who eat high-fibre diets are generally thinner than those who don't and less likely to put on weight. Here are some reasons why:
- Fibre-rich foods fill you up and keep you feeling full for longer.
- Fibre-rich foods take longer to chew, slowing down your eating and helping your body to recognise when it's full.
- Weight for weight, high-fibre foods usually have fewer kilojoules than low-fibre foods, so you can eat more of them.

Mood and energy

Adding more fibre into your diet may also help you feel less tired. A UK study at the University of Cardiff involving 139 people found that a modest 10 per cent increase in their levels of dietary fibre reduced feelings of fatigue and boosted their energy levels within just a couple of weeks. In the study, the increase in fibre was achieved simply by switching to a high-fibre bran cereal for breakfast each morning. The researchers suspect that one way fibre helps to lift mood and energy is that it speeds the removal of toxins from the body.

EATING 30g OF FIBRE

a day has been shown to halve the risk of breast cancer. One reason is that fibre lowers oestrogen levels in pre-menopausal women: experts believe that lower oestrogen levels reduce breast cancer risk. A second reason is that the higher level of antioxidants that come with eating a fibre-rich diet of fruits, vegetables and whole grains can help to lower cancer risk generally.

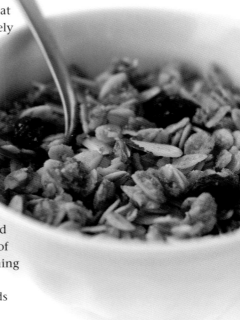

SOLUBLE FIBRE SOURCES:

- Oatmeal
- Oat and wheat cereals
- Lentils
- Apples
- Oranges
- Pears
- Oat bran
- Strawberries
- Nuts
- Linseeds
- Dried beans
- Cooked split or dried peas
- Blueberries
- Cucumbers
- Celery
- Carrots
- Potatoes

How you can get enough?

You might think that only boring foods are fibre-rich, but nothing could be further from the truth. You get fibre in strawberries, for example, and in grapes and other fruits. As a general guide, about 50 per cent of our fibre comes from cereals, about 20 per cent from vegetables and around 20 per cent from fruit and nuts. Some foods supply both kinds of fibre, just as many foods supply more than one vitamin or mineral.

Most of us don't eat enough. The average daily intake is 12–18g in the USA and 15–20g in Europe. Experts recommend between 25g and 35g a day, of which at least 6g should be soluble fibre. Children need less: ranging from about 12g for 4–6 years olds, to 20g for 11–14 year olds. Eating a variety of fibre foods is best. See left and right for ideas to get you started:

Easy ways to add fibre

If you have a good way to go to reach the recommended fibre intake, don't try to do it all at once. Some people will experience uncomfortable (potentially embarrassing) gassy side effects when they start enriching their diets with extra fibre.

The remedy? Go slow. One of the best places to start is with breakfast: people who eat high-fibre breakfast cereals are 80 per cent more likely to achieve their daily fibre target than those who don't. Then each week add more servings of fibre-rich foods. Lentils and legumes, such as black beans,

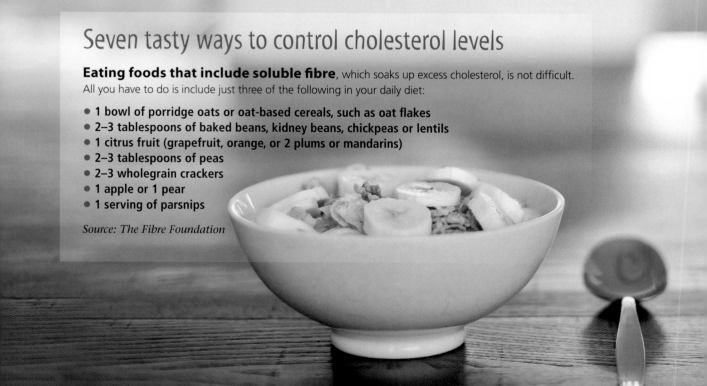

Seven tasty ways to control cholesterol levels

Eating foods that include soluble fibre, which soaks up excess cholesterol, is not difficult. All you have to do is include just three of the following in your daily diet:

- 1 bowl of porridge oats or oat-based cereals, such as oat flakes
- 2–3 tablespoons of baked beans, kidney beans, chickpeas or lentils
- 1 citrus fruit (grapefruit, orange, or 2 plums or mandarins)
- 2–3 tablespoons of peas
- 2–3 wholegrain crackers
- 1 apple or 1 pear
- 1 serving of parsnips

Source: The Fibre Foundation

kidney beans and chickpeas, are rich sources, so try lentil soups and beany stews. Fruits such as apples and pears are best unpeeled as they have more fibre with the skin. Get in the habit of reading labels to make sure you are choosing fibre-rich options. Here are a few examples of sensible food swaps for boosting your fibre intake:

✔ Choose this	Fibre/Serving	✘ Not this	Fibre/Serving
Bran flakes 40g	9.8g	Cornflakes 40g	0.4g
Porridge 40g	4.0g	Puffed rice cereal 40g	0.3g
Wholemeal bread 2 slices	3.2g	White bread 2 slices	1.4g
High-fibre rye crispbread 1	1.8g	Water crackers 3	0.1g
Blackberries, raw 140g	4.3g	Blackberry jam 15g	0.7g
Brown rice 180g	1.4g	White rice 180g	0.2g
Spaghetti, wholemeal 220g	7.7g	Spaghetti, white 220g	2.6g
Whole orange	2.7g	Orange juice 200ml	0.2g

Whenever you're preparing meals, think fibre. Here are eight simple ways to add that little extra into main meals and snacks:

1 Add fresh or dried fruit to breakfast cereal – extra points for prunes.
2 Replace white pasta with wholemeal varieties.
3 Leave skins on potatoes and fruits – that's where much of the fibre is.
4 Add chopped raw vegetables to wholemeal pita sandwiches.
5 Serve two vegetables and starchy potatoes or grains with dinner.
6 Add extra kidney beans and less mince when you make chilli.
7 Add lentils, split peas or beans to soups.
8 Try baked sweet potatoes instead of white potatoes.

Benefits at every age

There are so many delicious ways to include more fibre in your diet – and plenty of incentives. Fibre works at every age. Studies show that mothers who eat plenty of fruit and vegetables tend to have healthier children, who in turn are likely to develop her tastes. Adults will find that including plenty of fresh produce and cereals will help keep them fit and ward off the major diseases described above. And in older age, when you may become less active and when your gut may not function as effectively as it once did, dietary fibre will help relieve constipation and other bowel problems. For good health, giving your diet a fibre boost makes perfect sense.

INSOLUBLE FIBRE SOURCES:

- Wholegrain cereals
- Wheat bran
- Corn bran
- Seeds
- Nuts
- Barley
- Whole wheat couscous
- Brown rice
- Burghul
- Zucchini
- Celery
- Broccoli
- Cabbage
- Onion
- Tomatoes
- Carrots
- Cucumbers
- Green beans
- Dark leafy vegetables
- Raisins
- Grapes
- Fruit
- Skins of root vegetables
- Jacket potatoes

3 Good fats

Given its bad press, you might think that all dietary fat is bad for you. That is far from the truth. In fact, fat, in its many guises, is an essential nutrient playing a variety of vital, protective roles in your body.

Without fat, we would never survive – or indeed be born. It's vital from the earliest stages of foetal development; essential fatty acids, for instance, ensure that our eyes and brains develop as they should. Without fat, you would be unable to absorb vitamins A, D, E and K, because these need to be dissolved in fat before your body can use them (unlike the water-soluble B vitamins and vitamin C). Fat helps to maintain healthy skin and hair, and supports the body's defences against harmful viruses and bacteria.

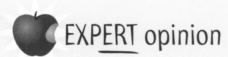 **EXPERT opinion**

A new link between taste and obesity

While our taste buds detect flavours such as sweet, sour or salty, scientists have discovered that we sense fat via a special protein on our tongues. This can influence how much of it we eat, says Dr Gary L. Went.

Gene variations mean that we have differing numbers of fat-sensing protein receptors. You might think if you have more, you'd be more aware of the taste and would eat more. In fact, the converse is true, says Dr Went, 'The lack of fat receptors appears to blunt the sensory response you get from eating certain foods, which leads to less stimulation of the brain's reward centres.' To try to get the brain's reward centre to light up, people with fewer receptors tend to eat more fatty foods. Meanwhile, for those people with more receptors, a small amount of fat goes a long way.

Dr Gary L. Went PhD *Professor of Medical Genetics at Ohio State University, USA*

Working for our wellbeing

The fats we eat include two – linoleic and linolenic fatty acids – which our bodies need but cannot make. These two fats, found respectively in foods such as olive oil and oily fish, help to control inflammation, help blood to clot, and are key to brain development. Fatty acids perform some remarkably intricate tasks in the body. They are chemical messengers that trigger reactions controlling growth, immune function, reproduction, and countless other necessary life processes.

Most of these go on inside our bodies without us being even vaguely aware of them. What can become all too visible are the subcutaneous reserves of fat that insulate the body, keeping it warm and cushioning our internal organs. Dietary fat

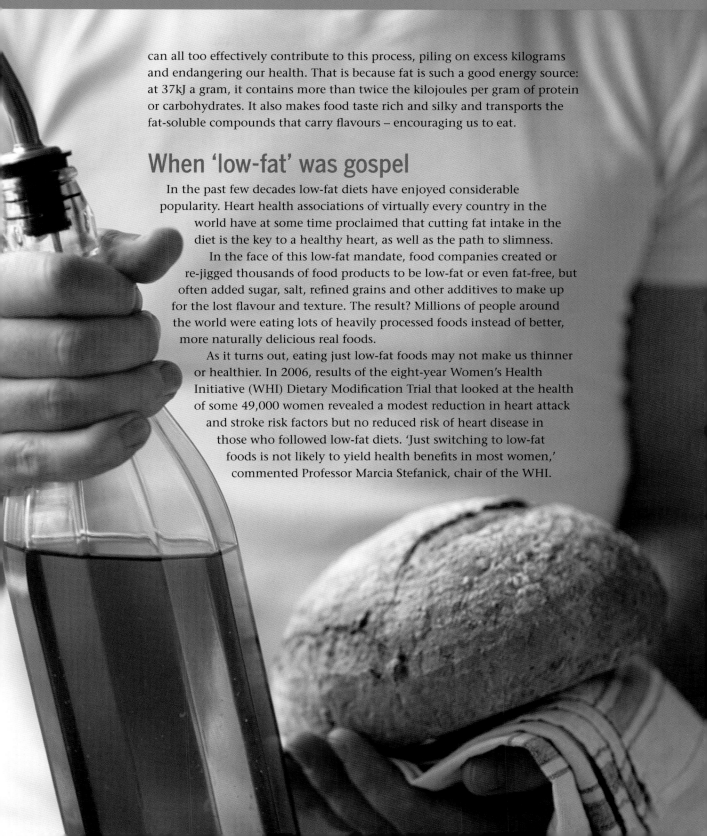

can all too effectively contribute to this process, piling on excess kilograms and endangering our health. That is because fat is such a good energy source: at 37kJ a gram, it contains more than twice the kilojoules per gram of protein or carbohydrates. It also makes food taste rich and silky and transports the fat-soluble compounds that carry flavours – encouraging us to eat.

When 'low-fat' was gospel

In the past few decades low-fat diets have enjoyed considerable popularity. Heart health associations of virtually every country in the world have at some time proclaimed that cutting fat intake in the diet is the key to a healthy heart, as well as the path to slimness.

In the face of this low-fat mandate, food companies created or re-jigged thousands of food products to be low-fat or even fat-free, but often added sugar, salt, refined grains and other additives to make up for the lost flavour and texture. The result? Millions of people around the world were eating lots of heavily processed foods instead of better, more naturally delicious real foods.

As it turns out, eating just low-fat foods may not make us thinner or healthier. In 2006, results of the eight-year Women's Health Initiative (WHI) Dietary Modification Trial that looked at the health of some 49,000 women revealed a modest reduction in heart attack and stroke risk factors but no reduced risk of heart disease in those who followed low-fat diets. 'Just switching to low-fat foods is not likely to yield health benefits in most women,' commented Professor Marcia Stefanick, chair of the WHI.

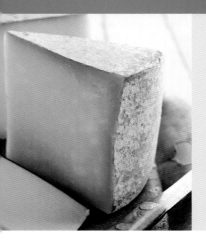

How much fat should I eat a day?

Adding up all the different sources of fat in your diet, health experts suggest that you aim for a fat total that comprises no more than 35 per cent and no less than 20 per cent of your daily food intake. For example, in a 8,000kJ per day diet, the daily fat content should be at least 43g but no more than 76g (1g fat = 37kJ, so 43g fat = 1600kJ, 76g fat = 2,800kJ). In a 10,000kJ per day diet, the minimum is 54g fat and the 95g is the top limit. A slice of buttered toast will have around 8g of fat, 50g of hard cheese around 17g, a small 100g fillet of salmon around 11g, and a large burger could set you back 38g, so it is quite easy to reach (or exceed) the limits. Ensure that the larger portion of those fat grams come from the healthy 'good' fats featured in this chapter.

➡ With all the different sources of fat in your diet it's quite easy to reach (or exceed) the daily limit.

A better approach

So why didn't the low-fat promise deliver the expected results? According to the School of Public Health at Harvard University in the USA, one reason is that dieters cut too much fat from their diet, excluding the good as well as the bad, and so lost the health-protection elements that come from fat. Another is that too often they replaced the lost fat kilojoules with kilojoules from refined carbohydrates such as white bread, white rice and potatoes, foods that can, over time, raise the risk of heart disease and diabetes as much as – or more than – eating too much saturated fat.

Health advice is now clear that some fat belongs in a healthy diet, but too much and the wrong kinds can lead to unwanted weight gain and many other health problems, from heart disease to diabetes. The trans fatty acids in hydrogenated fats, a food foe from Part 2 (*see* page 38), are dangerous to health and are best cut out of the diet altogether. Saturated fats should be kept to around 11 per cent of daily kilojoules – and enjoyed all the more for it. The fats you are about to meet in this chapter are the 'good' fats that should form the largest contingent of fat in your diet.

LOOK AT
nutrition labels to help you limit the amount of saturated fat you eat.
- High: more than 5g of saturated fat per 100g
- Low: less than 1.5g of saturated fat per 100g

What is a good fat?

The popular wisdom is that saturated fats, which tend to be solid at room temperature, come primarily from animals, either from meat or from dairy products such as milk, butter and cheese; eat too much of this fat and you may become susceptible to a cascade of chronic illnesses. Unsaturated fats – often liquid oils – are derived mostly from plant sources, with some from animals, especially fish, and have virtually the opposite effect on your health. These 'good fats' can lower blood cholesterol, ease inflammation, regulate heart rhythms and much more. There are two types of unsaturated fats: monounsaturated and polyunsaturated.

All the above is broadly true but the picture is a little more complex. In fact, even animal fats such as butter and lard contain some mono- and polyunsaturated fat, while olive oil and nuts, widely acknowledged to be good for health, contain some saturated fat alongside their impressive quotas of mono- or polyunsaturated oils.

Did YOU know ?

Food sources of good fats

Cooking oils aren't the only source of healthy dietary fats – some delicious foods are chock-full of them. So what are you waiting for? Here's a guide:

Healthy fat type	Foods containing high levels
Monounsaturated	Olives, peanuts, avocados, hazelnuts, pecans, pumpkin seeds and oily fish
Polyunsaturated	Walnuts, pine nuts, sesame and sunflower seeds, tahini paste and oily fish
Omega-3	Fish – especially salmon, trout, herring and sardines – walnuts, linseeds and chia seeds

The secret is balance and variety: some saturated fat is important for health, while it is also possible to eat too many 'good' fats as all types of fat are high in energy. Which is not to downplay their many health benefits when eaten in moderation. This is what they do.

Meet the MUFAs – monounsaturated fats

You'll find MUFAs (monounsaturated fats) in their greatest concentrations in olive, peanut and canola oils, as well as in avocados, nuts (almonds, cashews, hazelnuts, peanuts, pecans and others) and seeds (such as pumpkin and sesame). Making MUFA-rich foods your main source of fat decreases your risk of heart disease and may also help to normalise insulin and blood glucose levels.

A key MUFA component is oleic acid (omega-9), which bestows impressive health benefits on the oils and foods that contain it. For starters, recent scientific research suggests that oleic acid has the power to lower cholesterol, improving the ratio of 'good' to 'bad' cholesterol, and reduces your risk of heart disease. What's more, it has also been shown to block the action of a cancer-promoting gene called HER-2/neu, which is carried by 30 per cent of breast cancer patients. Adding to this beneficial effect is omega-9's apparent ability to enhance the effectiveness of drugs that target that same cancer gene. Olive oil is a particularly good source.

Avocados are an excellent source of MUFAs.

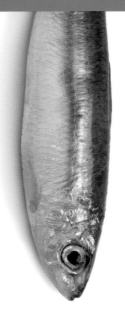

➡➡ PUFAs include omega-3 fatty acids, found in sardines.

Essential fatty acids – in nuts, seeds and fish

Polyunsaturated fats (PUFAs) include omega-3 fatty acids, found in greatest concentrations in pine nuts and walnuts, in certain oily fish (sardines, salmon, trout, herring, to name a few), and also present in various vegetables and fruits, from spinach and kale to avocado and chickpeas. Omega-6 fatty acids are found predominantly in vegetable oils, such as sunflower and safflower, and also in nuts and seeds. Both omega-3 and omega-6 are known as 'essential fatty acids' (EFAs) because they're essential for human health – but your body cannot make them, so you need to get them from food. Omega-3 and omega-6 fatty acids are crucial to the growth, development and function of your brain. They also regulate metabolism, maintain a healthy reproductive system, and keep your skin, hair and bones healthy.

Getting the ratio right

Good as both these types of fat are, nutritionists have identified one important problem. Our ancestors ate omega-6 and omega-3 fats in a ratio of 1:1. Because we now consume so many foods containing vegetable oils rich in omega-6 fats (check labels: they're in many processed foods) the ratio is closer to 15:1 or more.

Research suggests that an excessive intake of omega-6 fats may increase the risk of many serious diseases, including heart problems, certain cancers and autoimmune disorders such as rheumatoid arthritis. One study from the Center for Genetics, Nutrition and Health in Washington, USA, found that a reduction from 15:1 to 4:1 (omega-6: omega-3) PUFA fats was linked to a 70 per cent reduction in premature death from heart disease.

To improve your ratio, cook with olive or canola oils and eat plenty of omega-3-rich fish, such as salmon, trout or sardines.

Did YOU know ?

Omega-3s help strengthen bones, too

Scientists first became aware of the benefits of omega-3 fats after studying the Inuit people of Greenland. They eat a fatty diet of oily fish, whale and seal, yet appear to suffer far less than other populations from disorders such as heart disease and rheumatoid arthritis.

Now studies sponsored by the US space agency NASA have shown that one specific omega-3 fatty acid, eicosapentaenoic acid (EPA), found in salmon and other oil-rich fish, can also help to combat bone breakdown – a major effect of weightlessness in space. 'These results are very exciting and provide initial evidence that nutrition may be a key factor in mitigating bone loss in astronauts,' said Scott Smith, a NASA nutritionist. The agency believes their findings are equally valid for bone breakdown disorders such as osteopororis.

Olive oil – mainstay of the Mediterranean diet

The traditional diet of southern Europe – the diet of Greece, especially Crete, Italy, Spain and Mediterranean France – is renowned for its heart-healthiness. Study after study supports the benefits of eating the way people do in that sun-kissed part of the world. As well as plenty of olive oil, the Mediterranean diet includes lots of vegetables and fruits, legumes, whole grains, nuts and seeds, moderate amounts of dairy foods and of fish, poultry and wine, small quantities of red meat and few processed foods.

Golden-green olive oil plays a major role – in both the diet and its benefits, as a new Spanish study, published in the *American Journal of Clinical Nutrition* in 2012, confirms. Researchers from the Cancer Epidemiology Research Program in Barcelona examined the health of 40,622 people, aged 29 to 69, from five Spanish regions across a period of just over 13 years. During the period of the study, the people whose diets contained the highest amounts of olive oil were 26 per cent less likely to die from any cause and 44 per cent less likely to die from heart disease. What's more, general mortality reduced by 7 per cent and heart disease deaths by 13 per cent for each 10g increase in olive oil consumed.

The secret of its goodness

So what makes olive oil so good for us? One reason is that it's especially high in the key MUFA component oleic acid (*see* page 101), which appears to help lower 'bad' LDL cholesterol levels and combat inflammation. It may also help by reducing high blood pressure. In another 2009 Spanish study,

IN 3500BC

the early Minoan people of Crete were already using olive oil for cooking; the earliest olive oil amphorae date from this time. Some sources suggest that olives were cultivated in Canaan, present-day Israel, as early as 4500BC. The oil was used for rituals, medicines, fuel, soap-making and skin-care, as well as cooking.

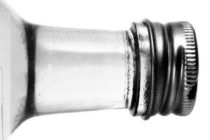
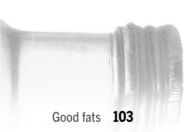

A guide to buying olive oil

- **Buy 'extra virgin'** – this refers to unrefined oil that comes from the first pressing of the olives. It has the freshest flavour and highest levels of phytonutrients, thought to help prevent disease and keep your body working as it should.
- **Choose dark bottles** – light and heat can quickly make oils go 'off', so dark bottles are best.
- **Seek freshness** – the fresher the oil, the higher its content of healthy compounds. Try to find oils that show the date of harvest, or at least a 'best before' date.
- **Use what you buy** – to maintain freshness, buy amounts that you'll use up quickly.
- **Experiment** – just like wines, olive oils from different regions vary in flavour, so try them out to find which ones you like best. If you're lucky you might find a shop that lets you taste different olive oils.

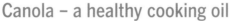

Did YOU know ?

Canola oil now comes cold-pressed

Some people worry that commercial canola oil production is highly processed: the oil is extracted from the seeds at high temperature, then bleached and deodorised to produce a neutral-tasting cooking oil. In recent years certain growers – in Canada, the UK and Australia, for instance – have begun producing more natural, cold-pressed canola oils. These are becoming increasingly available in supermarkets, and some food connoisseurs claim they rival olive oil in health benefits and flavour.

17 people with type 2 diabetes and 23 healthy people were given a diet rich in virgin olive oil for a month. At the end of the study, both groups showed measurably lower blood pressure.

Olive oil is rich, too, in antioxidants called polyphenols. These are the anti-inflammatory compounds that are proven to lower levels of C-reactive protein, the blood measurement used to assess levels of inflammation that indicate the risk of developing heart disease. Polyphenols may also restrict the growth of harmful gut bacteria that cause digestive tract infections. In particular, they hinder the bacterium *Helicobacter pylori*, now known to be the cause of stomach ulcers and other digestive woes.

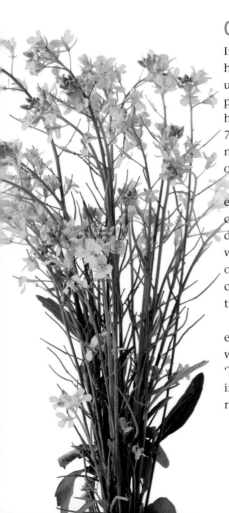

Canola – a healthy cooking oil

In about 40 years, since commercially viable strains were developed, canola has become the third largest oil crop in the world. Although now much is used in processed foods, canola oil is firmly in the 'good fat' camp. Sixty per cent of its fat comes from healthy monounsaturated oleic acid, and it has the lowest percentage of saturated fat of common cooking oils, at just 7 per cent (olive oil contains 14 per cent). It is also said to be the most nutritionally balanced cooking oil, with a far lower ratio of omega-6 to omega-3 fats than any other.

Recent Swedish research suggests that the oil may be particularly effective for lowering cholesterol levels. A team from Uppsala University compared the effects of two typically Western-style diets – one containing dairy fat, the other a spread made from canola oil. Fourteen men and six women, aged between 25 and 68 and in good health, followed one or other of the diets for three weeks. By the end of the study, the LDL (bad) cholesterol levels of those on the canola oil diet were 17 per cent lower than those on the dairy diet, as were their overall cholesterol levels.

Cholesterol-lowering effects of this magnitude are what you might expect to achieve by taking a statin drug. In fact, such dramatic benefits are within the grasp of most of us, suggests study co-author Dr David Iggman. 'The participants ate a rather normal Western diet that's moderately high in fat … This study shows what people can achieve when they actually replace saturated fats with unsaturated fats.'

How to choose the right healthy oil

When you're choosing cooking oils, it pays to appreciate the differences. Some oils are better suited to high-heat cooking such as searing or deep-frying (the least-healthy cooking technique, so use it only occasionally) because they can be heated to a high temperature without smoking. Other oils with a lower smoke point are better for baking or sautéing; others shouldn't be heated at all and are best used for dressings, dips and marinades. Some of these – particularly the specialty nut oils – are a little pricey, but can add a deliciously different flavour. Here's a round-up:

Oil	% Mono	% Poly	% Sat	Good to know
High smoke point (searing, browning, deep-frying)				
Almond	65	28	7	Special nutty flavour
Avocado	65	18	17	Smells sweet
Hazelnut	82	11	7	Strong and bold tasting
Palm oil	38	10	52	Very high saturated fat content
Sunflower	79	7	14	Choose brands with high oleic content
'Light' olive oil	78	8	14	Refined olive oil has a higher smoke point
Medium-high smoke point (baking, oven cooking, stir-frying)				
Canola	62	31	7	Good omega-6: omega-3 balance
Grapeseed	17	73	10	High in omega-6 fats
Macadamia	84	3	13	Rich flavour
Extra virgin olive oil	78	8	14	Best choice
Peanut	48	34	18	Best stir-fry oil
Medium smoke point (light sautéing, sauces, low-heat baking)				
Corn	25	62	13	High in omega-6 fats
Hemp	15	75	10	High in omega-3 (keep refrigerated)
Pumpkin seed	32	53	15	Some omega-3 fats
Sesame	41	44	15	Great for Asian cooking
Soybean	25	60	15	High in omega-6 fats
Walnut	24	67	9	Good source of omega-3 fats
Oils for dressings, drizzles, dips and marinades				
Extra virgin olive oil	78	8	14	Best choice
Linseed	65	28	7	Good omega-3 source (keep refrigerated)
Wheatgerm	65	18	17	Rich in omega-6 (keep refrigerated)

Source: Cleveland Clinic, Ohio, USA

4 Healthy lean protein
– why we need it

Many delicious foods supply the protein our bodies require. Understanding the unique range of other nutrients each one offers will help you to reap their health benefits and avoid any drawbacks such as unhealthy fats.

We call this important nutrient 'protein' but, in fact, it's not a single substance. There are at least 10,000 different kinds that play key roles in keeping our bodies working well. Proteins build and repair muscles, skin, bone, hair and every other body tissue. They make up the enzymes that enable us to digest food, produce the antibodies that fight off infections and disease, and help our muscles move and contract. Proteins transport life-giving substances such as oxygen around the body, and regulate the structure of cells. The list is practically endless.

A vital assembly line

Perhaps the most amazing thing is that your body makes all of these proteins, continually, from protein 'building blocks' known as amino acids. Like a great construction engineer, the body follows a 'blueprint' – or to be more precise, a genetic code – to string amino acids together to form different kinds of essential protein.

Scientists have identified more than 150 amino acids, 20 of which are known to be used by the human body. We produce some of these ourselves,

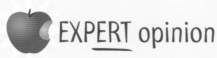

EXPERT opinion

How much protein do I need each day?

The daily requirement for protein varies with age, gender, pregnancy and breastfeeding, and from person to person, but is far less then most people imagine. These are the Australian and New Zealand recommended daily amounts:

AGE IN YRS	AMOUNT	WHICH COULD BE SUPPLIED BY:
1 to 3:	14g	1 egg + 35g hard cheese
4 to 8:	20g	60g lean mince + 100g pasta
9 to 13:	35–40g	70g canned tuna + 4 slices bread
14 to 18:	45–65g	150g roast turkey + 300ml low-fat milk
19 to 70:	46–64g	150g grilled steak + 200g yogurt
70 and older:	57–81g	200g grilled steak + 200g yogurt

NB *All meats, pasta and vegetables are cooked weight.*

but there are nine so-called 'indispensable' amino acids that our bodies cannot produce and must be obtained from the foods we eat. They are: histidine, isoleucine, leucine, lysine, methionine, phenylalanine, threonine, tryptophan, valine – names you may have noticed on ingredient labels. Your body cannot store amino acids efficiently in the way it does fats or carbohydrates, so it needs a regular supply.

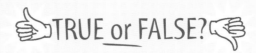

TRUE or FALSE?

All foods contain protein

TRUE! Even fruit supplies small amounts of protein. But only foods in the so-called 'protein group' supply it in quantities sufficient to support your body's ongoing needs. The group includes meat, poultry and eggs, dairy (milk, yogurt, cheese), fish, dried beans and peas, soy in many forms (tofu, tempeh, edamame), nuts, seeds and some whole grains, especially quinoa and buckwheat.

Where does protein come from?

We get our dietary protein from both animal and plant sources, and in two forms. 'Complete' protein sources supply all the indispensable amino acids, while 'incomplete' sources either lack one or more or don't have them in the right balance. Generally speaking, animal sources supply a complete set of indispensable amino acids and vegetable sources an incomplete set.

There are exceptions. Soybeans and quinoa are complete proteins, although both score lower than animal sources on the Protein Digestibility Corrected Amino Acid Score (PDCAAS), used by the World Health Organization to evaluate protein quality. Different plant foods – such as legumes and grains – can also be combined to supply a complete source of protein.

So both animal and plant protein sources provide good matches for our needs and protein deficiency is rare. But because protein foods come in different packages, what makes a difference to our health is the other nutrients each one contains.

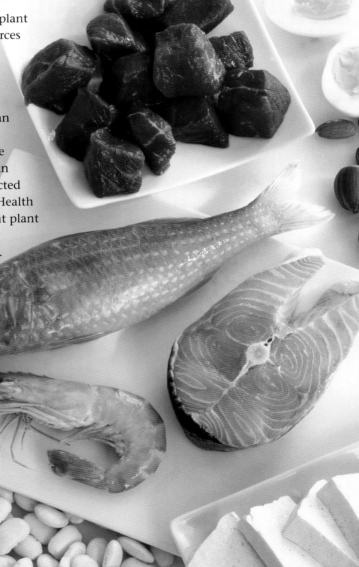

Your healthy meat guide

Not all meats are created equal. This handy guide shows the kilojoule and fat contents of some popular meats, alongside the protein contribution, per serving of 100g trimmed of excess fat.

Meat	kJ	Grams of fat (sat fat)	Grams of protein
Beef rump roast	740	5.5 (1.9)	32
Chicken (skinless white meat) roast	600	2.5 (0.8)	30
Duck (skinless) roast	770	9.5 (3.3)	24
Lamb leg lean roast	830	8.8 (3.5)	30
Pork loin lean roast	860	8.6 (3.2)	32
Turkey (skinless white meat) roast	650	4.0 (1.1)	30
Venison or kangaroo, roast	540	2 (1)	30

Source: NUTTAB, Food Standards Australia New Zealand (FSANZ).

Meat – the best-known source

GRASS-FED

beef is a healthier choice than grain-fed, according to the Mayo Clinic in the USA. Compared to grain-fed beef, it has:

- Less total fat.
- More heart-healthy omega-3 fatty acids.
- More conjugated linoleic acid, which may protect against heart disease and cancer.
- More antioxidant vitamins, including vitamin E.

Take, for example, one of the most celebrated forms of animal protein – red meat. A 175g rump steak contains about 40g of total protein, or nearly a day's worth. But with it, you also get 19g of fat, of which 8g is saturated fat – that's around a third of your recommended daily limit for saturated fat (the less healthy kind) – depending on your energy intake. Compare that to a piece of salmon of the same size, which gives you 35g of protein with a similar 19g of fat, only 3g of which is saturated fat. Then contrast both of these with one cup of cooked lentils with 18g of protein yet barely a gram of fat.

This offers a perfect illustration of why it's wise to include lean sources of protein in our diets. No one is suggesting giving up meat; in moderate-sized portions, it has much to contribute to a healthy diet. However, it is best to eat less red meat, although expert opinion differs on how much is safe to eat. While the World Cancer Research Fund suggests a weekly limit of 500g, at the more cautious end the Harvard School of Public Health in the USA says that red meat (beef, pork or lamb) should be restricted to just two 90g portions a week. The wisest course of action is to limit portion size, choose leaner cuts of red meat and not to eat it every day.

There's plenty of other fresh meat on the menu. As the chart above illustrates, turkey, chicken, venison and kangaroo all have much lower levels of saturated fats and fewer kilojoules than other meats. Game meats such as kangaroo and venison are also especially high in protein.

Other meaty benefits

As our ancestors recognised instinctively, meat is a highly nutritious food. It is a source of minerals such as iron and zinc and a good source of other minerals our bodies need. Half of the iron present in meat is haem iron which is much more easily absorbed than the non-haem iron in plant sources. Meat is also a good source of all the B-complex vitamins including thiamin, riboflavin, niacin, biotin, vitamins B_6 and B_{12}.

Incredible eggs

They are such an excellent all-round source of nutrition that eggs easily qualify as a 'superfood'. A single egg contains 6g of high-quality protein, containing all the amino acids we need, and 12 different vitamins and minerals, including the antioxidant selenium, vitamins B_2 and B_{12}, and the carotenoids lutein and zeaxanthin, which may reduce the risk of macular degeneration, a leading cause of blindness in older people.

Eggs are rich in choline and betaine, two substances that studies suggest reduce the 'markers of inflammation' in the body, including C-reactive protein, interleukin-6, tumour necrosis factor alpha and homocysteine. Each of these markers has been linked to chronic health problems, including heart disease, type 2 diabetes, osteoporosis and dementia. Choline in particular plays a role in memory enhancement and brain development.

So when an egg marketing scheme in the USA came up with the slogan the 'incredible, edible egg', for once the hype wasn't far off the mark. Most of us no longer need to limit egg consumption, unless advised to do so, as health experts concede that concerns about the effect on cholesterol levels were largely unfounded.

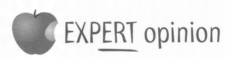

EXPERT opinion

Breaking the egg–cholesterol link

There is no clear link between eating eggs and the risk of heart disease according to Professor Maria Luz Fernandez. The cholesterol in eggs doesn't raise blood cholesterol for about 75 per cent of the population. What is more, she suggests, eating eggs seems to affect the way cholesterol works in the body, making it less likely to form plaque in the arteries. Eggs also contain the potent antioxidants lutein and zeaxanthin, which may protect against developing 'bad' cholesterol, according to a recent study at the University of Connecticut in the USA. 'I am pro-eggs,' says Professor Fernandez. 'They have no effect on heart disease and are loaded with nutrients and nutraceuticals.'

Professor Maria Luz Fernandez PhD *Department of Nutritional Sciences, University of Connecticut, USA*

Protein-rich fish: the pros and cons

We're frequently told that eating fish is good for us. White fish and shellfish of all types are low in energy, low in saturated fat, and more or less (depending on the type of fish) high in those extremely healthy fats, the omega-3s. Oily fish, such as salmon, are higher in energy as a result of their fats – but well worth eating as these fats, packed with omega-3s, bring their own special health benefits (*see* page 102).

Yet, as in so many areas of nutrition today, there's controversy about fish consumption for three key reasons. Some fish contain unhealthy levels of toxins, including mercury, PCBs (polychlorinated biphenyls) and dioxins. Certain fish, such as salmon, are intensively farmed in crowded pens that can pollute surrounding coastal waters and harm native wild fish populations. And many fish, particularly tuna, have been so overfished that their very existence is in jeopardy.

What health experts concluded

You may be wondering if the beneficial nutrients in fish counterbalance the danger of ingesting toxins. A number of scientists have studied this issue. In 2006, researchers at the Harvard School of Public Health in the USA embarked on a comprehensive analysis, combining available data on the health benefits of omega-3 fatty acids and the health risks of toxic mercury intake, PCBs and dioxin. They concluded that eating about 85g of farmed salmon or 170g of fresh mackerel per week reduced the risk of death from coronary artery disease by 36 per cent. They also calculated that eating fish regularly reduces premature death from any health-related causes by 17 per cent.

Researchers from the French Agency for Food, Environmental and Occupational Health Safety delved even further into the risks and benefits of eating fish. They studied 52 different fresh, frozen and canned fish and applied mathematical formulae to compare the nutritional profiles of each fish against its contamination with various toxins.

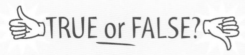

TRUE or FALSE?

Fish oil is a good source of omega-3s

TRUE! According to a New Zealand study, published in 2011, salmon oil capsules are just as good a source of omega-3 fatty acids as real salmon. Researchers from Massey University in Auckland randomly assigned 44 volunteers to one of four groups: one group got two 120g servings of salmon a week, while the others got either two, four, or six salmon oil capsules a day. At the end of the eight-week study, participants were found to have similar levels of omega-3 in the blood. However, when the researchers measured the levels of selenium, an important antioxidant, in blood samples taken from the volunteers, they found far higher levels in the group who ate the salmon compared to all the volunteers on capsules.

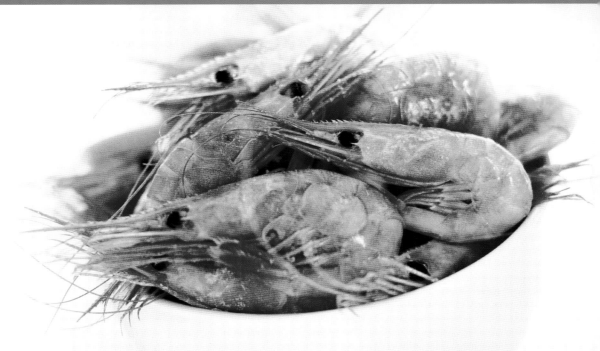

➡ All shellfish are high in protein, too.

How much should we eat?

After studying all the evidence, the researchers published their recommendations for healthy fish consumption in 2012. These turned out to be remarkably similar to those already espoused by many official nutrition organisations, including the American Heart Association, the UK Scientific Advisory Committee on Nutrition (SACN) and the Health Council of the Netherlands.

The researchers concluded that to benefit most from three key fish nutrients – vitamin D, omega-3s and the antioxidant selenium – while keeping within limits for potential toxins and minimising exposure to arsenic and mercury, we can safely eat two to three 150g serves each week of most types of fish sold in Australia and New Zealand. Fish that can have a high mercury content are mostly the large or very long-lived species such as tuna, swordfish, shark, orange roughy (sea perch) and catfish. Children under 12 and women of childbearing age should limit their intake of these fish to one serve per fortnight, with no other fish consumed that fortnight, and all other adults should stick to one serve per week, with no other fish consumed that week.

FRESH SARDINES

are richest in heart-healthy omega-3 fats, with a whopping 2000mg per 100g. Atlantic salmon is close behind with 1600mg per 100g.

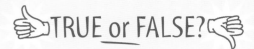
TRUE or FALSE?

'Live' bio-yogurt is much healthier

TRUE! Yogurt is a top source of bone-building calcium, protein and potassium, but its status as a superfood is down to the beneficial bacteria called 'probiotics' which are present in 'live' yogurt. These bacteria help to maintain the ideal balance of bacteria in the gut, and we're only just beginning to grasp how important this is for health and longevity. Yogurt with live, active cultures is particularly helpful for people with gut disorders, such as constipation, diarrhoea, irritable bowel syndrome, and the *Helicobacter pylori* infections that cause ulcers. What's more, these beneficial bacteria also enhance immunity. Finally, even people who are lactose-sensitive may be able to tolerate yogurt – so they don't have to miss out on the benefits of this calcium-rich dairy food.

Enjoy dairy foods

Among the most delicious sources of protein are the diverse cheeses, butter, yogurts, ice cream and milk that make up dairy products. Most are rich in bone-building calcium as well as vitamins A and D. But given that many are also high in fat, can they really play a starring role in eating well and living longer? The answer is 'yes' – in moderation. Here's why.

Together milk, cheese and yogurt are relatively low-cost foods that provide a unique package of essential nutrients. Milk is especially protective. In 2008, UK researchers analysed data from 324 studies of milk consumption and its links to heart disease, stroke, cancer and diabetes. Published in the *Journal of the American College of Nutrition*, the study was unequivocal – milk is good for you. The results indicated that drinking milk can lessen the chances of dying prematurely from heart disease by 10–15 per cent and stroke by up to 20 per cent. Two large European population studies also suggest that consuming cheese, yogurt and thick fermented milk such as cultured buttermilk and kefir may play a modest role in protecting against diabetes.

How much – and what kind?

The Australian Dietary Guidelines recommend about 3–4 portions of dairy products a day for most people over the age of 9, with adults and children over the age of 2 advised to eat lower-fat products whenever possible. Children under 12 months should not have cow's milk as a drink, but from one to three years about 500ml (2 cups) milk will supply their daily calcium needs. From age four to eight years, two to three dairy servings a day is about right. Each of the following counts as one serving:

- 250ml (1 cup) milk (skim, low-fat or full-fat)
- 200g (¾ cup) yogurt
- 40g (2 slices) hard cheese (cheddar, mozzarella, Swiss, parmesan)
- 120g cottage cheese or ricotta cheese

Milk in tea and coffee all counts towards an adult's daily intake, as do many other foods such as puddings made with milk, frozen yogurts or ice cream, and milk-based white or cheese sauces.

Soy: much more than a meat substitute

It can seem like the answer to a vegetarian's prayer; soy is not only rich in protein but also a good source of antioxidants, polyunsaturated fats, B vitamins and iron. What's more, eating soy can lower your cholesterol and protect the health of your heart. Tofu, a fermented soy food, is a staple of Asian cuisines which may explain why traditional Asian cultures have lower rates of certain chronic diseases. But in the West some soy foods (think vegie burgers and nuggets, for example) are highly processed, creating products that are very different from soybeans in their wholefood form. That's why nutritionally minded organisations recommend eating whole soy foods, such as edamame (whole soybeans), and traditionally fermented soy foods such as tofu and tempeh.

What if I'm vegetarian?

With thoughtful meal planning, vegetarians can get ample amounts of good-quality protein. Eggs and dairy products are good sources. Soy foods, nuts, seeds, whole grains, and legumes also contain plenty; include a variety of them to ensure you meet your quota. In fact, a balanced, varied vegetarian diet can be suitable for most people at any age – and can even meet the pressured needs of top athletes. Here are a few examples of important nutrients that plant foods supply:

● **Calcium** From dark green leafy vegetables, such as cabbage and broccoli, baked beans, soy milk, dried figs and calcium-enriched foods and juices.

● **Iron** As iron isn't as easily absorbed from plant foods, vegetarians need almost double the iron of meat-eaters. Dried beans, lentils, enriched cereals, broccoli, beetroot and dried fruit are good sources. Eating vitamin-C rich foods at the same meal enhances the uptake of iron.

● **Omega-3** If you're not eating fish or eggs, it's difficult to get enough of this essential fatty acid. Soybeans, walnuts, ground linseeds and canola oil are sources and a number of omega-3 fortified products are available.

● **Vitamin B$_{12}$** If you eat dairy products or eggs you will get enough B$_{12}$, which is essential for producing red blood cells and preventing anaemia. For vegans, sources include yeast extract spreads, fortified soy products and vitamin-enriched cereals, but supplements may be a good idea.

● **Vitamin D** Milk and eggs both supply some vitamin D, but the best source of the so-called 'sunshine vitamin' is just that – being outdoors in the sun. Vitamin D-enriched cereals, margarine, soy and rice milks can help those who don't get much sun exposure, or you could take a supplement.

● **Zinc** This is another nutrient that is not absorbed as easily from plant foods as from animal foods, but zinc can be found in whole grains, soy foods, legumes, nuts and wheatgerm.

5 Water, water...
and a little wine

Water is kilojoule-free and more or less tasteless, yet it is essential to all living things. Juices, milk and other beverages are helpful, too, and a little wine brings health benefits, while enhancing the pleasure of good food.

We can survive without food for weeks, but we can't last more than a few days without water. It's vital for health and makes up a surprisingly large proportion of our bodies. A new-born baby is around 75–80 per cent water but as we grow and age, the amount of water in our bodies decreases. The total varies from person to person; on average adult men are 60–65 per cent water and women 55–60 per cent. Levels also vary between body organs and tissues: the brain, for example, is around 80 per cent water, which is why it is so quickly affected by dehydration, while bones are just 10–15 per cent water. Muscle contains more water than adipose tissue (fat), so in a flabby, obese person, water may be as little as 45 per cent of body weight.

How much do I need?

Maintaining an adequate amount of water – in other words, keeping your body properly hydrated – helps to regulate body temperature and enables your body to dispose of waste efficiently, helping to prevent painful problems such as kidney stones and gallstones. Water is a lubricant that forms the basis of the mucus that lines and protects tissues throughout

2.5 LITRES
of water a day is the average amount that most adults take in, excreting enough moisture in sweat, respiration, urine and faeces to keep the body's water level constant.

the body. Pockets of water-based fluid act as shock absorbers for the body's organs, including the brain. In short, water is critical for wellbeing and healthy growth, with a role in countless biological processes.

A body in perfect balance will take in the amount of water it needs and excrete any excess consumed via sweat, respiration, urine and faeces. On average, adults take in and excrete about 2.5 litres. Having a highly efficient water-absorption and regulatory system, your body uses water not just from what you drink but also what you eat, along with a little released from your internal organs. Most people get about a litre a day from food.

So how much should we all be drinking? The guideline amount is about 1.2 litres a day, or about 6 to 8 glasses of 150–200ml each; suggestions for as much as 2.5 litres have no scientific basis. The truth is, the amount you need depends on your age, gender, body size, activity levels and a host of other conditions, including altitude and weather. The important thing is to ensure you stay well hydrated – for physical health and to keep your brain sharp and alert.

Did YOU know ?

The signs of dehydration

An obvious sign of dehydration is thirst and there are other signs that could alert you before you notice that you are thirsty:

- Feeling tired or lacking in energy.
- Starting to get a headache or feeling lightheaded.
- Not passing much urine or passing dark-coloured urine.

In addition, it is easy to mistake feelings of thirst for hunger and seek out something to eat, when what your body really wants is a drink.

Does it have to be water?

Milk – an important drink for children – is 88 per cent water and like others, including tea, coffee, fruit juice and herbal teas, counts towards your recommended daily intake of liquid. These drinks may also bring an added bonus in the form of vitamins, trace minerals or antioxidants. For instance, UK researchers from King's College, London, maintain that drinking three cups of black tea a day, but no more than eight cups, could help to protect against heart disease and tooth decay.

Coffee, too, has its benefits as a stimulant, but it's not a good idea to drink too much as it can also have a diuretic effect, increasing the amount of urine you produce. Soft drinks are often high in sugar and 'sugar-free' versions don't necessarily solve this problem, as the sugar is usually replaced by a load of artificial sweeteners. Alcohol is not recommended because it dehydrates the body rather than hydrating it.

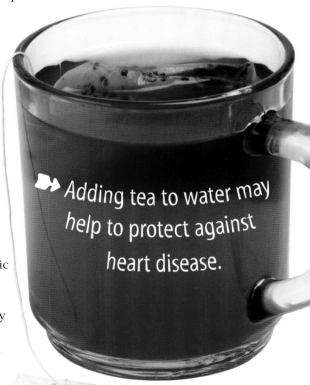

Adding tea to water may help to protect against heart disease.

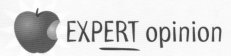

EXPERT opinion

Can I drink too much water?

Yes. Writing in the *British Medical Journal*, Dr Margaret McCartney says drinking more water than you need can impair concentration and cause sleep loss through having to get up in the night. In rare cases, drinking too much water too quickly causes hyponatraemia, a potentially fatal condition in which levels of body salts become dangerously diluted. A related problem, water intoxication, is most often seen in athletes or in infants given too much over-diluted infant formula. Health experts have suggested that advice to drink excessive amounts of water is spread by those with a vested interest and ignores liquid intake from food and other drinks.

Dr Margaret McCartney *UK family doctor*

For all these reasons, most health experts would recommend water above any other drink. Yet, according to metabolism expert Dr Stanley Goldfarb from the University of Pennsylvania, USA, there is no scientific evidence to support drinking extra water when you're not thirsty simply to boost health. 'There is no single study – and therefore no single outcome – that has led to these recommendations,' he says. In most cases, water is simply better for you than sugary drinks you might sip instead.

Bottled versus tap water

With fashionable labels, salubrious sources and a price point to match, bottled water presents a convincing healthy image. But is it really better than water from our taps? In most developed countries, tap water is perfectly good to drink. It undergoes treatment processes to meet safety and quality standards; some water authorities also add fluoride to reduce the risk of tooth decay.

Bottled water is usually either spring water, bottled at source directly from springs rising from the ground, or mineral water, which also rises from underground but then flows over rocks so it acquires more minerals before bottling. Bottled spring water must meet certain standards and may be treated to meet them. Mineral water is untreated, apart from removing debris. The various brands of both spring and mineral waters contain different types and amounts of minerals, depending on the source.

The bottom line, in the developed world at least, is that tap water is just as good as bottled – possibly better – although the taste may vary from region to region. If you don't like the taste of your local water, try using a water filter, or fill a couple of glass bottles with water from the tap and chill it in the fridge before drinking.

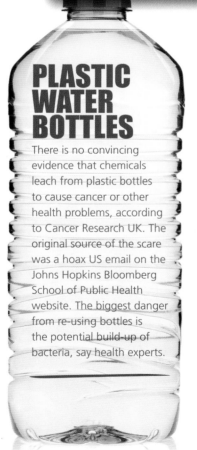

PLASTIC WATER BOTTLES

There is no convincing evidence that chemicals leach from plastic bottles to cause cancer or other health problems, according to Cancer Research UK. The original source of the scare was a hoax US email on the Johns Hopkins Bloomberg School of Public Health website. The biggest danger from re-using bottles is the potential build-up of bacteria, say health experts.

How healthy is fruit juice?

There is a huge choice of fruit juices on offer – some of them fortified with vitamins and minerals. Nutritionists sometimes suggest that a small glass of juice can even count as one of your seven-a-day fruits and vegetables, but be under no illusions. No matter which brand you choose, it will generally contain fewer vitamins, less fibre, fewer phytochemicals and more sugar than the fresh whole fruit it comes from. Yet juice is undoubtedly tasty and convenient, and healthy enough if the sugar content is not too high. For maximum goodness, try the following:

- Go for whole fruit juice – if the juice is made with the whole fruit, the skin included if appropriate, it will contain more health-giving properties. Shake the container well to disperse any bits of sediment before serving.
- Go for '100 per cent juice' – then you'll know you're not buying added sugar. But check to see if it contains fruits you weren't expecting. More expensive fruits, such as blueberries, may be 'stretched' with apple or white grape juice. This isn't always bad: cranberry juice, for example, is so tart it is often mixed with sweeter fruits to reduce the need for extra sugar. Avoid any juice drink that contains high-fructose corn syrup.
- Go for natural colour – juices made from deep purple, red and blue fruits such as grapes, cranberries, pomegranates and blueberries are rich in anthocyanins, which are antioxidant and anti-inflammatory.
- Dilute with water – adding still or sparkling water to fruit juice creates a more refreshing drink and slashes the sugar content.

Juice is good – but fresh fruit is better

A glass of fruit juice is a quick, easy way to get a blast of antioxidants, but whole fruit (with 'bits') delivers more. They both contribute towards the daily liquid your body needs.

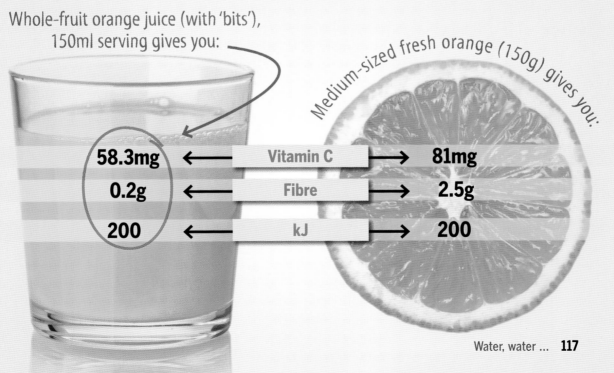

Whole-fruit orange juice (with 'bits'), 150ml serving gives you:

Medium-sized fresh orange (150g) gives you:

58.3mg	Vitamin C	81mg
0.2g	Fibre	2.5g
200	kJ	200

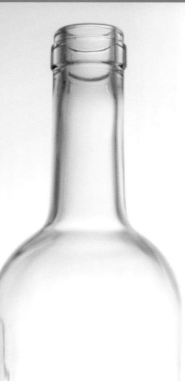

What's so good about wine?

Wine has been part of human culture and celebrations for thousands of years; the Bible miracle of turning water into wine for a wedding feast illustrates its importance. In Mediterranean countries especially, dinner without wine is almost unthinkable. Wine, in fact, is one of the elements suspected of contributing to the health and longevity associated with the Mediterranean diet.

The first study to suggest that drinking wine might be linked to a lower risk for heart disease began in Paris in 1967. Called the Paris Prospective Study, it tracked 7,453 middle-aged French police officers over eight years. The results showed that the men in the study, who submitted to medical tests for its duration, had just half the death rate from heart disease as American men – despite the fact that their diet was rich in saturated fats and that many of them smoked.

The French Paradox?

Soon we were calling it the French Paradox – that Frenchmen who enjoyed rich food, wine and cigarettes had healthier hearts than men elsewhere with supposedly better diets and lifestyles. In 1992, researchers from the French National Institute of Health and Medical Research published the results of a study in *The Lancet*, suggesting that the nation's legendary wine consumption had something to do with keeping French hearts ticking. They quoted the findings of other studies showing that 20–30g of alcohol a day – equivalent to two or three small glasses of wine – could cut the risk of coronary heart disease by 40 per cent. Their conclusion was that alcohol seemed to interfere with the clotting ability of blood platelets and that this might be how it helped to protect the heart.

Subsequent research had reported that moderate drinking of alcohol, not just wine, can lower the risk of heart disease. Research into other potential health benefits suggests it may also improve insulin sensitivity and help to combat inflammation. The key in all of this is

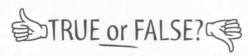

TRUE or FALSE?

Red wine is especially health-boosting

Probably TRUE! Recent research has focused on resveratrol, an antioxidant polyphenol compound present in the skins and seeds of grapes. Red wine has higher levels of resveratrol than white wine because the skins and seeds are left in the wine for longer at the initial crushing and fermenting stage. Resveratrol is the vine's defence mechanism against disease and may also help to protect our health in several ways. *Science Daily* has highlighted resveratrol's potential for 'decreasing the body's chronic inflammation response', implicated in many health problems including heart disease and diabetes. US research at Cornell University suggests the compound may also help to decrease plaque formation in the brain, which might protect against dementia.

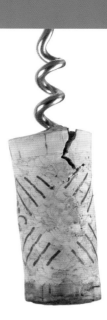

the term 'moderate'. Men and women who drink moderately seem on average to gain some benefits over both non-drinkers and heavy drinkers. They are more likely to be a healthy weight, to get the recommended 7 to 8 hours sleep a night, and to exercise regularly. But imbibe more heavily and any benefits quickly unravel. When it comes to wine and alcohol, a little is good – but a lot is not. As a general guideline, the World Health Organization suggests no more than two alcoholic drinks a day for women and three for men, with an absolute limit of four drinks on any occasion.

There is a further aspect to the French wine phenomenon. In Britain and elsewhere in the Northern Hemisphere, people often drink alcohol on its own and frequently drink to get drunk. But in French and Mediterranean culture, wine is a carefully chosen accompaniment to meals, drunk in moderation to complement flavours and enhance the pleasure of sharing good food with friends and family. That, too, may help to explain its heart-healthy reputation. As Dr Lionel Opie suggests in his editorial to *The French Paradox: Fact or Fiction?*, a series of papers published in 2008, wine alone does not explain it; 'the more Mediterranean, the better' might be a less mystifying and more accurate view, he says.

The eat-well message

The pleasures of such good food – and drink – and their outstanding benefits should now be becoming abundantly clear. Fruits and vegetables, high-fibre grains, 'good' fats, protein-rich foods, water and perhaps a little wine – with a minimum of additional processed products – are the basis of eating well, which can only enhance your health and quality of life for years to come. To double-check that you're getting all the nutrients you need, take a look at 'Are you missing out?', which follows.

➡ **Make it fresh** Researchers are unanimous on the superior nutritional quality of whole fruits and real vegetables compared to processed products.

➡ **Think fibre – it's not all boring bran** Getting plenty of fibre foods – whole grains, legumes and fresh produce – helps protect against diabetes, heart disease, cancer and more. Despite the 'bran' image, most fibre foods are delicious, too.

➡ **Yes, you can eat fat** In fact, it's essential and some of the tastiest foods – think olive oil and salmon – contain the healthiest fats, which benefit your body and your brain.

➡ **Protein matters** Meat, eggs, fish or a mixture of beans and grains are the cornerstones of a healthy diet. Add water, milk, a little wine or grape juice – here's to your good health!

Are you missing out?

It's not rocket science: you can live longer and improve your chances of avoiding chronic diseases by eating a healthy, balanced and nutritious diet.

Throughout our lives – in fact, even from before we are born – the foods we take in affect our health, strength, intelligence and longevity. Marion Nestle, professor of nutrition and food studies at New York University, USA, put it this way in her 2006 book *What to Eat*: 'Eating a food with sugar or trans fat is not going to kill you on the spot. Eating a particular fruit or vegetable is not going to provide lifetime protection against heart disease or cancer. It's what you habitually eat – and how much – that

The Healthy-Eating Plate formula illustrates the balance of key types of foods most people should aim for in a healthy diet. Eating these each day in the proportions suggested ensures a regular supply of all essential nutrients.

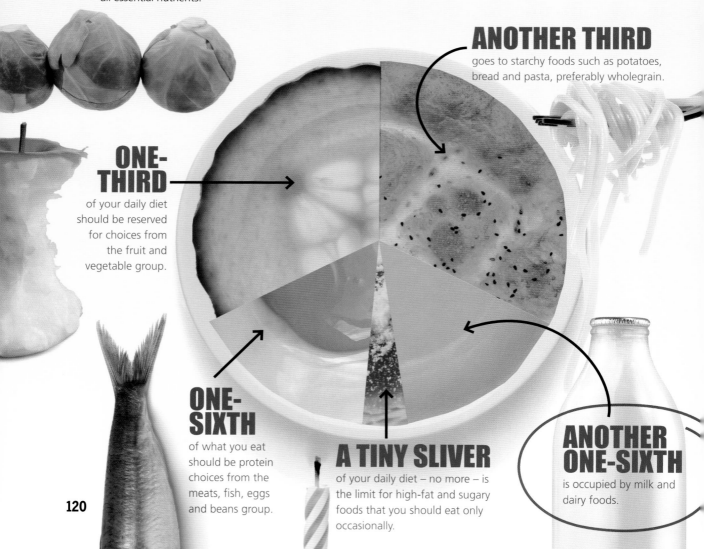

ANOTHER THIRD
goes to starchy foods such as potatoes, bread and pasta, preferably wholegrain.

ONE-THIRD
of your daily diet should be reserved for choices from the fruit and vegetable group.

ONE-SIXTH
of what you eat should be protein choices from the meats, fish, eggs and beans group.

A TINY SLIVER
of your daily diet – no more – is the limit for high-fat and sugary foods that you should eat only occasionally.

ANOTHER ONE-SIXTH
is occupied by milk and dairy foods.

matters.' She has this simple, sensible advice to offer: 'Eat less, move more, eat lots of fruits and vegetables, and go easy on junk foods.'

When you consider it from a cosmic perspective, there's something miraculous about the fact that the nutrients we humans require are abundantly found in the foods we (should) eat. But to get an adequate supply of those nutrients, we need to choose our foods wisely from the several different food groups and eat them in the proper proportions.

In Australia, the National Health and Medical Research Council (NHMRC) uses the plate diagram to help people consume the right balance of foods necessary for optimal health. This illustration (*see* left) makes it simple to picture what should be on our plates – and in what proportions – every day. By following the healthy-eating plate formula, you're likely to get your full complement of vitamins and minerals. But it's good to have a basic understanding of what these essential nutrients are. Let's take a look.

The big picture: macronutrients

Protein, carbohydrate and fat – relatively large molecular structures – are considered macronutrients. We require sufficient amounts of these to supply our energy needs.
- **Carbohydrates** These are our principal source of energy and provide about 50 to 60 per cent of our daily energy intake.
- **Protein** Your body uses protein's amino acids in many ways, such as fuelling growth and tissue repair. It can also be converted into carbohydrate or stored as fat. (*See* page 106.)
- **Fats** These give you a concentrated form of energy; but eat too much fat and it'll turn into … fat. Healthier fats are mono- and polyunsaturated fats, found mainly in olive and canola oil, nuts and avocado. Animal fats, from meat and dairy products, often have a higher proportion of the less healthy saturated

Did YOU know ?

Historic diseases are reappearing

If rickets and scurvy conjure images of Dickens' orphans and seafarers of yore, you may be shocked to find that both diseases are on the rise among children of ethnic minority groups in Europe and Australasia. 'Rickets was thought to have died out in the 1930s', reports Rebecca Dunn, spokesperson for the British Dietetic Association. 'However, the number of children under 10 admitted to hospital with the disease jumped by 140 per cent between 2001 and 2008.' Rickets is a bone disease which can develop when children get insufficient vitamin D. Scurvy, a disease caused by vitamin C deficiency, is also on the rise: 'The number of children admitted to hospital with scurvy between 2005 and 2008 increased by over 50 per cent.' Archaic diseases that put children in hospital in the 21st century are terrifying enough but only part of the story. Most of the diseases we battle today, such as diabetes, heart disease, cancer and their precursor conditions, including high blood pressure and high cholesterol, are partially due to lifestyle-related nutritional deficiencies, says Dunn.

fats. The trans fats found in processed food should be avoided as they have been linked to a host of diseases. You can read more about fats on pages 34–41 and pages 98–105.

The detailed picture: micronutrients

The nutrients you need in tiny amounts are called micronutrients. In some cases, as in vitamins, health experts know roughly how much of each we need for good health. The following tables illustrate the daily amounts suggested for adults (aged over 18 years) and some good food sources. In other cases, such as phytochemicals, it is not yet clear precisely how much we need.

NOTE: *If you're pregnant or breastfeeding, follow your doctor's advice about vitamins or other supplements as what you eat directly affects your baby, and requirements for young children are very different from those for adults.*

Vitamins

Vitamin	What it does	Good sources	Daily amount
Vitamin A (from retinols in animal products or pro-vitamin A carotenoids in plant foods)	Essential for vision; helps cells grow and develop normally; maintains healthy skin, tissue, teeth, hair and nails; supports the immune system.	Retinol: butter, egg yolk, cheese, milk, margarine, oily fish. Beta-carotene: orange and yellow fruits; orange, red and green vegetables, chilli, paprika.	Women: 700µg Men: 900µg
Thiamin	Helps to release and utilise energy from food, and is required for normal functioning of the nervous system.	Nuts, sunflower seeds, fortified cereals, bran, wheatgerm, oatmeal, potatoes, pork, oily fish, yeast extract.	Women: 1.1mg Men: 1.2mg (men >50 years 0.9mg)
Riboflavin	Aids growth and maintains skin, eyes and nervous system; helps the body release energy from food.	Lamb's liver, kidney, breakfast cereals, bran, egg yolk, milk, cheese, almonds, yeast extract, mushrooms.	Women: 1.1mg Men: 1.3mg
Niacin	Central role in metabolism and the utilisation of energy. Helps to maintain the health of digestive and nervous system.	Fortified cereals, bran, wheatgerm, wholemeal bread, lean meats, poultry, kidney, liver, game meats, fish, egg yolk, seafood, cheese, yeast extract.	Women: 14mg (>50 years: 12mg) Men: 16mg (>50 years: 16mg)
Pantothenic acid	Precursor of a coenzyme necessary for the release of energy from fat and carbohydrate and the synthesis of cholesterol.	Most foods. Higher concentrations in: liver, kidneys, meat, breakfast cereals, whole grains, egg yolk, nuts, avocado, dried fruits, milk.	Women: 4mg Men: 6mg
Vitamin B₆ (Pyridoxine)	Essential for the metabolism of amino acids and releasing glucose from body stores. Helps create haemoglobin, which carries oxygen in red blood cells.	Many food sources. The best include: wholegrain bread, nuts, sesame seeds, calf liver, salmon, poultry, potatoes, leeks, avocado, bananas.	Women: 1.3mg (>50 years: 1.5mg) Men: 1.3mg (>50 years: 1.7mg)
Biotin	Essential for breaking down and using fats in the body.	Chicken liver, kidney, cooked whole egg and egg yolk, nuts, plaice, soybeans, bran, wheatgerm.	Safe intake: 10–200µg
Folate	Works with vitamin B12 to form healthy red blood cells and maintain the health of rapidly dividing cells, especially in the nervous system of unborn babies.	Egg yolk, asparagus, beetroot, brussels sprouts, spinach, broccoli, fortified cereals, wholemeal or granary bread.	Women: 400µg Pregnant women: 600µg Men: 400µg
Vitamin B₁₂	Necessary for making red blood cells, maintaining the nervous system, releasing energy and processing folic acid.	All animal products, especially liver, kidney, molluscs, fish (pilchards, herring, sardines and kippers), eggs, Marmite.	Women: 2.4µg Men: 2.4µg
Vitamin C	Supports the production of collagen, a component of connective and fibrous tissues; promotes wound healing; prevents free radical damage and aids iron absorption from non-meat sources.	Berries, blackcurrants, kiwifruit, citrus fruits, pineapple, rockmelon, green leafy vegetables, broccoli, potatoes.	Women: 45mg Men: 45mg
Vitamin D	Helps the body to absorb and regulate calcium, a mineral essential for building healthy bones and teeth.	Oily fish, egg yolks, butter and fortified margarine, some fortified breakfast cereals, liver, cod liver oil.	Women: 5µg Men: 5µg Pregnancy, breastfeeding or age >50 years: 10µg
Vitamin E	An antioxidant that has a role in the immune system and helps to prevent cellular damage and chronic diseases, including heart disease and cancer.	Canola, cod liver, sunflower and safflower oils, wheatgerm, cereals, almonds, hazelnuts, avocado, egg yolk.	Adequate intake: Women: 7mg Men: 10mg
Vitamin K	Helps blood to clot and plays a key role in bone health and kidney function.	Kale, parsley, spinach, spring greens, broccoli, cabbage, brussels sprouts, canola, soybean and olive oils.	Adequate intake: Women: 60µg Men: 70µg

NB: Pregnant and breastfeeding women may need higher doses of some vitamins and minerals.

If I get too little?

Can affect sight, growth development and cause skin problems although deficiencies are rare in the developed world. Also linked to low fertility and poor immunity.

Severe weakness, muscle cramps, muscle wasting, tingling/loss of sensation in hands and feet, confusion, beriberi in extreme cases.

Mouth sores, swollen tongue, skin problems. May be associated with an iron deficiency and anaemia. Those who avoid dairy foods could have low intakes.

Diarrhoea, confusion and memory loss. Extreme deficiencies can cause pellagra where skin becomes dark and scaly when exposed to light.

Deficiencies are rare, but reports include burning feet syndrome, fatigue, insomnia, depression, vomiting, dizziness, muscular weakness, nerve and stomach disturbances.

General weakness, sleeplessness, peripheral neuropathy, personality changes, dermatitis, anaemia and impaired immunity.

Rare: scaly skin, hair loss, depression, raised blood cholesterol levels, conjunctivitis, loss of appetite and hallucinations.

Anaemia, abnormal red blood cells, impaired cell division, weight loss and intestinal upsets. Can cause birth defects.

Anaemia, degeneration of nerve cells and spinal cord, loss of balance, spastic weakness in lower limbs.

Bleeding from capillaries under the skin and gums, easy bruising, wounds are slow to heal and reduced immunity. If severe it could result in scurvy which can be fatal.

Bone weakness and abnormalities (rickets) in children. Osteomalacia and osteoporosis in adults, with pain, muscle weakness and bone fractures.

Muscle weakness and vision problems. Increased risk of some chronic diseases.

Prolonged bleeding before clotting of blood occurs. Possible osteoporosis.

If I get too much?

Over time, high doses can be toxic and have also been linked to certain birth defects so pregnant women or those trying to become pregnant are advised not to eat liver and to avoid supplements, including fish liver oil.

Chronic intakes result in headache, irritability, insomnia, rapid pulse and dermatitis.

High amounts might result in a harmless yellow discolouration of urine.

Hot flushes, nausea, diarrhoea, skin rashes and burning, palpitations, liver damage, impaired glucose tolerance and uric acid metabolism.

Very high doses may cause diarrhoea and other gastrointestinal disturbances, but no specific toxic side effects.

Taking more than 200mg can lead to sensory abnormalities such as loss of sensation in feet, arms and legs.

Unknown.

Large doses can inhibit zinc absorption. Taking more than 800µg a day could mask the symptoms of vitamin B12 deficiency.

Large doses have resulted in few, if any adverse side effects. Often used as a placebo in medical research.

More than 1g a day can cause stomach pain, diarrhoea and flatulence.

Thirst, loss of appetite, diarrhoea and possible calcium deposits in soft tissue such as kidneys, with risk of urinary stones.

Headache, fatigue, nausea, double vision, muscle weakness, gastrointestinal problems.

Can interfere with anti-clotting drugs.

Good to know

Can interact with many medicines so it is important to tell your doctor if you're taking supplements.

Cooking and preparing foods can destroy thiamin, so use freshly chopped vegetables in minimal cooking water.

Light can destroy riboflavin, so good food sources should not be stored in direct sunlight.

Eating milk and eggs can help remedy niacin deficiency as they contain tryptophan, which the body converts into a form of niacin.

Pantothenic acid in supplement form has many suggested uses, such as treating osteoarthritis, stress and conjunctivitis, but little scientific evidence to support them.

Safe maximum limit is no more than 10mg unless prescribed by a doctor. May interact with other medications.

Long-term use of antibiotics can inhibit the production of biotin by gut-dwelling bacteria, resulting in lower biotin levels.

Readily destroyed during food preparation and cooking in water. Adding vitamin C (in the form of lemon or other juice) reduces the loss of folate.

One of the few B vitamins that can be stored in the liver, with stores lasting two to five years.

Smokers require more vitamin C because nicotine and toxins in cigarette smoke deplete vitamin C levels in the body.

When exposed to sunshine, your body makes this vitamin, so a little sun each day tops up vitamin D which helps to keep calcium levels constant.

As this vitamin is fat-soluble, people who cannot absorb fat properly may develop a deficiency.

It is the chlorophyll in plants which supplies vitamin K; your gut bacteria also make it.

KEY: mg = milligrams, µg (or mcg) = micrograms

Minerals

Mineral	What it does	Good sources	Daily amount	Good to know
Calcium	Essential for building and maintaining bones, muscle contraction, nerve function, blood clotting and enzyme activity.	Dairy foods, small fish eaten with bones, bread, tofu, almonds, leafy green vegetables, dried figs, sesame seeds, tahini.	Women: 1000mg (>50 years: 1300mg) Men: 1000mg (>50 years: 1300mg)	It's the body's most plentiful mineral and works in concert with vitamin D and K and minerals magnesium and phosphorus.
Chromium	Works with insulin, the hormone that regulates blood glucose. It allows glucose to enter cells, where it's used to produce energy.	Fish, meat, poultry, nuts, potatoes, cereal products, broccoli, lentils, legumes and spices.	Adequate intake: Women: 25µg Men: 35µg	A deficiency of this micronutrient is extremely rare as it is widely distributed in food sources.
Copper	Component of many enzymes with key roles in pigmentation of hair, skin and eyes, making haemoglobin, development of brain, immune system and bones.	Liver, walnuts, almonds, cashews, brazil nuts, sunflower and sesame seeds, crab, oysters, whole grains, bran, wheatgerm.	Women: 1.2mg Men: 1.7mg	A deficiency is rare but it can cause anaemia, changes in bones, hair pigment, decreased skin tone and neurological problems.
Fluoride	Reduces tooth decay by combining with minerals in enamel to become more resistant to erosion, inhibits bacterial enzymes, and increases remineralisation.	Fluoridated water, fortified toothpastes and mouthwashes, tea, seafood, some bottled waters.	Adequate intake: Women: 3mg Men: 4mg	If you don't live in an area where fluoride is added to the water supply, ask your dentist if a supplement is necessary.
Iodine	Your body uses iodine to make thyroid hormones, required for healthy growth, metabolism, protein synthesis and connective tissue.	Seafood, seaweed or seaside plants (as seawater contains iodine), also milk and cereals. Some countries enrich table salt.	Women: 150µg Men: 150µg	Deficiencies reduce the amount of thyroid hormone produced and can lead to a slow metabolism (due to underactive thyroid), and goitres (neck swellings).
Iron	Iron is an oxygen carrier in haemoglobin in the blood which transports oxygen from lungs to tissue, and to myogloblin in muscles. It is also a component of enzymes for various processes.	Liver, offal, shellfish, red meat, egg yolk, dried beans, dried fruits, poultry, tuna, green leafy vegetables, peas, nuts, whole grains.	Women: 18mg (>50 years: 8mg) Men: 8mg	Low levels lead to iron-deficiency anaemia. Those at risk include menstruating women, vegans and people with gastro-intestinal disorders who cannot easily absorb iron from food.
Magnesium	Essential roles in bone development, nerve transmission, muscle contraction and protein synthesis; activates enzymes and regulates levels of other key nutrients.	Nuts and seeds, whole grains, wheatgerm and bran, soy flour, bread, legumes, tofu, hummus, leafy green vegetables, herbs, dried fruit.	Women: 320mg Men: 420mg	Deficiencies are rare if consuming a varied diet. Some research is indicating it might help to lower high blood pressure. However, excessive amounts will cause cathartic diarrhoea.
Phosphorous	Helps in the formation of bones and teeth; essential for metabolising fats and carbohydrates, and is an essential component of cell membranes.	Protein-rich foods, including grains, nuts, dairy products, egg yolk, crustaceans, meat, poultry, fish, legumes, tofu, yeast extract.	Women: 1000mg Men: 1000mg	Deficiencies are rare as the mineral is present in many foods. Excessive supplementation can cause diarrhoea and upset the gastro-intestinal tract.
Potassium	Helps to maintain fluid balance; essential for heart function and digestion as it helps muscles contract and nerves to function.	Dried fruits, nuts, seeds, beetroot, spinach, avocado, bananas, rhubarb, blackcurrants, grapes, potatoes, vegetables, legumes, fish.	Adequate intake: Women: 2800mg Men: 3800mg	Symptoms of dangerously low potassium include muscle weakness and cramps, low energy and an irregular heartbeat.

...continued

Mineral	What it does	Good sources	Daily amount	Good to know
Selenium	Essential for the proper functioning of the immune system and thyroid gland.	Brazil and cashew nuts, sunflower seeds, kidney, lamb's liver, shellfish, squid, fish, lentils, meat, egg yolk, mushrooms.	Women: 60µg Men: 70µg	Selenium is an antioxidant and may help protect against cancer by shielding cells from DNA damage caused by free radicals.
Sodium	Necessary to regulate blood pressure and volume; essential for helping muscles and nerve function.	Crustaceans, shellfish, offal, eggwhite, meat, spinach, beetroot, celery, milk. Sodium is added to many processed foods.	460–920mg Maximum intake: 2300mg	Sodium is added to many foods – check labels. There is 0.4g sodium in every 1g of salt (sodium chloride).
Zinc	Essential for breaking down nutrients, growth and reproduction, healthy immune function and making DNA and RNA.	Calf liver, offal, beef, crab, lobster, quorn, oysters, wheatgerm, nuts, Parmesan cheese, egg yolk.	Women: 8mg Men: 14mg	People who don't get enough may suffer symptoms including loss of taste sensation, poor appetite, diarrhoea, vomiting and poor wound healing.

KEY: mg = milligrams, mcg (or µg) = micrograms
Source for daily vitamin/mineral amounts: UK Reference Nutrient Intakes (RNIs) and NHS Choices

Other healing nutrients

Plant foods are powerhouses of nutrition because they contain energy, fibre, vitamins and minerals, plus literally thousands of other health-sustaining compounds. These 'phytochemicals' give plants their colour, aroma and flavour and help them resist attacks from insects, disease and other dangers. Now scientists are learning how they also protect human health (*see* page 87).

● **Anthocyanins** are flavonoids responsible for the red, purple and blue colours in many fruits, vegetables and cereal grains. They may help prevent cancer, diabetes, cardiovascular and neurological diseases.

● **Carotenoids** include more than 700 fat-soluble nutrients that produce the orange, green and red colours of carrots, pumpkins and many other vegetables and fruits. They include beta-carotene (a precursor for vitamin A), lutein and lycopene, all of which are important for vision. Lycopene, found in tomatoes, may also help to protect against prostate cancer. In general, all the carotenoids are antioxidants.

● **Catechins** belong to the well-studied group of flavonoids found in tea, grapes and apples, which are known for their potent antioxidant power and may protect against a variety of malignancies. For more about tea, *see* page 293.

● **Isoflavones,** found in soy, chickpeas and other legumes, and lignans in linseeds and whole grains, seem to mimic the action of oestrogen and may play a role in protecting against hormone-dependent breast and prostate cancer.

● **Lutein** is a carotenoid found in dark green leafy vegetables and some fruits. It is thought to protect the eyes from sunlight damage and may help prevent the eye disease known as age-related macular degeneration and reduce the risk of developing cataracts.

● **Resveratrol** is found in the skin of grapes and is present in wine. Among the many studies that have highlighted its benefits is Spanish research in 2012, which revealed that among those at high risk of heart disease, moderate red wine drinking appeared to improve cholesterol levels, heart rate and blood-glucose levels. (*See also* page 118).

Control those portions

Working out how much we should be eating to get the nutrients we need without piling on the kilos is no easy task. Many restaurants serve hugely over-sized platefuls; friends or family who overeat can influence us, too.

You can scrub your diet free of fast, junk and processed foods, but you still won't enjoy that zenith of vibrancy or energy if you don't eat food in proper proportions and portion sizes. Dietary balance is key to good health.

As the obesity epidemic increases across the developed world, both governments and food manufacturers have acknowledged that most people are getting portions and proportions horribly wrong – with disastrous results for their health.

Portion sizes

The best way to rectify the balance is to get to know the number of daily portions you should aim for from the various food categories, which include cereals, breads, meats, fish, grains, dairy, fruit and vegetables.

If you're a normal, moderately active, healthy adult, the following guidelines will ensure you meet your needs for energy and nutrition. If you're overweight, you'll need to trim your portion sizes so that you reduce your energy intake safely, possibly working with a doctor or dietitian. People who are inactive, older or shorter (especially postmenopausal women) need to eat less food generally, because they have a slower metabolism, which makes it easier to gain weight.

You don't have to stick to single portions of the different foods listed here. What's important is to keep within the suggested daily portion limits. Most people eat much more than they think they do, which is why they put on weight. So keep it real: measure your portions until you have a sense of how much food is appropriate for you.

Meat, fish and other proteins

3 portions a day

At least one portion a week should be oily fish (salmon, herring, mackerel, sardines)

Examples of portion sizes:

LEAN MEAT = size of a deck of cards
Raw: 100g   Cooked: 65g

FISH = size of a cheque book
Raw: 115g   Cooked: 100g (or small can)

EGGS = 2 medium

BAKED BEANS = ½ tin
5 tablespoons

LEGUMES = 1 heaped handful
4 tablespoons   (lentils, chickpeas, split peas)

NUTS = 1 small handful
2 tablespoons

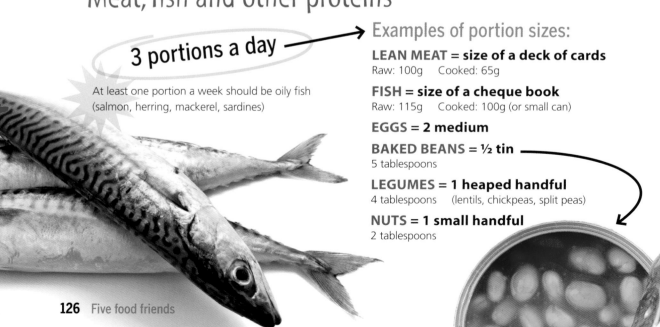

Fruits and vegetables

At least 7 a day ... preferably more.

150g of any fruit or 75g of any vegetable:

MANGO, PINEAPPLE OR PAPAYA = 1 cup diced Or any large fruit

APPLE, PEAR, ORANGE, BANANA, PEACH = 1 Or any medium-sized fruit

KIWIFRUIT, PLUMS OR MANDARINS = 2 Or any small fruits

GRAPES OR BERRIES = 1–2 handfuls

FRUIT JUICE OR SMOOTHIE = 1 small glass
125ml (no added sugar); just one serving of juice or smoothie a day

PEAS, CARROTS, CORN, CABBAGE, BROCCOLI, etc. **= ½ cup**

SALAD GREENS = 1 cup

Grain (cereal) foods

8–10 portions a day

Opt for wholegrain breads, pasta and cereals.

Examples of portion sizes:

BREAKFAST CEREAL = 30g (¼–⅔ cup)

BREAD = 1 slice

PASTA (cooked) **= ½ cup**

RICE (cooked) **= ½ cup**

PITA OR FLATBREAD OR BREAD ROLL = ½

SCONE OR CRUMPET = 1

CRACKERS = 3 small

Dairy

2–4 portions a day Choose lower-fat options when possible.

Examples of portion sizes:

MILK = 1 cup (250ml)

YOGURT = 1 tub (200g)

HARD CHEESE = size of small matchbox (40g)

COTTAGE CHEESE OR RICOTTA = ½ cup (120g)

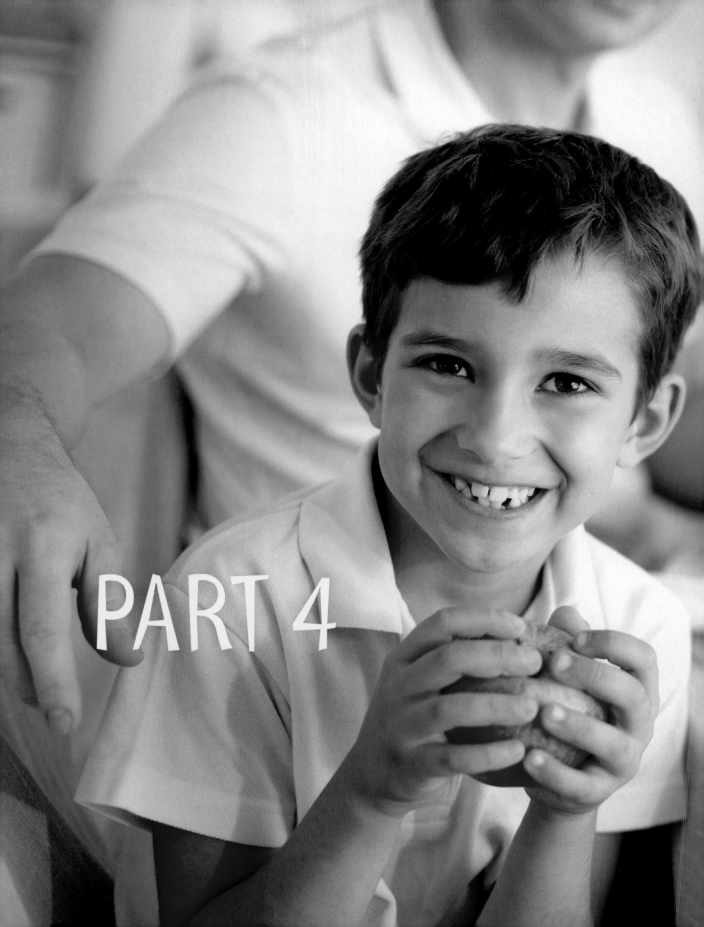

PART 4

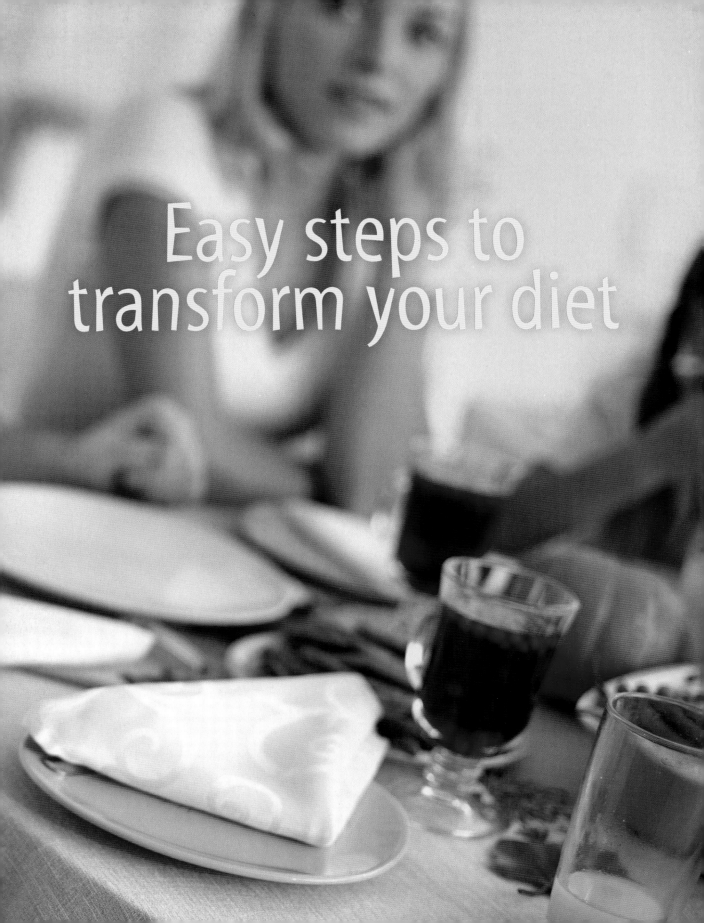

Easy steps to transform your diet

The good food habit

From the earlier chapters of this book, you will already have gleaned a wealth of information about what goes into our food today and what makes a healthy or unhealthy diet. While theory and examples are all very well, the trick is putting all that knowledge into practice. Here's how.

This section is your practical good food guide as you shop, cook, manage your daily meals, grapple with special dietary needs or embark on weight loss. It is not about rigid formulas or prescriptive meal plans. What is important is to recognise that so much of what is seductively packaged and pitched as 'delicious' – think cupcakes, rich ice cream, sugary doughnuts or sizzling cheeseburgers – is often poor quality and almost certainly not conducive to good health. The challenge is to look beyond profit-making lines to find foods that truly nourish and sustain, and then to ensure they become part of our everyday lives.

First steps

With food so readily available, it's easy to be 'reactive', eating whatever comes our way. The first step is to take control.

▶ **Getting started** Back in Part 1, you answered the 'Food and you' quiz, designed to reveal your current shopping and eating habits, with a few tips on how to improve them, if necessary. Here you'll find some home truths about the way many of us now eat and you'll discover fresh incentives to make changes if necessary. You'll also discover what health experts say we should be eating at different times of life, plus tips on keeping track of your diet and some simple ideas for healthy food swaps in everyday meals.

▶ **Shopping for quality** You might ask, what constitutes 'quality' in food? Obviously, a product should be both safe to eat and nutritious. Less obviously, quality food is not necessarily costlier or more time-consuming to prepare than less wholesome food. Fruit and vegetables, when in season, for example, are not only at their best in terms of nutrients and taste, but cheaper too. You'll discover the best outlets for different foods and how to navigate the confusing minefield of labels and nutrition information on packaged products.

▶ **Home-made is best** aims to put you in the driving seat for a diet filled with variety, based on whole, healthy, unprocessed foods. Cooking doesn't have to take up hours of your time – and it puts you in charge of how much salt, sugar and fat is in your food. You'll see the benefits of a well-stocked larder and discover plenty of mouth-watering ideas for time and money-saving everyday meals.

Through the day

We need good fuel to function well in our waking hours. Getting the amounts and balance of nutrients right helps us feel our best.

▶ **Breakfast review** What nutrients does your body need after its overnight fast? What happens to your body (and your brain) if you just snatch a 'little something' on your way to work, or skip breakfast and nibble biscuits to compensate? The chapter outlines the best breakfast options – including those that take minimal time to prepare – to help you feel alert and keep you going during the morning.

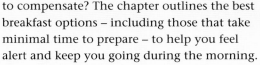 **Healthy snacks** Filling up between meals with sweet, salty or fat-filled snacks can make you pile on the weight, so this chapter looks at more nutritious ways to plug the hunger gap. It also provides some clear psychological insights into why we might be reaching for that chocolate bar or biscuit tin – snacking is not always about hunger.

Your midday meal In today's world, it's easy to rush lunch, postpone it or even miss it out completely. Here you'll find a delicious and versatile selection of healthy options to choose from – including packed lunches – that can all be quickly and easily prepared.

Delicious dinners For many of us, this is the day's key meal. Whether you take it early or late, it's often the time when you eat well and relax, share a meal with a friend, sit down with the family or celebrate a social occasion. This chapter is packed with tasty ideas for preparing quick, nutritious dishes that everyone will enjoy.

Tailored to your needs

For varying reasons we can't always eat whatever we want to. Here's how to manage different dietary requirements – and enjoy good food.

Special diets More and more people have to restrict what they eat – often as a result of allergies or intolerances. With a little forethought and planning, most special diets can be easily accommodated with meals that supply all the nutrients required. Vegetarian and gluten-free are among those discussed.

Effective weight control Crash diets are not the answer for people who are overweight or obese. You'll find out how to identify a weight problem and its health implications, how to prepare yourself mentally for change, and where to get the best information. You'll get the low-down on popular diets and also discover – unsurprisingly – that lifestyle changes, small portions and balance are among the solutions for long-term success.

1 Getting started

Eating well is not about drastic change. It's about first taking stock to see if your everyday diet is up to par. Then – if necessary – you can tweak it gradually in many different and enjoyable ways to benefit your health, whatever your age.

When you answered the 'Food and you' quiz questions in Part 1 of this book, and then looked through the comments on your specific choices, did you have a sneaky feeling that, if this were your school report, the overall assessment might be 'could do better'? Whatever your score, everything you've now learnt about modern food production will no doubt have inspired you to take a fresh look at your approach to everyday eating and how it might affect your health and perhaps the health of your family, too.

Why good nutrition matters

All too often, we're lulled into a sense of false security by food companies and advertisers, trusting that because most food is 'safe' – in the sense that it won't make us ill in the short term – then that must also mean it's 'good' for us.

Despite media headlines, many people are still unaware of the dangers of poor nutrition. This is why you need to know:

➡ **Study after study** links poor nutrition, especially eating too many artery-blocking fatty, sugary foods to a host of major diseases, including diabetes, heart problems and cancer.

➡ **Your eating habits** influence those around you – your partner, your children, even a dependent parent. By encouraging a respect for good food, you promote their health and wellbeing as well as your own.

One recent survey by food company Organix of 1,500 UK parents of young

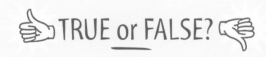

TRUE or FALSE?

You can eat much the same at any age

FALSE! For optimum health, our bodies need varying amounts of nutrients at different stages of our lives, according to 2011 research at the University of Lisbon in Portugal. What we eat throughout life may significantly affect how long we live and our quality of life as well, according to a 2012 study by Polish researchers. They suggest that nutrients such as B-group vitamins, antioxidants and polyunsaturated fats are likely to play 'a significant role' in the prevention of neurodegenerative diseases such as dementia. (*See also* page 134.)

children found that 28 per cent never checked the nutritional value of the foods they served. More than a fifth let their children choose what they wanted to eat and a similar number believed that 'a child grows out of any bad eating habits as they get older'; 27 per cent conceded that their kids preferred sweets, cakes, crisps and pizza to healthier foods.

Focus on food

But parents aren't the only ones who appear to be struggling to find time to concentrate on food. We eat on the run, we eat at our desks, we snack as we travel and many of us watch TV with our evening meal. For some, eating around the table as a family is now a special event when guests come round, rather than the norm.

The danger of eating and drinking in such a distracted way is that we're barely conscious of what we consume (*see* Over 200, below) and eat badly or overeat as a consequence. We may also be rushed and unfocused as we shop. Who, you might ask, has time to read nutrition labels when buying foods or to shop around to find good ingredients and then cook them?

In the 21st century, when so much unhealthy food is so readily available and the consequences of consuming it day in, day out are so dire, the answer has to be 'you'.

➡ **A fifth of parents let their children choose what they wanted to eat.**

Making changes

Examining your thoughts about food and your eating habits (*see* Keeping track of what you eat, page 136) and understanding their significance are first vital steps. But making changes – if you need to do so – should be a gradual process. Your age and current state of health may suggest the sort of tweaks that would help; *see* Eat right for your time of life, pages 134–135, which highlights different nutritional needs at various life stages. Start by making small, healthy day-to-day food swaps and you'll be much more likely to stick to them, so they will have a bigger, more long-lasting effect.

OVER 200

'food decisions' are made every day by the average American, says Dr Brian Wansink, author of *Mindless Eating*. Most people believe they make no more than 15, he adds. The rest are often made almost unconsciously. 'If we knew why we eat the way we do, we could eat a little less, eat a little healthier and enjoy food a lot more.'

Continued on page 136

Eat right for your time of life

In general, good food is good food, but your body has different nutritional needs at different stages of your life. It makes sense, therefore, to tailor your diet to ensure that you meet those needs – it can minimise risk factors for disease, prevent unwanted weight gain and help to enhance your health and wellbeing.

Childhood – Once weaned, babies need a full range of nutrients in small, easily digestible portions.

➡ As they grow and get more active give them vitamin- and mineral-rich cereals and starchy foods, vegetables and fruit, high-protein foods such as poultry, meat, fish and legumes and dairy foods. **Use whole milk up to the age of two.**

➡ **Limit salty, sugary or fatty foods and sugary drinks such as soft drinks and juice** to protect them from becoming overweight and the health problems that brings, including childhood and future diabetes. **Establish good habits now and they'll have them for life.**

Adolescence – To fuel their growth spurt at puberty, teenagers need more of most vitamins and minerals. It is also now that they lay down stores of minerals such as calcium and iron for later life.

➡ **Energy needs from 11–18 years increase** a boy's go up by nearly 2000kJ per day, while a girl's increase by just under 1200kJ.

➡ **Protein:** boys require 13g more between the ages of 11–18 years as they grow, and girls need around 4g more than younger children. **Girls also need more iron-rich foods as their menstrual cycle begins.**

➡ **Four servings of milk, cheese and yogurt a day** will ensure teenagers get sufficient calcium and phosphorus. They need **two to three portions of meat**, **fish** or alternatives to meet extra iron requirements, plus **plenty of fruit and vegetables** and nutrient-dense snacks, such as fortified cereals and bread.

➡ **As appetite increases at this age, resisting the temptations of fast food** is crucial – for good health, and to keep weight under control.

In your 20s – Surveys suggest that this age group eats less healthily than older adults.

➡ High intakes of high-fat, high-sugar and high-salt foods plus excessive alcohol consumption will lead to obesity, raised blood cholesterol and blood pressure levels as well as diabetes.

➡ Regular exercise several times a week is important now and **a nutritious diet that includes plenty of calcium** (dairy foods, bread, tofu, almonds and green leafy vegetables) as the body is still building bone; ensuring you get enough calcium in your twenties helps to combat osteoporosis in later life.

➡ **Women should eat plenty of iron-rich foods** such as meat, eggs, dried fruit, green leafy vegetables (for folate, too) and iron-fortified cereals; around 10 per cent of women in Australia and New Zealand have low iron levels.

In your 30s and 40s – With career and family responsibilities, activity levels often decrease, while stress and fatigue can prompt poor food choices.

➡ Men aged 35–49 are most likely to exceed the recommended daily alcohol limit. This can lead to higher blood pressure and weight gain.

➡ From the age of 35–40 bone mass and density start to decrease. **Eating foods rich in vitamin D** (eggs and oily fish), **calcium** (dairy foods and green leafy vegetables) **and protein foods** can combat the decline.

➡ After 40, type 2 diabetes is more common, too; risk factors include excess weight, especially around the abdomen. To avoid this and other health problems, **eat oily fish, nuts and legumes** for protein variety, and get plenty of high-fibre wholegrain foods. **Eating more potassium-rich fruit and vegetables** will help to combat high blood pressure.

In your 50s and early 60s – Both sexes are more susceptible to the cardiovascular damage that cholesterol-clogged arteries can cause. Good nutrition now is vital for a healthier old age.

▶ Most men develop high blood pressure between the ages of 35 and 55, raising their risk of heart attacks, stroke, and kidney and eye damage.

▶ Excess salt (more than 6g a day) is linked to high blood pressure and stroke risk. **Cut back on processed foods**, (they account for 75 per cent of total salt intake), **and foods high in saturated and trans fats**.

▶ For women, the risk of cardiovascular disease rises sharply after the menopause. Muscle mass also decreases and the loss of oestrogen encourages fat deposits – especially around the abdomen.

▶ The rate of bone loss accelerates, too, as oestrogen levels fall. A healthy diet plus more physical activity will help to counter the natural loss of muscle and bone mass and control weight, too.

▶ **Eat more 'good' fats, whole grains, nuts and fresh produce**, which also supply the antioxidants, B-group vitamins and polyunsaturated fatty acids identified in a 2012 Polish study as essential factors for maintaining brain health and minimising the risk of conditions such as dementia.

At 65 and beyond – In older age you are more vulnerable to infections and other ailments and conditions. Certain nutrients can help.

▶ **Eat plenty of fruit and vegetables** for their infection-fighting vitamin C content, to help counter high blood pressure, to control your weight and to combat diabetes and heart disease.

▶ **You will need more vitamin D** to strengthen bones against osteoporosis; oily fish and fortified cereals are good food sources. **People over 65 should also take a vitamin D supplement**.

▶ **Eating plenty of fibre, including fresh produce and whole grains**, helps combat constipation and digestive problems which often occur in older age.

▶ **Non-starchy vegetables, such as leafy greens**, 'probably' protect against some cancers of the mouth, throat, voice box, oesophagus and stomach, according to the World Cancer Research Fund and American Institute for Cancer Research. The phytonutrient lycopene in tomatoes may also protect against prostate cancer.

▶ **Older adults should drink 1–2 litres of liquid a day** as thirst decreases but the risk of dehydration, which can cause mental confusion and other physical problems, is higher.

Fertility & pregnancy

INFERTILITY AFFECTS AROUND 15 PER CENT OF YOUNG COUPLES IN AUSTRALIA AND NEW ZEALAND – men and women in equal numbers.

▶ Being over- or underweight is a factor in women. A low intake of fruit and vegetables can increase the risk of a low sperm count in men. Smoking and excess alcohol can affect fertility in both sexes; women should also avoid alcohol during pregnancy.

DURING PREGNANCY you need **foods rich in iron, folate, calcium and vitamin D**. You should eat a variety of starchy foods, fruit, vegetables, legumes, dairy products, lean meats, some oily fish and well-cooked eggs.

▶ In the first 12 weeks, **you should take a folate supplement** to safeguard the development of your baby's central nervous system and to prevent neural tube defects such as cleft palate, spina bifida and brain damage. **Throughout pregnancy a vitamin D supplement is also advised**.

▶ **Iron-rich foods**, such as lean meat, are recommended throughout and will fuel the increase in blood cells and blood volume in the later stages; you will also process more calcium to meet your baby's growing needs.

▶ **Getting enough iodine (good sources include seafood and seaweeds) is important** as a mild deficiency has been linked to lower IQ levels. By around 30 weeks, pregnant women need an extra 1500–1900kJ a day in the second and third trimesters but 'eating for two' is not advised; excessive weight gain (beyond the healthy range of an additional 10–13kg) can affect the health of mother and unborn child.

Did YOU know ?

Tastes can change

If – as hard as you try – you can't bring yourself to like a healthy food, don't give up. Dr Linda Bartoshuk of the University of Florida Center for Smell and Taste in the USA has three tips for tricking your taste buds. Bring out the sweetness, or add a little fat, she says, since both set off pleasure signals in the brain. Or try social cues. 'Eat with someone else who really enjoys it, or with someone who you admire and like. All of these things can make the food seem more appealing.' The tips, she adds, are useful for combating children's food fads, too.

RDI VALUES ON LABELS

are a generalisation. Unless otherwise specified on the packaging they are based on an average-sized woman doing an average amount of physical activity. Individual requirements for kilojoules and nutrients differ from person to person.

Get the read-the-label habit

As you start to make changes, you will need to know precisely what you're eating. With so many processed foods on the market, it may not be immediately obvious. Labels vary from country to country but there is a strong move in Europe and the USA towards 'at-a-glance' guidance, which is useful if you're short of time. This can take the form of traffic light colour coding, highlighting whether a food is high (red), medium (amber) or low (green) in fat, saturated fat, sugars and salt. You will also see 'Percent Daily Intake' values which indicate what percentage the nutrients in the food (sugar, fat etc.) represent of recommended daily requirements or maximum daily intake. Just remember, as it's not stated, that those figures cited for fat, sugar and salt are percentages of a daily limit, not of a recommended amount. For more on food labelling, *see* page 144.

Keeping track of what you eat

The very best way to monitor what you eat is to keep a food diary for a minimum of three consecutive days and preferably for up to a week. Always include at least one day at the weekend when eating habits tend to be slightly different. Doing this just once a year with the aim of making nutritious adjustments will boost your diet and long-term health immeasurably. Everyone should try it and it is especially helpful if:

- You want to lose weight. Keeping a record can help you meet your target intake and ensure that you are eating a complete and balanced diet.
- You're an emotional eater and want to identify what foods you eat and the moods that prompt you to eat them.
- You have an allergy or food intolerance and need to pinpoint whatever might be causing the adverse reactions you experience.
- You're an athlete and keen to monitor what you eat and drink in order to boost your diet and maximise your performance.

Your diary should list the whole spectrum of your eating habits over each 24-hour period at work and at home, meals in, meals out and any snacks in between. Record every piece of food and every drink you consume and when you have them. Be sure to write down everything, including 'treats'. Note how a food is cooked – grilled or fried, for instance – and the rough portion size of what you eat or drink. Jot foods down as soon as possible, rather than later, when you may easily – and conveniently – forget the details, amounts and those unforeseen and unnoticed extras such as a surprise slice of cake at an office birthday celebration or the 'corner' of a sandwich that your child left unfinished.

Always keep your food diary handy; you might go for a notebook which slips into a pocket or bag (you can always transfer jottings to a larger space later on), or use your smartphone or tablet computer and download a food-diary app. These diary days are enough to give a clear snapshot of your eating and drinking patterns and put you in a great position to see at a glance where simple and beneficial adjustments can be made to correct nutritional balance.

Highlight some of the things you can change straightaway.

Swap:

sugar (on breakfast cereal or porridge)	**FOR**	dried fruit or blueberries
biscuits (with morning coffee)	**FOR**	wholegrain toast topped with banana
potato chips	**FOR**	extra vegetables
cheesecake	**FOR**	rice pudding or low-fat yogurt with berries

Cut:
- Everyday wine with the evening meal; have at least two alcohol-free days a week
- Portion sizes (though not of vegetables and fruit)
- Chips – replace with brown rice or new/baked potatoes
- Processed meat – replace with fresh meat or fish

Add:
- Extra crunch to sandwiches with mixed leaves, tomatoes, grated carrot and cucumber
- Side salad to dishes like pasta or jacket potato
- Side orders of vegetables as extras with a meal
- Wholegrain products wherever possible

Remember your aim is a diet that is:
1 **Complete** – with foods from all the different food groups.
2 **Balanced** – each food group on your 'daily plate' should be in the right proportion, adjusting for individual needs.
3 **Varied** – you should regularly eat different foods from each group.

It is impossible to overstate the importance of eating well to promote life-long health and longevity. With the expert advice and information in these pages, we can all find ways of making improvements. You may be surprised at how easily attention to labels and ingredients becomes second nature, or how quickly you discover small tweaks that make a big difference to the taste and goodness of the foods you eat every day.

2 Shopping for quality

Whether you're entertaining, shopping for your evening meal or collecting a week's supplies, for your health's sake, you should get the best quality you can afford. Here's how.

If you're short of time and on a tight budget, shopping for healthy food and preparing it might feel like a luxury. But given how important good nutrition is to a long and healthy life – and, conversely, how much damage junk food can cause – it is worth buying and cooking with good-quality ingredients. What many of us forget – as we grab a ready meal – is that you can eat superbly without spending a fortune or half the day in the kitchen.

Many delicious, healthy foods (including eggs, whole grains and root vegetables) are low-priced, while other good but pricier foods can be used in small ways to supplement a dish and still make the overall meal surprisingly affordable. Rather than focusing solely on the pick-up price of food, decide if a food really represents value for money.

This need not be time-consuming. Once you get into the 'eat-well' habit, you'll know exactly what you're looking for much of the time. Then you'll be in the best position to resist marketing ploys – alluring snacks and baked goods or the buy-one-get-one-free or two-for-one 'bargains'.

How do you know a food is good?

'Quality' is one of the most abused words in the English language. Frankly, anyone who wants to sell you anything will use it as an assurance to get you to pay more – and what food producer is going to say their food isn't quality? So what are the hallmarks of genuinely good food?

➡ **It should be healthy**, nutritious and a pleasure to eat.
➡ **It should be safe and as fresh as possible** – with minimal chemicals added at the growing or processing stage.
➡ **If processed**, it should be made from wholesome natural ingredients.
➡ **If the food is fish or animal-based**, the wellbeing of the creatures is important, too. Mass-produced fish or livestock are often nutritionally inferior, more susceptible to disease and often frequently dosed with antibiotics in a bid to keep them healthy.

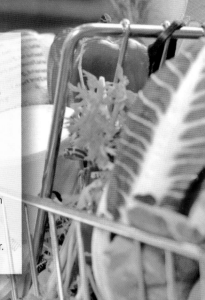

Five ways to resist the siren call of supermarkets

1 **Never shop when you're really hungry;** you're much more likely to succumb to tempting treats that you wouldn't otherwise have chosen.

2 **Shop with a friend** to make the most of buy-one-get-one-free or similar bargain foods, that you might otherwise waste or eat too much of.

3 **Look up and down shelves** when you're choosing what you want; supermarkets sometimes put better priced foods slightly out of reach.

4 **Don't buy prewashed, packaged salad** or pre-cut vegetables unless you're up against the clock. They are expensive, pre-cutting reduces the nutrients and they soon deteriorate when the packaging is opened.

5 **Take a bottle of water** and have a drink while you wait in the checkout line. It will distract you from any tempting confectionery; our brains often confuse thirst and hunger.

Our food system should be capable of producing genuinely high-quality food. But food production in the 21st century has become such a massive, global, industrialised business that freshness and nutritional quality are not something that can be taken for granted.

Where we live and time constraints mean that many of us have little choice where we shop. But, when you can, it's worth seeking out local foods, markets or farm produce. Instead of a supermarket swoop, locate a local farmers' market, to buy fresh eggs, fruit, fresh meat and other produce – and taste the difference.

Getting the best

Supermarkets

Most of us do the majority of our food shopping in these one-stop shops of convenience – drive in, whizz around, pay the big bill, then load up the car and go home. Supermarkets stock up to 80,000 different product lines, offering a range of qualities, but because these chains are tied into centralised buying, which requires large volumes of product, they rely on big companies as suppliers. So, with some notable exceptions, the majority of foods they stock are of the standard, mass-produced sort.

MULTIBUY offers may not be bargains. In a year-long survey the UK consumer body Which? examined 115 popular products from five major supermarkets and compared 300,000 prices. About one in ten products actually increased in price when they became multibuys, while others were almost permanently discounted.

Assessing quality – convenience foods

Whatever the price, your best guide to the quality of a processed food is the listed ingredients. If you don't want to cut convenience foods out of your diet, select those with:

- **Shorter ingredients lists** By law, the ingredients in a food product must be listed by descending order of weight, so anything that appears near the top of the list will form a bigger part of the product than those towards the bottom.
- **A good percentage of their main ingredient** If an ingredient forms part of the name of the food – 'meat pie', for instance – or is emphasised on the label in words or pictures, the label must also give a percentage for the amount of that ingredient, for example 'steak 32 per cent'. These percentages give you a clear idea of whether the food is value for money. A fish pie, for instance, may not seem such great quality when you see that it contains only 14 per cent fish, padded out with water, milk powder, potato and various starches.
- **Few – if any – unfamiliar additives** Although most are safe and some are essential, some you may want to avoid; see Part 2, chapter 4, pages 64–71, for further details.

When buying a 'meat pie', meat should be top of the ingredients list...

5 TOP TIPS

to make sure you enjoy good food, even on a tight budget:

1 Buy the best quality possible for the foods you eat most.

2 Save money on basics by buying generic, rather than branded products.

3 Seek out local fresh produce whenever possible.

4 Buy meat from the butcher and fish from a fishmonger.

5 Exclude all junk foods.

The buying power of supermarkets allows them to command low prices from their suppliers, but the pursuit of low prices does not always make for well-motivated suppliers. Smaller farmers and growers often complain that the unreasonably low prices demanded by supermarkets – often below the actual cost of production, especially for a product such as milk – is putting them out of business.

Thanks to their huge buying power, supermarkets can offer consumers price deals that smaller food retailers cannot afford to match. But when it comes to high-quality fresh food – fruit, vegetables, meat, fish, cheeses, eggs – they often charge more than independents, such as greengrocers, fishmongers and butchers.

Supermarkets are skilled in offering promotions and price deals that sound fantastic and pull customers in, but if you stop to examine them, they may not be the bargain they're cracked up to be (*see* Multibuy, page 139). So keep a cool head and only go for deals that really do stack up on foods that you actually want.

Markets

Some towns and cities still have **traditional markets**, outdoors, indoors or both. Fruit and vegetable stalls are often the main draw and can be very good value. Unlike supermarkets, where freshness is often maintained by refrigeration, greengrocer stallholders typically buy from a wholesale market, then aim to sell the fresh produce they buy to retail customers that same day. As stallholders have only modest overheads, and also work on volume turnover with lower associated costs, they can often sell good-quality fruit and veg for significantly less than supermarket prices. However, produce offered at bargain-basement prices is likely to be on its last legs, so it's important to watch what you're getting.

Meat in markets is more variable, often emphasising low prices and quantity, so they can save you money but sometimes at the expense of quality. Some markets also have a scattering of specialist food stalls selling cheese, for example, or bread, olives, herbs and spices, or tea and coffee. These can be attractive both in terms of quality and price, but sample them or buy small quantities first to make sure you are happy with what's on offer.

➡ Farmers' markets bring you face to face with the people who grow, rear or make the food they sell.

A newer type of market is the **farmers' markets**. These offer a pleasant alternative shopping expedition and are good places to connect with small producers of high-quality food, especially if you want free-range and organic meat, and seasonal fruits and vegetables. They aim to bring you face to face with the people who grow, rear or make the food they sell.

Prices are variable – sometimes lower than the supermarket equivalent, especially for organic eggs or fresh fruit and veg, and sometimes higher, so it's important to compare like with like. Sausages may be more expensive, for instance, because the meat comes from a traditional breed of pig that is less 'productive' in terms of the amount of meat it yields, but could be far tastier – and not have the additives associated with mass-market sausages.

Independent shops

If you are lucky enough to have a main street with a traditional butcher, greengrocer, baker or fishmonger, you may find that these specialists are in a position to offer you

Eat with the seasons

We've become so used to fresh produce being available all-year round in supermarkets that we tend to forget that most fruit and vegetables are seasonal. You should buy seasonally when you can because:

- **Produce tends to be fresher**, not least because it often comes from closer to home. An expedition to a fruit farm to pick berries, or events like town harvest festivals, can make a memorable and fun family outing.
- **Fruits and vegetables are cheapest and tastiest** at the peak of their growing season. Some, such as berries, show a definite seasonal curve – not quite sweet enough to start with, rising to a taste peak, then falling off into sourness again. The art is to eat as many as possible when plentiful and at their seasonal best.
- **Seasonal fresh produce is likely to be more nutritious**. When researchers at Montclair State University in New Jersey, USA, compared the vitamin C content of locally grown broccoli in season with broccoli imported out of season, they found that the latter had only half the vitamin C. Another study, published in the *Journal of Agricultural Food Chemistry*, found that the levels of health-promoting anthocyanin pigments increased more than fourfold as blackberries went from underripe to overripe.
- **Meat and fish also have seasons**, which can affect availability and taste. Spring lamb will have a milder flavour and paler colour than the richer-tasting meat from more mature lambs slaughtered in the autumn. Some fish, such as mullet, loses its 'muddy' taste in summer when it moves from estuarine waters to the sea.

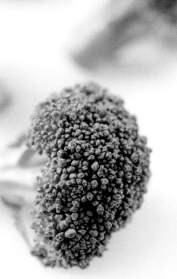

exceptional quality and value. In rural towns, traditional butchers usually source their meat as close as possible to the area, and if you want a specific cut of meat, they will have the expertise to provide it – and the knowledge to offer advice. Fishmongers have disappeared from main streets in some places, but in many places the gap has been filled by mobile fishmongers who work out of refrigerated vans. They turn up at a certain time each week and are well worth seeking out, often offering quality fish at less-than-supermarket prices. Some urban and rural areas are sprouting small bakeries that produce bread using traditional methods.

Fruit and vegetables can be cheaper from a greengrocer than a supermarket, and may be more local as greengrocers buy from the nearest wholesale market.

Many people have discovered that the most convenient way of all to buy food is with **home delivery**. With the growth of internet shopping, supermarkets now supply a growing proportion of their customers through home delivery schemes, but many independent traders, such as greengrocers and butchers, also deliver to the door. A lot of interesting, useful, high-quality food can be bought from small food companies or farmers, either on the internet or by phone. It can be a good idea to get

➥ Broccoli imported out of season was found to have only half the vitamin C of home-grown seasonal broccoli.

together with a couple of friends to make it more affordable. Organic box schemes, where customers receive a weekly delivery of fresh organic fruit and vegetables, are now a well-established way to buy organic food at reasonable prices.

Food co-operatives are another option that is growing in popularity, as they keep prices low by taking advantage of the cost savings of buying in bulk. These local organisations may charge members a fee to join and are usually run on a not-for-profit basis.

Why organic may be best

The jury is still out on whether organic foods have measurably more nutrients in terms of vitamins than foods produced by conventional farming (*see* Food News, top right), but there is general agreement that organic produce reduces exposure to pesticides, chemicals and antibiotic-resistant bacteria.

In organic farming, antibiotics can be used only to treat cases of illness; they cannot be used routinely to prevent infection as commonly happens with factory-farmed animals. Only five pesticides are approved for use on organic crops, and these may only be used in very limited circumstances. By contrast, conventional farmers have more than 300 pesticides at their disposal and use them routinely. Organic foods rarely contain pesticide residues, whereas around a third of all conventionally produced food, and almost 40 per cent of fruit and vegetables, is contaminated with small traces.

Few additives, too

Organic symbols on processed foods flag up that the food is less likely to have chemical additives you might wish to avoid. Organic food processors can use only 32 additives and these must come from natural sources, such as vitamin C from lemon juice. So organic versions of processed foods will not contain undesirable additives, such as artificial flavours and colours.

In contrast, 329 chemical additives are permitted in non-organic food. Some of these are the subject of furious debate on health grounds (*see* Part 2, chapter 4, pages 64–71). No one really knows what the long-term effect of these chemicals on our bodies will be.

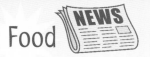
Food NEWS

The 'Stanford study'

In autumn 2012, a team at Stanford School of Medicine in the USA made headlines by reporting that their scientific review had found 'no strong evidence that organic foods are significantly more nutritious than conventional foods'. Critics condemned the research as 'junk science', pointing out that the team used a narrow definition of 'more nutritious' as only 'containing more vitamins and minerals'. The study also ignored the fact that many people eat organic foods to reduce their exposure to pesticides and antibiotic-resistant bacteria – a nutritional benefit not refuted by the Stanford study. A UK review of research in 2011 had concluded there was clear evidence of higher levels of certain nutrients in organic foods.

FOOD ALLERGIES

may be increasing as a result of high levels of common dichlorophenol-containing pesticides, according to Dr Elina Jerschow from the Albert Einstein College of Medicine in the USA. Her 2012 study revealed a clear association between the two.

The language of labels

Wherever you're buying it, to be sure that a food is really good, you have to look behind fancy packaging and clever wording to identify the essential facts. Learn to spot the words that may give a product a halo of quality but guarantee no such thing – and make a point of ignoring them.

Many familiar terms seen on food packaging may have no legal definition whatsoever. Watch out for: 'artisan', 'traditional', 'pure', 'handmade', 'fresh' and 'farmhouse'. Some products do live up to the promise, but you can't take that for granted. Similarly, a front label may feature mouth-watering pictures of food, or idyllic images of green fields and happy animals. Be sure to read the small-print ingredients label on the back which contains the harder facts.

Many food manufacturers are well-practised in placing phrases on their packaging to suggest that the product has a healthy nutritional profile, which may not be the case. A product with a 'low fat' label might sound healthy, but that product could be loaded with sugar.

'No added sugar' sounds promising, but a food or drink with this on the label may contain an artificial sweetener that might be controversial for various health reasons (*see* pages 70–71). The phrase 'as part of a balanced

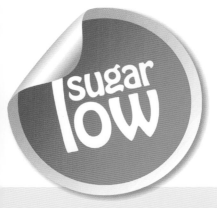

What does 'high' or 'low' actually mean?

In Australia and New Zealand, government health guidelines provide the following definitions:

Total fat	**High:** more than 20g of fat per 100g	**Low:** 3g of fat or less per 100g (or 1.5g or less per 100ml liquid
Saturated fat & trans fat	**High:** more than 5g of saturated fat per 100g	**Low:** 1.5g of saturated fat or less per 100g (or 0.75g or less per 100mL liquid)
Sugars	**High:** more than 15g of total sugars per 100g	**Low:** 5g of total sugars or less per 100g (or 2.5g or less per 100mL liquid)
Salt	**High:** more than 1.5g of salt per 100g (or 0.6g sodium)	**Low:** 120mg sodium or less per 100g

Source: NHS Choices website

diet' might suggest that you can eat a product freely but strictly means that you must take its ingredients and kilojoules into account. 'Supplies your energy needs' is just a clever way of saying that a food contains kilojoules: it certainly doesn't mean that it's a particularly healthy food.

Finally, remember that a higher price doesn't always equal better taste or quality. If you have any doubts, buy a few different brands, strip off the packaging and do some blind tasting to test your choices objectively.

Promoting good nutrition?

Across the world there are many different labelling regulations, some legal, some voluntary. The World Health Organization recommended a compulsory front-of-pack food-labelling system to help consumers make healthy choices more easily. This was strongly opposed by food manufacturers and retail groups and the result was a variety of voluntary systems in different countries. In Australia and New Zealand, the ingredients list and nutrition information panel are tightly regulated by Food Standards Australia New Zealand (FSANZ). There is also a set of FSANZ rules about the information on the front of the pack, for example, claims that a food is low in fat, or good for your heart. But other aspects of food product labelling are not regulated, and can be very confusing.

- **Serving size:** the nutrition information panel gives quantities of nutrients per serving as well as per 100g. Sometimes the 'serving' is an amount that the manufacturer has chosen, such as half a tub of yogurt, or eight corn chips, which may not be the usual amount that people would consume. This can create a misleading impression of the nutritional value of the food.

- **Percent daily intake values:** the nutrition information panel may show per cent daily intake values per serving, for a variety of nutrients. Sometimes these are displayed on the front of the pack as well. Again, as these are expressed per serving, they can be misleading. If your serving size is different from the manufacturer's amount, all the percentage values would be different for you. Also, it is not clear to the consumer what the daily intake amounts are.

In the case of energy, the daily intake value is 8700kJ, which is considered to be the 'average' adult energy intake. If your energy intake is different from this, then the energy percentage value would be different for you. The other nutrients are mostly expressed as a percentage of the recommended maximum limit, not your required amount for good health. For instance, the daily intake value for salt is 6g, much more than the ideal amount to consume. A food labelled '10% RDI' for sodium might not sound very salty, but this amount in a small serving size could vastly exceed sodium recommendations.

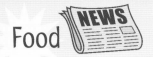

Food NEWS

The case for honesty and tighter controls

In 2013, a variety of food scandals highlighted the need for stricter industry controls. Pork was found in beef and halal meat products. Most explosively, processed beef products in the UK and Europe were found to contain up to 100 per cent horse meat. The discoveries, which involved major supermarket chains and food manufacturing companies, caused a furore, with European ministers calling for labels that clearly define the source of all meat in processed foods. The scandal has rocked consumer confidence. As France's agriculture minister, Stéphane Le Foll, commented, we should know what we're eating. 'There has to be a correspondence between the container and what's in it. It's about respecting something quite simple: what is written on the label has to conform to what is in the product.'

'QUALITY ASSURED'

is a label that foods such as Scotch beef, Welsh lamb or British pork may carry. Such labelling schemes are designed to inspire consumer loyalty and help farmers to market their products, which must conform to a list of requirements that help promote food safety and traceability. Such labels are probably but not necessarily a guarantee of superior quality.

The importance of freshness

One of the most important defining characteristics of high-quality food is its freshness. Some foods, such as biscuits, chocolate, cereals and dried pasta or legumes, can be kept for months if stored correctly, usually at room temperature. For more perishable foods – meat, fish, dairy products, eggs, fruit and vegetables – freshness can be critical. But how fresh is 'fresh'? Two labels set out to make it clearer:

● **Use By** – this date label appears on foods that are sold chilled or frozen because they are highly perishable and could give you food poisoning if you ate them after the stated date. Foods that come into this category include chicken, soft cheese and cooked cold meats. The date assumes that you will store the product according to the instructions on the packaging. Once you open a food with a 'use by' date, you need to follow any instructions on the packaging such as 'eat within one day of opening'.

● **Best Before** – this date label appears on less perishable foods, for example, lentils, pasta, rice and canned tomatoes. When the date is passed, it doesn't mean that the food will poison you if you eat it, but it is an indication that it could be past its prime. For instance, biscuits might become a bit soft or stale. Dried fruit might lose its fruity freshness and become hard and sugary. Old legumes might take far longer to soften.

Two other date marks, 'Display Until' and 'Sell By', often appear on food packaging. These are not aimed at customers – they are instructions for the guidance of shop staff to assist stock rotation.

You shouldn't use any food or drink after the 'use by' date, even if it looks and smells fine, but there are exceptions. You can freeze a food up until the date and thereby extend its life quite safely. If you do this, it's important to follow any instructions on the pack, such as 'cook from frozen' or 'defrost thoroughly before use and use within 24 hours'. Certain foods need not automatically go into the rubbish bin after the 'use by' date, provided that they are well cooked or baked.

While both 'use by' and 'best before' dates are helpful, bear in mind that there are different types of freshness:

● **Naturally fresh** describes foods, such as fruits and vegetables, that have been recently harvested. There is a relatively short window of opportunity to enjoy them. Usually you will buy/harvest them close to their source and quickly eat them while at their best – a matter of hours, rather than days.

● **Stored fresh** describes perishable fresh foods that have had their natural shelf-life and availability extended by the use of technology. For instance, fresh apples and pears may be picked in autumn and stored at cool temperatures in air modified by removing the oxygen, then they're sold as fresh produce until the new season's crop arrives. A 'stored fresh'

BISIN, a byproduct of harmless bacteria, has been hailed as a potential future super-preservative for meat, dairy and eggs, in theory allowing them to stay fresh for years. As yet no bisin-preserved products are on the market.

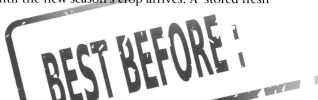

apple may be softer, less crunchy and more 'mealy' than the naturally fresh equivalent. Grapes can also have their life extended after picking; being stored and treated with chemical fumigants, such as sulphur dioxide, which can leave a detectable dank smell on them.

● **Chilled fresh** describes fresh foods sold in chiller cabinets. The aura of freshness helps them to sell for more than frozen, canned or dried equivalents. But it's worth remembering that many chilled products have a surprisingly long shelf life. Milk will often have a 'use by' date for ten days in the future. To extend shelf life, many chilled processed foods may contain chemical preservatives that would not be in naturally fresh food.

➤➤ Fruit may be picked in autumn, stored, then sold as fresh produce until the new season's crop arrives.

● **Frozen fresh** may have a more down-market image, but when you compare like with like, frozen food tends to have fewer additives than the chilled equivalent. In nutritional terms, there's a strong argument that food frozen when truly fresh – such as freshly picked peas, for example – will be nutritionally superior to a chilled or even fresh equivalent, which may hang about on the shelf for days or even weeks.

● **Processed fresh** describes chilled processed convenience foods, such as fruit yogurts, ready meals, sandwiches and desserts. These sell as fresh, but some of the ingredients may not exactly fit that bill. Many chicken-based ready meals, for example, contain chicken that the food manufacturer bought frozen and sometimes pre-cooked. Eggs in convenience foods are rarely freshly shelled; instead, manufacturers use liquid pasteurised egg, or egg powder reconstituted with water.

3 Home-made is best

Cooking doesn't have to be complex – you don't need a chef's skills or repertoire. It's simply about combining good basic ingredients to provide tasty, balanced meals that will always be healthier than highly processed foods.

COOKING can enhance the antioxidant content of some vegetables. Tomatoes, spinach and older carrots are among those that supply more antioxidants when freshly cooked than when they are eaten raw.

The pressures of modern life can make us feel that cooking is simply too time-consuming. As a result, many of us eat out more, and ready-prepared convenience foods become a larger part of our diet. However much you enjoy a restaurant meal, or like the quick option of a ready meal or takeaway, eating mostly home-made food, cooked freshly from unprocessed raw ingredients, is by far the better option – for your own and your family's health throughout life.

Simple home cooking will almost certainly taste better and save you money. It may take a bit of initial organisation but eating this way can be almost as quick as heating up a ready meal and often far more enjoyable. It just means centring your diet on vitamin-rich fresh produce, protein foods such as lean meat, low-fat dairy, fish and eggs, combined with wholegrain cereals and legumes to supply all the nutrients your body requires.

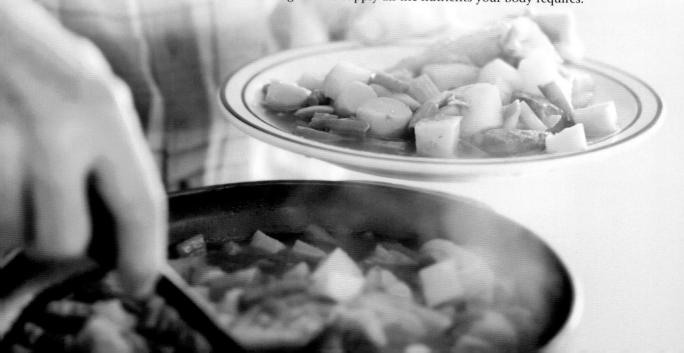

➡ A fresh egg looks quite different from an old egg, which will be runny, with the yolk breaking into the white ...

Fresher and healthier food

Cooking at home from scratch using mainly unprocessed ingredients reduces the time it takes for your food to travel 'from field to fork', so it will almost certainly be fresher than the ready-made equivalent. Most ready-made, shop-bought food is produced in a factory, and each ingredient may be subject to a production process that involves treatments, such as pasteurising, freezing, blast chilling, sterilising, and then packaging, storage and distribution. All these stages in the creation of a convenience food mean that it is no match for food home-cooked from fresh ingredients.

By handling foods in their whole, original form, you can ensure that each ingredient you use is good quality. For instance, if you cook a fresh fish fillet, or a whole fish, its freshness will be more obvious from its appearance and smell. If you buy pre-battered or breadcrumbed fish, it is far more difficult to judge. When you crack an egg for yourself, you can check that it is really fresh: the yolk will stand up to attention, supported by a thick, cloudy jelly-like white. It looks quite different from an old egg, which will be runny, with a tendency for the yolk to break into the white. An old egg will also float when placed in water, while a fresh egg will sink.

Know what you're eating

Preparing most of your own meals puts you in charge of their content, giving you every incentive to eat better. If you rely on takeaways and convenience food, it's much easier to eat badly.

This is why people who eat a lot of ready meals, takeaway and restaurant food often find it hard to control their weight. Although a few convenience food brands aimed at healthy eaters do make a point of emphasising that they are full of fruits and vegetables, the vast majority of convenience foods are top-heavy with fat, salt and carbohydrates. A cottage pie ready

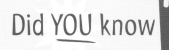

Did YOU know

Cooking gave us big brains

New research suggests that we owe our large brain size to the fact that our early ancestors learned to cook. By cooking raw food, humans were able to take in and digest far more kilojoules in a short space of time, and the spare energy they gained fuelled the development of their brains. It also saved them huge amounts of time that could be spent in other ways. The research, from the Institute of Biomedical Sciences in Rio De Janeiro, Brazil, supports an earlier theory put forward by British primatologist Richard Wrangham, who believes that the invention of cooking was crucial to our evolution. You could say it was cooking that made us human.

Did YOU know ?

Safe and sound?

Many food additives and processed ingredients have been in the food chain for a relatively short time, so they do not have a long track record of being safe and beneficial for human consumption. Regulators require proof of safety (such as independent test results and toxicological reports) before products can be used in food production. Most are supplied by the manufacturer, but other evidence may also be considered. Controversial items or ingredients include certain artificial food colours that may be linked to ADHD, hydrogenated fats and high-fructose corn syrup, described on labels as isoglucose or glucose-fructose syrup. (*See also* page 64.)

meal, for instance, may contain at least a third of your salt and a fifth of your fat for the day. Takeaways are often laden with fat – fish and chips, for example, or fried chicken – with few or no vegetables.

Even up-market restaurant meals tend to be fatty and protein-centric, featuring steak or fish dishes with carbohydrate content (potatoes, rice or pasta) that is minimal or refined, or both, and often cooked in additional fat. Whole grains, and fresh fruits and vegetables almost always play second fiddle.

If you only eat food that's not home-cooked once in a while this is not so important, but if such food forms the backbone of your diet, there can be negative consequences for your health.

SNEAKY SALT

lurking in ready-prepared or processed foods, takeaway and restaurant meals accounts for around 75 per cent of the salt in the average Western diet, say health experts. If that's what you usually eat, your taste buds will be used to the salty taste but your health could suffer. Eating too much salt is strongly linked to high blood pressure. When you do the cooking, you control how much salt you add and it's much easier to cut back, and add herbs and spices to enrich the flavour instead.

Avoid the additives

The scale and nature of factory methods for manufacturing convenience foods are qualitatively different from home cooking. Processing can remove a lot of the character of individual ingredients and can affect their flavour, leaving them tasting rather bland and in need of pepping up. This is something you can easily test yourself – compare a home-made wholemeal muffin with seeds and oats to a classic shop-bought English white muffin; the difference will be clear.

Processed foods routinely contain commercial additives that no home cook would use. Check a few product labels; you'll find artificial flavourings, colourings, sweeteners, preservatives and a legion of emulsifiers, stabilisers, thickeners, gelling agents, acidity regulators, anti-caking agents, anti-foaming agents, bulking agents, carriers and carrier solvents, emulsifying salts, firming agents, flavour enhancers, flour treatment agents, foaming agents, glazing agents, humectants and modified starches. (*See also* page 64.)

All this is because these foods are produced on an industrial scale to supply the supermarket chains and other food outlets and have to be transported and stored for some time before they are consumed. Food additives help to keep processed foods safe to eat and looking good for longer than fresher ingredients. You will very rarely find commercial additives in home-made food.

Three good reasons to cook

Convenience meals are almost always inferior to home cooking. Here's why:

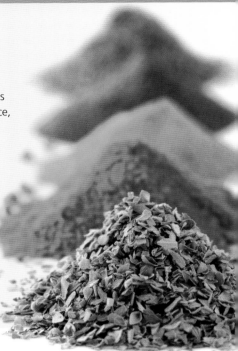

● **Lower-quality ingredients** Large retailers of own-label convenience foods and the manufacturers who supply them are keen to get the cheapest production price, which can drive down the quality of ingredients. There's also less incentive to use the best because they're destined to be turned into composite products with multiple ingredients, so the difference won't shine through.

● **Synthetic unnatural flavours** Many processed foods use ingredients developed especially for processing, such as a commercially made lemon extract instead of fresh lemon juice, either because they are cheaper or because they work better when large-scale production equipment is used.

● **Similar tastes and texture**s Different ready meals often share similar flavours and textures because a relatively small number of large-scale food manufacturers supply the major retailers. Much the same additives and ingredients are used, often ones designed for mass production, to save both money and time.

Cooking to save money and time

If you are not in the habit of cooking regularly, getting geared up to do so can seem daunting. Assembling the ingredients you need for a recipe might, at first, seem off-puttingly expensive, especially in a single or two-person household. If your kitchen is not stocked with the basics, it might cost, for instance, around $50 – much more than the price of a ready meal or takeaway – just to buy what you need to cook a meal for two.

Don't be put off. As you build up your pantry (*see* page 153), you'll soon find that you're spending much less, and getting significantly better value, than you would if buying convenience food. There is no need to buy everything at once. To minimise cost and effort, do it in stages, perhaps buying a new spice as you try out a new recipe. With your new collection of standby food essentials, and a few tried-and-tested recipes under your belt, you will always be able to put together healthy, affordable, cooked meals.

Beyond the basics

Supplement your pantry stocks with fresher, more perishable foods (fruit and vegetables, meat, fish) either weekly or as you need them. Buy a pot of fresh coriander to enliven a simple soup made from your store of legumes,

GROW YOUR OWN HERBS

at home to add fresh flavour to your cooking. It's easy and cheap to do so. On an indoor windowsill you can have parsley, basil and coriander. If you have a little outside space you could grow mint along with rosemary, thyme, tarragon and bay. The simplest way is to buy herbs in small pots from a nursery, or common herbs in pots from supermarkets. Then invest in a bag of compost, transfer them to bigger pots and watch them grow.

tomatoes, onions and garlic – and launch your home herb farm (*see* left). Supplementing pantry staples such as rice and chicken stock with just two additional items – some fresh parmesan and an onion, for example – you can make a tasty and nutritious risotto.

As you explore new recipes and buy new ingredients, your initial store will soon grow to reflect your personal tastes and eating habits. Having basics to hand plus more interesting items such as specialty oils, exotic seasonings and spices will expand your capacity to provide instant and interesting healthy meals.

Home cooking also saves money by enabling you to take full advantage of foods in season. Newly ripe fruit and vegetables, especially if locally produced, can be far cheaper than out-of-season imports. In a market, or at the greengrocer's, the seasons are visible in the food on display, with new arrivals flagged up at different times of year. What's on offer will remind you, for instance, that, spring is the time to buy fresh asparagus, or that late autumn is when the mandarin season comes into full swing.

Processed food is much the same all year round. If you always head for the processed food shelves, the ebb and flow of seasonal harvests, and the ripe nutrients that they bring, will pass you by.

Easy dishes to make quickly from scratch

Using some of your pantry basics plus a few fresh ones, you can make many quick, healthy meals. Look at the Healthy-Eating Plate on page 120 to check that you get the right balance of nutrients. Here are some ideas:

- Eggs: boiled, poached, scrambled or as an omelette. For a Spanish-type omelette on a potato base, add cooked potato cubes, mushrooms, chopped herbs and cheese.
- Chopped tomatoes with capers, anchovies and fresh herbs, served with some canned tuna or cooked chicken on warm pasta or bruschetta.

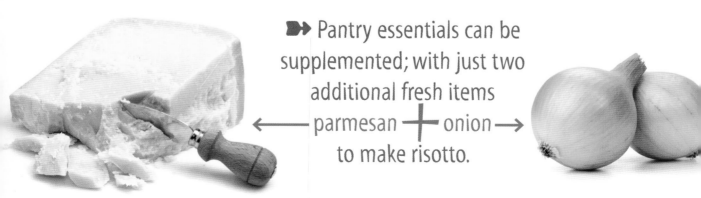

➧ Pantry essentials can be supplemented; with just two additional fresh items ⟵ parmesan ✛ onion ⟶ to make risotto.

Pantry standbys

Keeping a good stock of standby foods is invaluable on days when you've been unable to get to the shops as planned, need something to stretch yesterday's leftovers or when unexpected guests drop in. With these handy ingredients, plus any home-grown herbs, you'll always have the makings of a healthy, speedy and inexpensive meal.

Here are some suggestions and where to store them; the choice of course, is up to you.

In the fridge

Parmesan, reduced-fat **tasty cheese**
Low-fat natural yogurt and low-fat **crème fraîche**
(check 'use-by' dates)
A selection of **mustards**
Chilli paste
Thai curry paste

In the freezer

Frozen vegetables – peas and leaf spinach; also green beans, corn, broad beans, edamame beans
Salmon, **chicken**, **lean mince**, small packs of **prawns** – individual portions are best as they can be quickly defrosted
Home-made stock
Chillies and **herbs** (coriander, basil, mint)
Frozen yogurt and **sorbets**
Ready-to-roll **pastry**
Wholegrain **sliced bread**, **flatbreads** and **rolls**
Frozen berries – often great value compared to fresh and you can just use the amount you need

● **Build up your store** bit by bit with nutritious items that will keep – dried and canned foods kept at room temperature, frozen foods and longer shelf-life items in the fridge or freezer.

In the cupboard

Canned **tuna, sardines, mackerel, salmon**
Canned **tomatoes** and **tomato puree,** salt-free concentrated **tomato paste**
Assortment of **legumes, canned corn**
Artichokes, anchovies, **sun-dried tomatoes** (in oil)
Capers, gherkins
White wine, **red wine** and **balsamic vinegars**
Tabasco, Worcestershire sauce
Olive oil, **extra virgin olive oil**, **canola oil**
Sesame oil, **soy sauce**, **Chinese rice wine** and **Chinese vinegar**
Dried herbs and **spices**, **black pepper**
Flour (wholemeal, plain and self-raising), **cornflour**
Assorted dried **pasta** (spaghetti, lasagne sheets, penne etc.), **couscous**
Egg and **rice noodles**
Brown and white **rice**, **oats**
Lentils, **split peas** and **dried beans**
Nuts and **seeds** (such as walnuts, almonds, brazils, poppy seeds, pine nuts, sesame seeds)
Tahini paste
Wholegrain **crackers**
Honey
Reduced-fat **coconut milk**
Onions, **garlic**, **potatoes**
Canned fruit in their own juice
Dried fruit (such as sultanas, raisins)

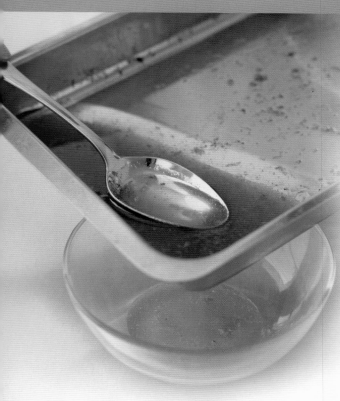

Top tips to get the best out of good food

You want your cooking to be as and healthy as possible. Here's how to retain flavour and nutrients:

1 To reduce the loss of water-soluble vitamins, microwave or steam vegetables, rather than boiling them; bake or roast vegetables such as carrots, parsnips, onions, capsicums or pumpkin or quickly stir-fry chopped vegetables using a splash of liquid and minimal oil.

2 Bake fish in a foil parcel, microwave or steam to ensure it retains its moistness, natural flavour and nutrients.

3 Roast or grill meat and poultry and where possible use the nutritious cooking juices in a gravy or sauce. An inexpensive gravy separator jug, with a spout rising from the bottom, can be a great help to skim the fat off the juice from a roast.

4 To minimise the fat in roasted meat, especially for fattier cuts such as lamb or pork shoulder, cook the meat on a rack above the roasting pan to allow the fat to drain out.

➡ Skim off the fat and retain the juices for a gravy.

- Baked or microwaved potatoes in their jackets with protein fillings such as baked beans, tuna, ricotta or cooked mince, served with a salad or other vegetables.
- Smoked fish, such as trout, baked, grilled or poached, and served with a poached egg, spinach and potatoes or crusty wholegrain bread.
- Grilled meat or fish, served with two or three quickly cooked vegetables, pepper and any herbs you have to hand.
- Stir-fried vegetables (you can buy them frozen) with noodles, prawns, chicken or meat plus herbs and spices. There are dozens of variations.

Start-then-leave-alone dishes

Slow-cooked, one-pot casserole and stew dishes are simplicity itself. They can take several hours to cook, but are quick to prepare so don't take much time. To make a simple stew, you need only to brown the meat (already trimmed and cut up by the butcher) with chopped onion, add herbs and aromatics, water, wine or other liquid such as chopped canned tomatoes, then cover and put it in the oven to cook. Give it a stir from time to time and add other vegetables, such as carrots or mushrooms, as cooking progresses so they don't overcook, then finally add pepper and herbs to taste towards the end of cooking. To make life really simple, put some potatoes into the casserole or to bake in the oven alongside.

Slow-cooked dishes of this type allow you to use more economical lean cuts of meat, such as stewing steak, shin of beef, neck of lamb, or lean diced pork, which many find have more flavour than expensive prime cuts. Vegetarian one-pot meals, such as baked beans, or a spicy chickpea and vegetable stew, are equally low-effort, producing cheap and delicious food that is particularly welcome on a cold winter's day.

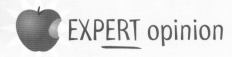

EXPERT opinion

'Intuitive' healthy eating

'Beyond the science … I can say quite categorically that my experience with literally thousands of individuals tells me that a diet based on natural, unprocessed foods including meat, fish, eggs, nuts, seeds, fruits and vegetables very often leads to significant benefits for health that can be transformational.

'To my mind, healthy eating is intuitive – it means consuming foods that sustained us during lengthy periods of our evolution. These are the foods that have genuine capacity to nourish and sustain us, not the processed, often-chemicalised foods that the food industry tries to pass off as healthy.'

Dr John Briffa BSc (Hons) MB BS (Lond), doctor, *author and leading authority on diet and health*

Time-effective cooking

Putting home-cooked meals at the heart of your diet doesn't mean you must cook from scratch every day. With a bit of forethought and organisation, one stint of cooking can feed you and your family up to three times. A big Sunday roast is an obvious candidate; leftovers are easily revamped into different meals (*see* page 156).

Periodically, set aside a morning or afternoon, or a couple of hours twice a week, when you generate food that will serve more than one meal, then chill or freeze the rest. If you're making cottage pie, for example, cook double the ingredients and freeze half – either with its mashed potato topping, or add that next time.

Concentrated bursts of cooking can save a huge amount of time and effort later. If you can organise yourself in this way, and remember to take things out of the freezer when required, with

➡ Sunday roast leftovers can be easily revamped into different meals …

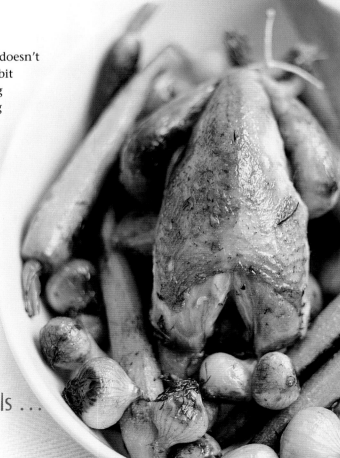

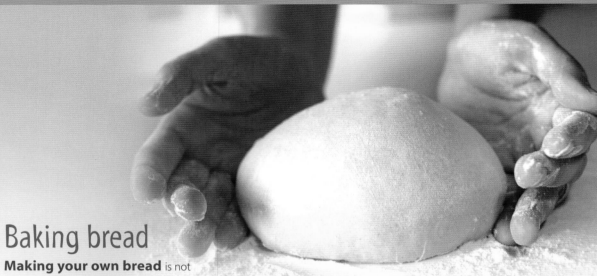

Baking bread

Making your own bread is not
only a healthy option – it saves money. For plain leavened bread, you need just you need just three ingredients –
flour, water and yeast. Salt is also typically added to help the bread rise uniformly (with no big air pockets) but the
quantities in commercial breads and ready-made bread mixes are unnecessarily high. From one 1.5kg bag of bread
flour, for roughly the price of a small shop loaf, you can make about six. Baking bread is not as time-consuming
as you might think. It involves short bursts of effort and while the dough rises you are free to do something
else. Make a batch once a week or so, keep one loaf out fresh and freeze the rest till you need it. Or if you have
a bread machine hidden in a cupboard, dig it out and get into the habit of making a loaf as you need it. Once
you've mastered the basics, you can experiment with different flours and added ingredients. But if making your
own bread is not for you, then perhaps you might want to seek out a local bakery making high-quality bread.

minimal reheating you will always have something nice and home-made to
eat. Leftovers can always be served up again in the same form as first time,
or tweaked to make a different meal.

Here are a few ideas for using one basic dish to produce further meals –
with practice, you'll discover many more.

● **Beyond the Sunday roast** A traditional roast dinner can generate
many further possibilities. At its simplest, leftover roast meat can be used
for weekday lunches in sandwiches or salads, reducing the amount of salty,
processed meat you eat. Or a small amount of chicken can go a long way
in a risotto. Once the carcass has been picked clean, that can be simmered
with vegetables and aromatics to make stock for soup or to use as a base
in another casserole. If you have leftover lamb you can make a tasty curry,
or use leftover beef, plus a can of tomatoes and red kidney beans to make
a quick chilli con carne. Or try meat patties: blitz the meat in a food
processor, dip in egg and breadcrumbs, then brush with a little olive oil
and fry on a griddle.

Did YOU know ?

Acrylamide

Be careful when grilling, frying, roasting or barbecuing foods. The chemical acrylamide can be produced if meat, cereals and vegetables are overly browned or blackened. Because acrylamide has the potential to cause cancer, Food Standards Australia New Zealand recommends trying to eat less acrylamide.

- **Reinventing leftovers** Leftover risotto, for example, dressed with a little lemon juice or balsamic vinegar, extra salad vegetables or cooked meat for more protein, makes a tasty packed lunch.
- **Soups and stews** Similarly, any chunky vegetable soup can be eaten over one or two days, or on the second day you could turn it into a stew. Add a grain, such as pearl barley or spelt, some fresh green leaves (spinach or finely shredded cabbage) and/or fresh herbs, then drizzle it with olive oil and serve it with grated parmesan cheese as a vegetable stew. Include cooked meat to make it more substantial or soybeans as a vegetarian option.
- **Same main item, different presentation** Make a big stew and serve it up with mashed potatoes and cabbage, then freeze the leftover stew to be brought out later and topped with pastry to make a pie. Meanwhile, any leftover potato and cabbage can be added to a soup or mashed together and used as a topping for a fish or meat pie.
- **Make different dishes from the same ingredients** Using minced meat plus a few of your pantry basics, you could try the following:

1 Mix together minced meat, chopped onions, parsley, eggs, any fresh herbs you fancy, plus spices and pepper. Take one half of the mixture and form it into patties or burgers that you grill or fry, and serve with hot vegetables or salad in a wholemeal bun, with pickles on the side. With the rest of the mixture make meatballs and cook them gently in a bubbling tomato sauce made with lightly sautéed onion and garlic, olive oil and canned tomatoes or passata. Chill or freeze the meatballs in tomato sauce and serve them with pasta on another day.

➡ Make a Bolognese-style sauce …

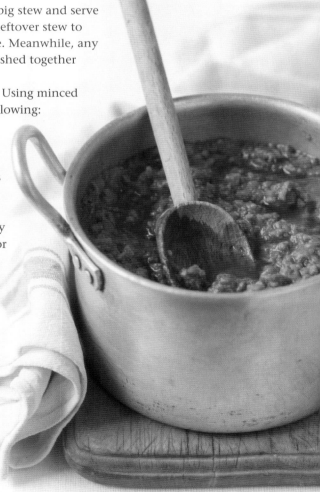

2 Or use the mince to make a Bolognese-style sauce. Serve half with spaghetti for dinner and put the other half into a lasagne to serve with a fresh green salad another day. Or flavour half the sauce with a touch of cinnamon, then roast eggplant halves (30 minutes in a hot oven). Fill them with the mince mixture and bake (covered) for 10 minutes until the eggplant is very soft and the filling is bubbling hot.

4 Breakfast review

Every morning we break our nightly fast. We need plenty of liquid to rehydrate our bodies plus nutrients that supply lasting energy. Here's the low-down on how best to start your day.

When you get up in the morning, it may be ten or 12 hours since you last ate or drank. Your blood glucose will be at a fasting level. Without sustenance your body has to call on its energy reserves, and you may feel tired despite your sleep and possibly unwell. Breakfast provides an effective supply of dietary glucose to fuel the start of your day.

Top up your tank

Liquid is the first requirement. You lose moisture every time you exhale – breathe on a mirror to see the effect. Moisture also escapes through your skin. Overnight, this all adds up to about a mugful. In addition, the body has been making urine as it deals with consumption from the previous evening. To process and excrete a dinner with a high salt content, especially if accompanied by alcohol and followed by caffeine, requires another mug or two of water from the body. To replace all this:

➤ **Start with a glass of water**, before moving on to your preferred morning drink, such as tea or coffee, juice or milk.

➤ **Most adults need to drink** at least 1.2 litres of liquid through the day; you should drink around a third of that within an hour of getting up.

➤ **Drink something you like**. Research suggests that, when asked to drink more water and cut down on soft drinks and other beverages, people drank less fluid altogether. But limit caffeine drinks to no more than five a day.

No excuse not to eat

Most health experts recommend a breakfast that gives you at least 1200kJ and some say much more. Not everyone feels hungry first thing in the morning and many of us are in a rush. But lack of time is no reason to skip breakfast as there are now so many quick, healthy options to choose from.

BREAKFAST SKIPPERS

lose out in at least three different ways, according to research. They have:

- Poorer eating habits for the rest of the day. They tend to have a higher BMI and a larger waist measurement.
- An insufficient intake of vital nutrients – in particular vitamin C, iron, protein, calcium and fibre.
- Reduced attention and concentration levels. Children who don't eat before school make more mistakes in mental arithmetic and have slower memory recall.

By contrast, a morning meal reinforces both physical wellbeing and feelings of self-worth.

It takes just a few minutes to:
- **Eat a bowl of cereal**
- **Down a drinking yogurt**
- **Munch a slice of wholegrain toast and peanut butter**

… and you really don't need to feel hungry to do so.

What breakfast should supply

A bigger breakfast will sustain you for longer. Try to think of it on a plate, with representatives from your 'food friends': complex carbohydrates, protein, dairy foods, fats and fruit or vegetables. Aim for a combination of these to supply the energy and range of nutrients you need to keep going through the morning.

Foods that keep you feeling full

What you choose really does influence your eating all day:

✗ **Highly processed carbohydrate foods** – such as sugary cereals – have a high GI (glycaemic index). They are quickly digested, giving a rapid rise in blood glucose but don't keep you feeling full.

✓ **A low-GI breakfast** takes longer to digest, helping you feel full for longer, and the passage of glucose into the bloodstream is more gradual. Low-GI foods tend to be rich in protein and include whole grains, seeds and nuts.

You might think that by eating little or no breakfast, you're saving kilojoules for the day. That's not how hunger works. Breakfast is the meal that most successfully regulates the hunger-stimulating hormone ghrelin, keeping levels low, which reduces hunger and food cravings throughout the day. This was shown clearly in one 32-week Israeli study of a group of clinically obese people on a low-energy diet; those who ate a good breakfast had lower levels of ghrelin than those who didn't and also lost more weight.

A number of studies now conclude that eating a balanced breakfast is important for weight control, as well as general wellbeing.

Did YOU know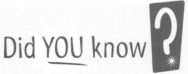

Your morning habits affect theirs

If you're a parent, don't set a bad example. Finnish research shows that, if parents go without breakfast, their children are more likely to do so. Teenagers tend to be the worst offenders: UK research found that 29 per cent of adolescents skip breakfast, while the US National Health and Nutrition Survey put the American figure at 31 per cent.

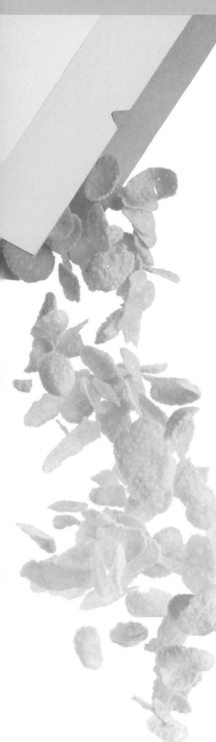

Breakfast cereals – what do they offer?

People in as many as 140 countries now start their day with breakfast cereals. But many of these products contain alarmingly high sugar levels as the UK's consumer organisation Which? reported (*see* page 60). The organisation also criticised the nutrition information on packaging as complicated and confusing. For example:

- If a cereal product is low in salt or sugar, or high in fibre, is made with whole grains, or has added vitamins and iron, these are prominently positioned on the box.
- Less desirable details tend to be tucked away in a small-print nutrition label; when 'low salt' isn't mentioned, there may be as much as 0.5g per 30g serving, or 1.7g per 100g, which experts consider unhealthily high.
- Nutrition analyses of different brands are calculated in different ways – some use dry weight, for example, while others add in the milk to represent a real serving. This makes them difficult to compare.

Most of us choose packet cereals for convenience. They can be a perfectly healthy option, too. Just make sure you opt for wholegrain, low-sugar/low-salt products and avoid those which are heavily processed.

➡ Add almonds to cereal – they keep you feeling full and may help lower blood glucose, too.

Better options – muesli and porridge

They may take a little longer to prepare and eat but many oaty cereals provide better, longer-lasting sustenance. If the ingredient list is short and simple, you can see at a glance what the product is made from and know exactly what you are getting.

● MUESLI

Raw rolled oats mixed with nuts, seeds and dried fruits supply a rich variety of nutrients, especially when combined with the protein and calcium of milk or yogurt. Oats are slow to digest, and with the protein and fibre of nuts, provide a lasting feeling of fullness. Muesli is rich in vitamin E and essential fatty acids, plus the beta-glucan in oats helps keep blood cholesterol levels low. But check the nutrition labels, especially of sweetened and toasted muesli varieties, as these products can be high in fat and kilojoules. Overnight soaking can make muesli easier to eat.

▶ Muesli – best served with live (probiotic) yogurt and fruit.

▶ 100ml portion of live yogurt contains
- 4.8g protein
- 162mg calcium (16 per cent RDI)
- 0.3mg vitamin B_{12} (12 per cent RNI)
- Friendly 'good' bacteria to enhance gut health.
- Soy yogurt is a useful and tasty option for those who are sensitive to dairy foods; soy protein is reported to have cholesterol-lowering effects.

▶ Add berries and fruits – seasonal fruits have both the best taste and nutrient content.
- Blueberries contain lutein and zeaxanthin, which can help maintain good eyesight.
- All brightly coloured fruits contain helpful phytochemicals: try raspberries, strawberries and cherries in summer; apples, pears, bananas or stewed apricots and prunes in winter.
- Frozen berries are a nutritious alternative when fresh are out of season.

▶ Porridge – best with milk and fruit.

● WHOLE OAT PORRIDGE
Whole rolled and steel-cut oats are a rich source of beta-glucan, a soluble fibre that removes cholesterol from the intestine, and also supply vitamin E, which neutralises damaging free radicals (*see* page 85). Buy them in preference to instant oats, which are more processed and have a higher GI, making them less filling. Whole and steel-cut oats benefit from overnight soaking.

▶ Preparing porridge with milk improves the protein quality of the porridge, as well as adding calcium.
- Soy milk is a healthy, tasty alternative to cow's milk: it contains calcium and protein, is low in fat and may help reduce 'bad' LDL cholesterol levels.

▶ Try these toppings – for extra nutrients.
- Seasonal berries and fruits add vitamins and phytochemicals and further enhance the fibre content.
- Manuka honey, believed to have antibiotic qualities, adds natural sweetness.
- Walnuts crumbled on top add vitamin E, essential fatty acids and a satisfying crunch.

Breads and buns – choose the best

Wholegrain seeded breads vs white bread

Many of us enjoy toast at breakfast; it's warm, it smells good as it cooks and holds toppings well. So what type of bread should you toast? Eating whole grains may help to prevent heart disease, but shop-bought wholegrain or seeded breads are not necessarily the healthiest choice.

➤ **Wholegrain wheat bread** with lots of seeds supplies protein with a rich mix of fibre, essential fatty acids and vitamins A, D and E. However, many breads and rolls – including some of the best-looking seeded varieties – also contain much more salt than you would add to a home-baked loaf.

➤ **White bread** lacks the fibre of whole grains, but is still nutritious. By law in Australia, all bread flour must be fortified with the B vitamins thiamin and folate to replace those lost in the milling process. With white as with wholegrain and wholemeal bread, salt levels vary.

➤ **Which is best?** The ingredients label of a shop-bought loaf – white or brown – is your best guide. If the bread contains more than 1g salt per 100g, some health experts say it's too high. If you have the time and the inclination, bake your own and take control of the salt level. Bread-making machines work well – just beware of the temptation to eat a newly baked, aromatic loaf all in one go.

What to spread on bread

● IS BUTTER A SIN?

Many people still consume unhealthy amounts of saturated fat each day, which can contribute to heart disease. Butter is one particular source, so this may be where you should cut back if necessary.

Health experts suggest that fats should supply no more than about a third of our total daily kilojoules, and that saturated fat should make up at most a third of total fat. That's a suggested maximum of less than 50g of butter a day, with no saturated fats from any other sources such as meat.

Butter is the gold standard for taste and 'melt in the mouth' sensation, but if you tend to eat too much saturated fat, consider these alternatives – most have a buttery taste, with fewer kilojoules, less fat and less saturated fat:

- Olive and sunflower oil-based spreads.
- Light, fat-reduced spreads. These can help to reduce overall fat intake. Margarines may be supplemented with vitamins A, D and E.

CRUMPETS & PASTRIES

may be a delicious holiday or weekend treat, but they aren't a healthy choice for every day.

- Crumpets could be a good option but for the 1g salt per crumpet – more than in a regular packet of crisps.
- They're low in fat, too – but only if you leave out the pats of butter that traditionally melt into a hot crumpet.
- Croissants taste divine, but again the high butter and salt content makes them for special occasions only.
- Danish pastries are also quite high in fat and usually high in sugar, too.

All figures are per 10g serving

	KJ	Total fat	Saturated fat	Monounsaturated fat	Polyunsaturated fat
BUTTER Only ingredient is milk, can have added salt	300	8.1g	4.9g	2.0g	02.g
BUTTER, LIGHT, SPREADABLE Blend of butter and oil, reducing sat fat content	200	6.0g	2.4g	2.3g	0.8g
IMITATION BUTTER Very similar to light spreadable butter	200	5.9g	1.8g	2.9g	1.0g
LIGHT IMITATION BUTTER Very low fat	140	3.8g	0.9g	1.9g	0.8g
POLYUNSATURATED VEGETABLE OIL MARGARINE A reasonably priced healthy product	160	4.5g	1.0g	1.1g	2.3g
LIGHT POLYUNSATURATED VEGETABLE OIL MARGARINE The lowest kilojoule and fat content	120	3.0g	0.7g	0.8g	1.5g
OLIVE OIL-BASED MARGARINE Best source of monounsaturated fats	200	5.6g	1.4g	3.0g	1.5g

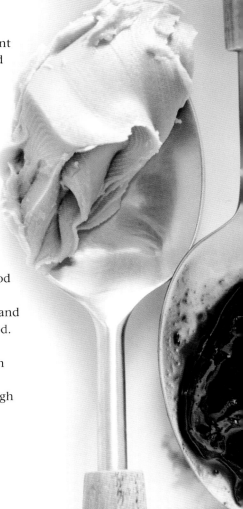

- Cholesterol-lowering spreads may be helpful for people with raised blood cholesterol. The light versions are better still for those who want a low-kilojoule spread. They are not suitable for those with low blood cholesterol levels or children.

WHAT ABOUT OTHER SPREADS?

Additional spreads are often a question of individual taste; some have a few nutritional benefits but most have drawbacks, as well:

➡ **Jam** brings sugar but only a trace of vitamins – look out for high fruit content varieties. Some reduced-sugar jams use concentrated grape juice to add sweetness.

➡ **Honey** has more fructose than regular jam, which gives it an intensely sweet taste. You need only a little.

➡ **Low-fat ricotta** is high in protein and calcium, and low in fat. Commercial ricotta may have added salt, however – check the label. Other spread alternatives such as hummus, or mashed avocado, are good choices as they add fibre and good fats.

➡ **Peanut butter** and other nut butters improve the protein quality and quantity when added to bread, producing a nutritious and satiating food. Look for low-salt and low-sugar varieties.

➡ **Hazelnut chocolate spread**, like peanut butter, increases protein quality, but it also adds sugar and saturated fat. Best used sparingly.

➡ **Yeast extract spread** is a rich source of B vitamins, but is very high in salt. Fortunately, it has so much flavour that even the thinnest smear is enough.

➡ Look for low-sugar peanut butter and jam.

BREAKFAST EGG IDEAS:

- If you're feeding several people, cook an omelette and add extra ingredients such as grated cheese, parsley, mushrooms or tomatoes.
- Delight hungry teenagers with breakfast pancakes – savoury with a cheese and mushroom filling, or sweet, with berries or other fruit.
- If you have a waffle iron or waffle maker, serve up potato waffles with poached eggs and spinach.

The cooked breakfast – what to embrace and what to avoid

Eggs are a good choice ☑

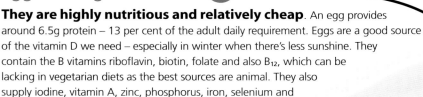

They are highly nutritious and relatively cheap. An egg provides around 6.5g protein – 13 per cent of the adult daily requirement. Eggs are a good source of the vitamin D we need – especially in winter when there's less sunshine. They contain the B vitamins riboflavin, biotin, folate and also B_{12}, which can be lacking in vegetarian diets as the best sources are animal. They also supply iodine, vitamin A, zinc, phosphorus, iron, selenium and some omega-3 fats.

With about 280mg cholesterol per egg, there has been concern that eggs raise blood cholesterol levels. Various scientific studies are challenging this.

➡ **One 12-week UK study** found that people on a low-energy diet who ate two eggs a day not only lost weight but also reduced their blood cholesterol levels.

For most healthy people, the dietary intake of cholesterol, especially from low-fat foods such as eggs, has little impact on blood cholesterol levels.

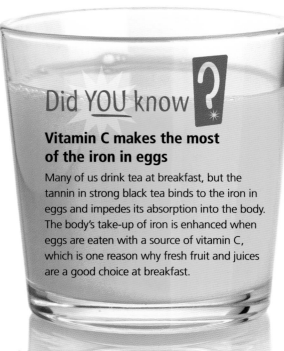

Did YOU know ❓

Vitamin C makes the most of the iron in eggs

Many of us drink tea at breakfast, but the tannin in strong black tea binds to the iron in eggs and impedes its absorption into the body. The body's take-up of iron is enhanced when eggs are eaten with a source of vitamin C, which is one reason why fresh fruit and juices are a good choice at breakfast.

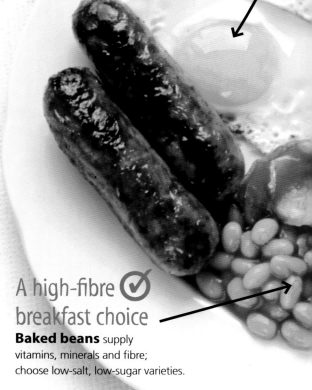

A high-fibre ☑ breakfast choice

Baked beans supply vitamins, minerals and fibre; choose low-salt, low-sugar varieties.

☑ Boiled, poached, fried or scrambled

Eggs are also particularly good at increasing satiety – feelings of fullness – and decreasing hunger, according to a review of recent research published in *NHD*, a magazine for professional dietitians. One or two eggs served with a piece of wholegrain toast make an excellent breakfast, but don't add extra salt.

Boiling or poaching eggs adds no extra kilojoules (except for those in a drop of oil if you are using a poaching pan). Frying does increase the kilojoule count, so it's best to use a non-stick frying pan and a little olive oil. For scrambled eggs, mix one or two eggs with a drop of milk and cook with a little oil in a non-stick pan, then serve on wholegrain toast.

Avoid hash browns and fried bread ✗

Imagine soaking a small sponge in fat, then frying it. Hash browns and fried bread are like starchy sponges full of fat – best avoided.

Limit breakfast meats, sausages and bacon ✗

The World Cancer Research Fund reports a link between eating processed meat and increased risk of bowel cancer. They recommend that meats that have been smoked, cured or had preservatives added, such as ham, bacon and some sausages, should be restricted in the diet. A healthier breakfast choice is a little grilled salmon or trout. Alternatively, add smoked salmon to scrambled eggs – keep the serving small to limit salt intake.

Grilled tomatoes

Other good cooked choices: ☑

Sautéed mushrooms

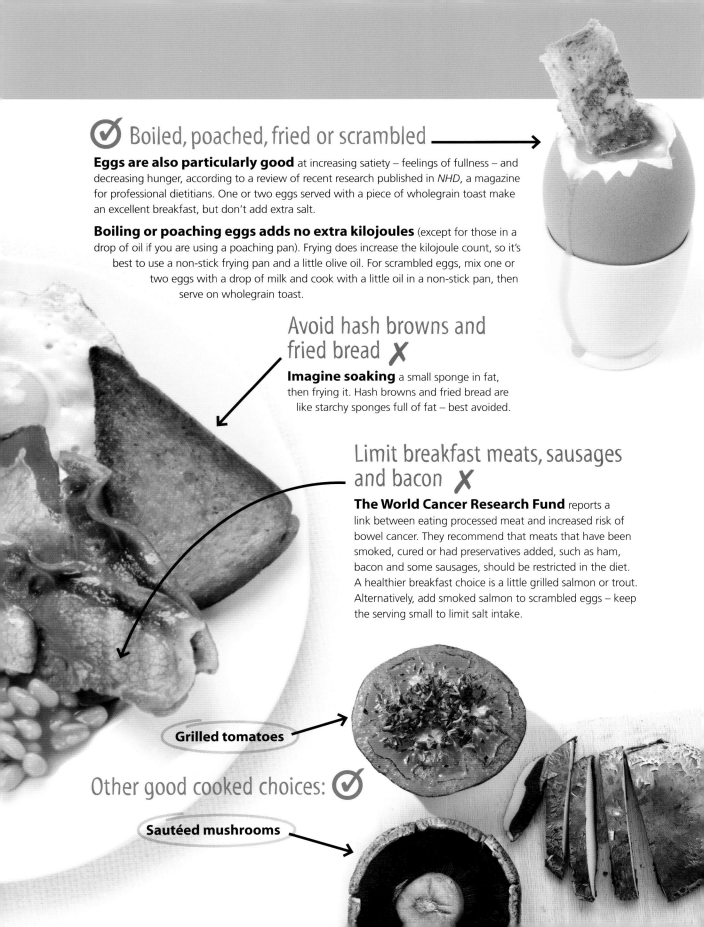

Breakfast beverages

Tea

Popular in many countries across the world, tea is often the single biggest contributor to our daily fluid intake. Black tea has some caffeine to help wake us up and also contains disease-fighting molecules called catechins, although levels are higher in green teas. Two other phytochemicals are present in trace amounts – theobromine and theophylline, which are used medicinally to treat asthma and other respiratory diseases. Many studies have been carried out on the possible role of tea in reducing rates of cancer, but results have been inconclusive.

A recent UK study reported that young men given a cup of black tea de-stressed and relaxed more quickly after undertaking challenging tasks than those who drank a tea substitute. In times of stress, it seems, a cup of tea can have a calming effect – at breakfast or throughout the day.

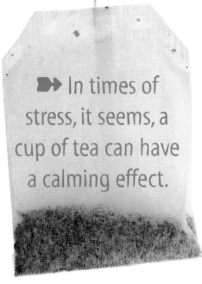

➡➡ In times of stress, it seems, a cup of tea can have a calming effect.

Coffee

Over the years, the reputation of coffee has swung from good to bad and back again. Recent favourable studies suggest that the benefits of consuming up to five cups a day may be:

- A lower risk of developing Parkinson's disease and dementia.
- Better bowel mobility, which may help to prevent constipation.
- Better cognitive performance, especially in later life.

It seems that drinking some coffee is good for most of us. But not all; pregnant women are advised to avoid it as caffeine passes through the placenta and lingers in the developing baby ten times longer than in an adult.

Many people also get 'coffee jitters' if they drink more than a few cups of strong coffee. The caffeine can produce sleep problems if drunk later in the day.

The espresso brewing method produces the best-quality coffee with not too much caffeine, lots of taste and the highest yield of antioxidants. Plunger coffee comes

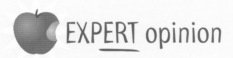

EXPERT opinion

Drinking coffee can protect the brain

Caffeine or coffee may be linked to a reduced risk of dementia, according to Dr Gary Arendash, co-author of a US research study. 'Moderate daily consumption of caffeinated coffee appears to be the best dietary option for long-term protection against Alzheimer's memory loss.' he says. 'Coffee is inexpensive, readily available, easily gets into the brain, and has few side-effects for most of us. Moreover, our studies show that caffeine and coffee appear to directly attack the Alzheimer's disease process.'

Dr Gary Arendash *Research Professor, University of South Florida, USA*

second for quality, with more caffeine. The hotter the water and the longer the beans or granules are immersed, the more caffeine is available.

Milks and yogurts

Dairy products contribute important nutrients to the breakfast meal. A cup of milk alone or in a bowl of cereal supplies about 8.5g protein – around 16 per cent of daily protein needs – and about 40 per cent of daily calcium needs, plus riboflavin, pantothenic acid, vitamin B_{12}, phosphorus and iodine.

Young children under two years should have whole milk, especially if they are very active. Reduced-fat or skim milk is a better option for adults who have to be more careful with the energy and fat content of their diets. Other available milks and milk-products include:

● **Soy milk** The fresh chilled varieties have a pleasant taste and come sweetened or non-sweetened. The contents are about 5 per cent soybeans, with added calcium and vitamins. A cup of soy milk contains around 6g protein. Some people with an intolerance to the natural sugar in cow's milk (lactose) find soy milk a useful alternative.

● **Yogurt** This is made by heating and cooling milk, then adding a bacteria culture which ferments the lactose into lactic acid. As a result of the slightly denatured protein, the reduced amount of lactose and the presence of a bacteria culture, many people find yogurt easier to digest than milk.

● **Yogurt-type drinks** are sold as a daily nutrient boost in small individual bottles. Some contain acidophilus strains of bacteria to increase the population of friendly bacteria in the gut, and some contain plant sterols with cholesterol-lowering properties.

Juices – the fresher the better

They make a refreshing start to the day and are a good source of vitamins, minerals and phytochemicals; one serving can count as one of your recommended seven-a-day fruits and vegetables. However, most juices contain more than 400kJ per 250ml glass, as well as acids that erode the teeth, so keep the glass small or drink them diluted. These are the choices:

● **Freshly squeezed:** gives you the most antioxidant vitamins.
● **Not from concentrate:** pasteurised juice with a shelf-life of up to 30 days.
● **From concentrate:** made from juice that has been pasteurised and evaporated, frozen and shipped, then reconstituted and packaged.

BREAKFAST ON THE RUN

can still be nutritious. Always have a drink, then take breakfast food with you. Many cafés now sell takeaway yogurt, muesli and porridge pots, plus tea and coffee. But a breakfast packed at home will almost certainly be cheaper – and probably healthier. A few portable suggestions:

● A small handful of walnuts or almonds, or four brazil nuts.
● A few dried prunes or apricots.
● A yogurt – probiotic or soy, if preferred.
● A small peanut butter wholegrain sandwich.
● A fruit smoothie.
● Pita bread filled with ricotta and berries.
● A piece of fruit plus a drinking yogurt.

5 Healthy snacks

Eating something between meals can be a perfectly normal part of a healthy diet. Just be careful what it is and why you feel you need it – emotions can play a role.

It's natural to feel hungry between meals, which may be 5 hours or much more apart. A medium-sized meal takes 1 to 2 hours to pass through the stomach, before continuing along the small intestine. Blood glucose rises soon after eating but within a few hours falls back to its normal level and the brain begins to signal hunger. The best type of snack plugs the gap so we reach our next meal ready for food but not ravenous.

We may dismiss feelings of hunger when distracted by an absorbing activity. But if we do, the body has to draw on other energy reserves to supply glucose to our brains and tissues, which can make us feel tired. If the gap between meals is too great, our brains know we need energy and hunger can become so intense that we eat too much at the next meal. Healthy snacks between meals can help to keep hunger under control.

➡ A snack is effectively a 'mini-meal'. It doesn't have to be big, but nutritionally it should be healthy.

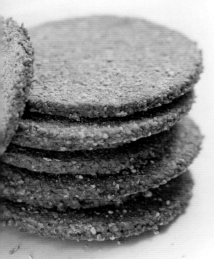

Who requires a snack?

A typical daily snacking schedule might be breakfast / SNACK / lunch / SNACK / dinner. The urge to snack will hit at different times depending on individual patterns of activity or stages in life.

● **Early risers** – Anyone who eats breakfast around 7am, especially those who do physical work, will need a substantial snack mid-morning.

● **Late diners** – If lunch is around 1pm, anyone who will eat dinner later than 7pm may need something late afternoon to avoid the hunger-driven temptation to pick at anything available.

● **The young** – Children don't eat large meals and need healthy snacks throughout the day to maintain their high energy and nutrient levels.

● **Adolescents** – Even though teenagers might eat lots at mealtimes, the growing body makes high demands on energy and nutrients, so regular healthy snacks are essential.

● **The very active** – Fit, sporty adults who take a lot of exercise need to boost energy and nutrient intake between meals.

By contrast, retired people may well eat breakfast later, followed by smaller but more frequent meals and an earlier dinner. Unless they are very active during the day, an appropriate snack could be as light as a nutritious drink or piece of fruit.

What's the difference between a snack and a treat?

A treat should be eaten only infrequently, perhaps as a 'reward' for a job well done, or as an occasional indulgence. By contrast, a snack is effectively a 'mini-meal'. Nutritionally it should make a healthy contribution to daily energy requirements and dietary needs.

A good starting point to help distinguish snacks from treat foods is to look at their fat, sugar and salt content. A healthy snack should not contribute so many kilojoules to your recommended daily intake that there aren't enough left over to allow for proper meals. A treat food will often be disproportionately high in fat, sugar or salt. If offered a treat you can't resist or in a situation when it would be rude to refuse, make sure you share it – with as many people as possible.

ONE IN SEVEN cases of stomach cancer in the West could be avoided if people ate less than 6g salt a day, according to the World Cancer Research Fund. Many snacks, such as crisps, are very salty.

Treat or snack?

	KJ per portion	Total fat	Saturated fat	Carbs	Carbs as sugar	Fibre	Salt
2 MILK CHOCOLATE BISCUITS	650	8g	4g	21.6g	9.2g	1g	0.1g
2 WHOLEGRAIN CRACKERS	350	3.6g	0.8g	12.2g	0.2g	1.6g	0.36g
40g BAG OF CRISPS	700	9.6g	1.2g	24g	0.2g	1.8g	0.6g
10 ALMONDS (20g)	450	10g	1g	4g	0.5g	2.3g	0g
JAM DOUGHNUT	1500	18.3g	9.2g	55.4g	18.1g	2.7g	0.3g
BANANA	400	0.4g	0.1g	27g	14g	2.3g	0.01g

Four tips for sensible snacking

A snack is satisfying when it produces feelings of satiety and passes slowly through the digestive system. Top nutritionists recommend:

1 Protein – from foods such as cheese, eggs, hummus or peanut butter *or*

2 Fat – preferably 'good' fats such as those in nuts or avocados *or*

3 Complex carbs – from snacks such as wholegrain crackers or bran muffins *plus*

4 A pause for 20 minutes after snacking so your brain can register the effect.

What makes a good snack?

What you choose to snack on matters. It not only affects your appetite and what you eat at mealtimes, but can also influence how effectively you function throughout the day. A good snack will do three things:

- **Boost your daily nutrient intake**
- **Plug a hunger gap**
- **Give you a feeling of wellbeing**

A stick of celery might help with the first, but it leaves you unsatisfied and doesn't get you through to the next meal. Treats may fail on all three counts as any mouth-feel and taste satisfaction may be disappointingly short-lived. Sugary treats are also digested very quickly so you're soon feeling hungry again. Then you eat more, setting a dangerous precedent.

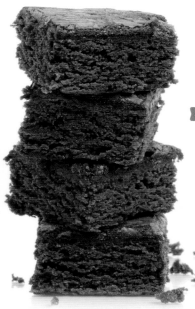

➡ Sugary treats spend little time in the stomach.

Blood glucose highs and lows – the dangers

When foods are quickly digested and absorbed as glucose, it creates a rapid rise in blood glucose. The biscuits, sweets and other refined carbohydrates that produce this effect are described by nutritionists as having a high glycaemic index (GI).

When blood glucose increases:

- The body secretes insulin which encourages the cells in muscles and the liver to take up the glucose, bringing blood levels back to normal.
- Feelings of lethargy can occur as blood glucose falls. Regular sweet drinks and snacks can result in a yo-yoing cycle of high and low blood glucose levels, while not achieving any real feeling of satiety.
- A pattern of surging blood glucose levels without enough exercise to use the glucose and prevent the excess being converted into fat is a major risk factor for developing diabetes.

Healthy quick bites

Below are some examples of snacks that meet all three 'good snack' conditions – they are nutritionally sound, they help fill a gap and they're delicious enough to be satisfying, too. First is a category that you might not suspect could be good for you.

● BAKERY GOODS

These get a bad press but scones and English-style muffins are low in fat and the wheat flour is a source of protein, calcium and B vitamins. Go for home-baked and use some wholemeal flour; processed versions usually contain too much salt. The basic ingredients – milk, flour and butter – supply essential nutrients, and you control the fat, sugar and salt content:

➠ **Homemade scones** can be sweet or savoury: sultana, cheese and chive, date or pumpkin. They are best eaten the day they are made, but freeze well, too.

➠ **Banana loaf, malt loaf, sultana and bran muffins** are further examples of healthy home-baked snacks. The loaves can be sliced and frozen in batches; muffins also freeze well.

● FRUIT

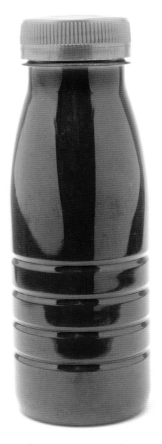

A couple of pieces a day add the sweetness we often crave and help us achieve our daily requirements for vitamin C, folic acid and fibre, plus important phytochemicals. Where possible, buy fruit in season; it tastes better and has more nutrients. Wash fruit to remove dirt and pesticide traces. **Apples, pears and bananas** are good staples. Easy-peel **mandarins** are practical and packed with vitamin C. In winter, **oranges** are at their best: sweet and delicious and well worth the effort of peeling. **Red grapes, berries and cherries** pack a terrific antioxidant boost. Orange and red-coloured exotic fruits, such as **papaya, mango and rockmelon,** are rich in carotenoid phytochemicals that aid good eye function.

➠ Mandarins are easy to carry.

● LIQUID SNACKS

There is a tasty variety of smoothies and drinking yogurts available, but always check the contents as some are sweetened and contain too much sugar and unnecessary additives.

➠ **Smoothies** which contain the whole fruit pulp rather than just the juice have plenty of fibre. A small daily whole-fruit smoothie can count as one of your recommended seven-a-day fruit and vegetable portions.

➠ A daily smoothie counts as one of the recommended seven-a-day.

Hearty snacks

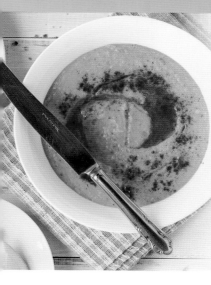

If you get home late in the afternoon and go out again to play sport or take part in an activity that will delay your evening meal, you need a substantial snack to keep you going for a few hours. Here are some suggestions:

- Pita bread toasted and filled with hummus plus tomato or grated carrot.
- Two wholegrain crackers with ricotta or cottage cheese.
- An apple and a small handful of nuts.
- A glass of low-fat milk and a small bran muffin.
- A small wholegrain roll with lettuce and tuna or hardboiled egg.
- Hummus with sticks of carrots, celery, capsicum, cucumber, broccoli or cauliflower.
- Low-fat drinking yogurt with a banana.
- Slice of wholegrain toast spread with peanut butter or low-fat cheese.

➡ **Drinking yogurts** can be pure yogurt or a mixture of yogurt with juice. They tend to be easily digested, provide valuable calcium and phosphorus, and the high protein content helps us to feel full. But again, check labels to avoid additives, flavourings and excessive sugar.

➡ **Probiotic drinking yogurts** have strains of acidophilus bacteria added to help maintain the population of beneficial bacteria in the intestine. Intestinal bacteria keep the gut healthy and provide certain essential fatty acids as well as two thirds of our daily intake of vitamin K.

➡ **Milky drinks**, such as lattes and cappuccinos, can feel satisfying even when made with low-fat milk. But beware the fashionable hijacking of this healthy snack through the addition of unnecessary sugar, syrup or cream.

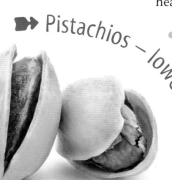

➡ Pistachios – lowest in fat.

● **RAW NUTS**

Raw nuts are highly nutritious so just a few make a healthy snack. A handful of mixed dried fruits and nuts, well wrapped and carried in a lunch box or handbag, provides an excellent portable snack. Nuts contain essential unsaturated 'good' fats, plus phytosterols that inhibit the absorption of 'bad' LDL cholesterol. A number of studies suggest that they help heart health.

➡ **Brazil and cashew nuts** are particularly rich in selenium, which is essential for healthy thyroid function.

➡ **Pistachios** are the nuts lowest in fat and highest in protein.

➡ **Nut spreads** such as peanut or almond butter make a great snack on wholegrain crackers or a small piece of wholemeal or rye bread.

WARNING: The dangers of nut allergy have led some schools to adopt a no-nut policy to avoid a potential medical emergency, so this is not a snack to take to school.

Avoid the snacking danger zones

With tempting snacks all too readily available, it's easy to succumb despite our best intentions. Here are a few of the most common snack-traps and simple ways to arm yourself against them or, at least, mitigate their effects.

DANGER ZONE ONE: Peer-pressure snacking

Sharing food and drink with friends and family at home or work is one of life's most pleasurable rituals. Yet, when unhealthy, highly tempting foods are so readily available it can have an unwelcome impact on health. In one piece of UK research 64 per cent of office employees felt that co-workers brought too many cakes and treats into the office, 24 per cent said they couldn't resist them and 14 per cent felt pressured to join in eating them. It feels rude to refuse, so if everyone is sharing a celebration cake or packet of biscuits, you join in, even though you might be trying to watch your weight and know that this is not the healthiest choice. Can you buck the trend for treats without causing a riot?

● **Timetable the treats** While an everyday biscuit or cake habit is unwise, a complete absence of food treats at work seems unfriendly and unnecessary. As a compromise, try to encourage healthy snacks as the norm, with treats being kept, say, for Friday afternoons or, better still, for more special occasions.

● **Turn peer pressure into peer support** An online survey by the Australian Psychological Society found that people are more successful at making changes to poor eating habits when they seek help from friends and family. Getting a few key allies to support you in a quest to include healthier foods is likely to be more successful than tackling the issue alone.

● **Make the first move** At work or at home, be the first to introduce a selection of healthy snacks to nibble on, such as:

● Strawberries, grapes, peaches, figs or apricots in season.
● Pistachios or other nuts.
● Small packets of dried fruit.
● Wholegrain crackers.

Once a daily habit of healthy snacks is established, a treat will be appreciated all the more. Encourage home-made cakes and muffins, as they will probably contain healthier ingredients. More indulgent offerings, too, are perfectly acceptable – once in a while and in small portions.

64% OF PEOPLE

in one UK survey said that co-workers brought too many cakes and treats into the office.

DANGER ZONE TWO: Snacks with alcohol

Most of us know we should eat something when we're drinking alcohol. The problem is that healthy snacks are seldom available in bars. Most bar snacks are salty – a deliberate ploy designed to make us drink more. If salted crisps and nuts are the only options, limit the portion size by sharing and don't make them a habit. If you are serving drinks at home, or whenever the place or situation allows:

SWAP THE BAD GUYS ...

- **A 50g serving of salted roasted peanuts:** 1200kJ, 53 per cent fat (9.5 per cent saturated; dry roasted have slightly less fat) and 0.5g salt.
- **A 50g bag of crisps:** 17g of fat (around 10 per cent of your daily fat limit). **Plus:** you'll probably eat more as the fatty salty taste of crisps is compelling and crisps, being low in protein, are not filling.
- **Root vegetable crisps:** healthier image but similar energy, fat and salt content.
- **Corn chips with salsa:** high in kilojoules and fat (a 50g serving contains 900kJ and 10g fat).

... FOR THE GOOD GUYS

- **Raw peanuts:** high in protein, magnesium and zinc, more B vitamins and iron, no salt and less fat than salted, roasted versions.
- **Nuts in shells,** such as pistachios and raw peanuts: slower to eat as you have to shell them and a good source of essential fatty acids.
Plus: in one US study, when two groups were given shelled or unshelled nuts to eat, those who had to shell their nuts ate 50 per cent less but felt equally satisfied. The pile of empty nut shells also gives a visual reminder of the quantity consumed.

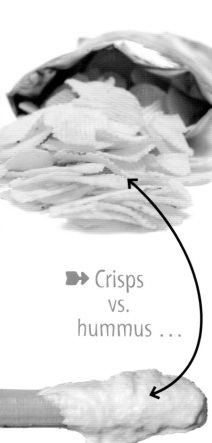

➡ Crisps vs. hummus ...

... let the good guys win!

- **Hummus with vegetable sticks:** 400kJ per 50g serving and all goodness – protein and fibre from the chickpeas, blended with olive oil. Serve with strips of carrot, celery, cucumber and capsicums. Check the contents of supermarket brands, as some are higher in salt and fat, or make your own. Reduced-fat supermarket versions contain around 400kJ per 50g.
- **Edamame beans (soft young soybeans):** high in protein and fibre, and a good source of thiamin, folate and iron. They are best bought frozen, then the green soybean pods can be briefly blanched. Like nuts, these beans

need to be shelled from their pods, so are quite fun to eat. Edamame can also be bought as a baked salted snack – a 50g serving has 20g of protein and 7.3g fibre, but also comes with 0.5g salt.

GOOD NEWS AND BAD NEWS

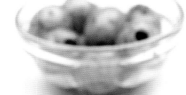

- **Olives** are rich in good monounsaturated fat, but most are very salty: a 15g serving, around 2–3 olives, contains 0.8g salt, or 13 per cent of the maximum daily limit.
- **Pretzels** are low in energy but are almost pure carbohydrate with few useful nutrients. Like most salted snack foods, they have too much salt.

➡ Olives contain healthy fats but most are also very salty.

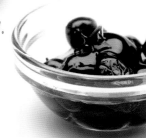

- **Popcorn** is low in energy and high in fibre, but has a high GI so it is quickly digested and not a suitable snack for diabetics on its own. A 22g portion of supermarket salted popcorn has 500kJ and 0.4g of salt. Home-made popcorn is better as you control the salt level, and the type of fat. Microwave popcorn, though, is high in harmful trans fats.

DANGER ZONE THREE: Just got home and starving

A particular snacking danger zone occurs when we are hungry enough to eat a full meal but have to wait. One of the commonest times for this is arriving home from a day at school or work. Dinner may still be a few hours away, so raiding the fridge is common practice – and the hungrier we are, the less careful we are about what we eat. We want instant gratification, so healthy snacks need to be available fast or the temptation to pig out on biscuits, salty crackers or chocolate is too hard to resist.

PLAN AHEAD

- **Pack a snack**. If you carry a healthy snack to eat shortly before leaving work, or even on the way home, you will avoid arriving home feeling ravenous and a cup of tea or piece of fruit will be enough.
- **Stock up on healthy snacks**. Make sure the fridge always contains easy snacks such as drinking yogurt, hummus and carrots, or ricotta cheese to spread on wholegrain crackers. Always have fresh fruit available.
- **Plan what you will eat**. If you get home without any idea of what you are going to snack on and start roaming the cupboards for anything edible, it is all too easy to eat too much of the wrong stuff. It is better to

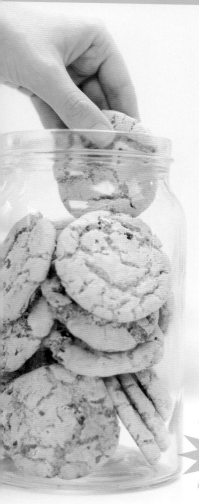

know in advance what the snack is going to be. Children and young people especially benefit from being told what to go for. If they know, for example, to help themselves to a post-school snack of a bowl of cereal, or a drinking yogurt, or a piece of wholemeal toast with peanut butter, this removes a large part of the anxiety caused by feeling hungry. They can be quickly satisfied and move on to other activities.

● **Don't bring the bad guys into the house**. If crisps and biscuits are in the house, they're going to get eaten and ruin best intentions of snacking well. High-fat, salty and sugary foods can be irresistible when arriving home hungry. Think of them as treat foods that are bought in small quantities for specific occasions, not as a regular feature in your pantry.

● **Don't mistake thirst for hunger**. When we arrive home from a day out anywhere, it's likely that we're thirsty and to avoid fatigue we need to rehydrate rather than eat. Our brains can often confuse these two needs. A glass of tap water is perfect, perhaps followed by a smoothie or drinking yogurt. Tea is great to help de-stress; a cup of coffee is also fine as long as it is large enough to quench thirst.

● **Beware of opportunist snacking**. As many mums know, children's teatime leftovers can be a dangerous temptation. When the kids leave tasty morsels on the plate, it is easy to justify polishing them off as 'avoiding waste'. Don't eat for the sake of it, or feel you have to eat up leftovers. Plan to have a small snack-sized share or have a healthy alternative to hand.

DANGER ZONE FOUR: 'Need a lift' nibbles

These moments can occur when we aren't even hungry – the urge to eat is a 'substitute' desire. It could stem from feeling a bit unsettled, or perhaps bored, or having to wait for something or someone. A snack fills the gap and a treat affords a bit of short-lived pleasure. But when 'need a lift' nibbles become too regular, they can become an unhealthy habit. Avoid the danger by training yourself to switch to an alternative.

BUCK THE BOREDOM NIBBLES BY:
● **Drinking something not associated with snacking**. Try chilled fizzy water, a calming peppermint tea, or an infusion of hot water with a slice of fresh ginger and lemon.

● **Performing a substitute mood-raising activity**. Get some exercise: do ten squats, or lie on the carpet and do ten tummy crunches. Alternatively phone a friend, switch on the radio, listen to music, or do a bit of personal pampering such as moisturising your hands.

➨ If there are biscuits in the house, they are likely to get eaten and ruin the best intentions.

- **Sucking a mint or chewing gum**. The action of sucking has a calming sensation that is hard-wired into the brain from the earliest moments of infancy. When you are an adult it can still bring relief from tension. The sweet mint flavour can also reduce cravings for other foods.
- **Banning unhealthy treats from the house**. If you do this, you won't be presented with irresistible temptation. If you must eat, go for something chewy such as dried mango or apricot.
- **Postponing the nibble**. Decide what you're going to nibble on, but put off actually doing it for 15 minutes. There is a good chance that the desire will subside, especially if you get effectively distracted by some activity.

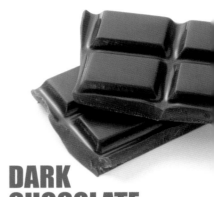

DANGER ZONE FIVE: Night-time munchies

FEELING HUNGRY AT NIGHT CAN HAPPEN WHEN:
- **Dinner is eaten very early**
- **The evening meal wasn't substantial enough**
- **You've been very active and need to top up your energy**
- **You have digestive problems and can only eat small portions**

Night-time snacking doesn't have to be a danger zone, but can be if the nibbles are unhealthily high in fat, sugar or salt. When you eat early then relax at home in front of the television, you're probably aware that TV food commercials or even cookery programs are a potential snack trigger. Don't succumb to an urge that is not a need – or make sure that you eat fruit or something equally healthy rather than crisps, biscuits or cakes. Dark chocolate can be an occasional treat (*see* right).

If your day-time eating is disordered this can also lead to 'grazing' behaviour – snacking on bits and pieces here and there, and never gaining a clear picture of the amount of food actually eaten. A nourishing evening meal – eaten several hours before bedtime to allow digestion but not so early that you become hungry again – is the best way to stay feeling full.

Those whose lives are very active may need a substantial snack in the late evening, despite an earlier evening meal. Ideal snacks at this time are foods such as a bowl of cereal or wholegrain toast that supply the energy you need but won't keep you awake.

For others the classic hot milky drink is comforting. The protein helps you feel full while natural sugars add a little sweetness. Home-made cocoa is better than drinking chocolate, as you can control the amount of added sugar; ready-prepared chocolate drink powders often have more sugar and less cocoa. Skim or low-fat milk keeps the kilojoule count down.

DARK CHOCOLATE

can be a satisfying snack because Its bitterness, countered with just enough sweetness, makes it pleasant but not so sweet that you want to eat the whole bar. Two squares of dark chocolate with a low-fat cappuccino tastes like total indulgence, while being packed with nutrients. Studies suggest that dark chocolate in small quantities can help to boost heart health; the European Food Safety Authority agrees that cocoa flavonoids help to improve blood circulation.

Are 'light' or mini-snack treats healthier?

Food marketers know that many of us are health and weight conscious. So it's not surprising that a number of 'treats' have undergone a 'low' or 'light' makeover, reducing their fat and kilojoule content. The table (right) shows a range of regular treat items followed by 'lighter' equivalents, selected to be as closely matched as possible in type and portion size.

Take a look. Do these apparently slimline products justify the 'healthy' claims made for them? The answer for all of them appears to be 'no'.

- **Energy:** With a reduction in kilojoules of around 10 per cent most are not much 'lighter' than the regular version – but may be more expensive.
- **Fat:** The energy reduction usually comes from cutting the fat content: except for the chocolate chip cookies, most of the lighter versions contain around half the fat. The lighter cereal bar is the star in terms of overall fat reduction but others show a significant reduction in saturated fat.
- **Carbs and sugar:** In all cases, with the exception of the cookies, the carbohydrate content is slightly higher in the light version and in some cases the sugar content has gone up too. These increases help to maintain the palatability and portion size of the treats while reducing their fat levels. So while being lower in fat, these 'light' treats can be intensely sweet and are not suitable for those who need to monitor their blood glucose levels and want to achieve a healthier diet.
- **Fibre:** The fibre content is greater in most of the 'light' versions – probably to increase their bulk for few kilojoules, but still a healthy addition.
- **Salt:** There is no significant difference in salt content – but muffins and crisps tend to be high in salt anyway. Consumers aren't always aware that foods such as shop-bought muffins add so much to our daily salt intake.

Is small beautiful?

Some small cakes and treats are sold not as 'light' or 'reduced fat', but as being small enough to be 'guilt-free'. This might be true if we could guarantee eating only one small portion, but inside a tub of bite-sized chocolate cakes there may be 20 small pieces and it's our decision how many we eat. By their very nature treats tempt to have 'just one more'. Such packaging is clever marketing: it's easy for us to justify buying the pack because we are going to share them with colleagues or family. But you can be sure that these are seldom eaten in solitary tiny portions.

Other treats are packaged to decide portion size for us – some biscuits, for example, come in pairs, while cakes and slices are individually wrapped with the kilojoule content prominently displayed. This is designed to

OVER 9,000

new snack foods were launched between 2008 and 2012 in the USA and most of them were in the 'healthy' cereal/energy bar category, according to a recent Mintel survey.

Treat foods v. 'Light' versions

	Kilojoules	Total Fat	Saturated fat	Carbs	Carbs as sugar	Fibre	Salt
BLUEBERRY MUFFIN	790	8.5g	0.8g	25.6g	12.g	0.6g	0.5g
BLUEBERRY MUFFIN (LIGHT)	785	3.8g	0.3g	35.2g	18.2g	1.0g	0.4g
2 CHOC CHIP COOKIES	420	4.6g	2.4g	13.4g	6.6g	0.6g	0.2g
2 DOUBLE CHOC CHIP COOKIES (LIGHT)	360	3.5g	0.9g	11.6g	4.4g	1.8g	0.1g
CARROT CAKE SLICE	560	6.0g	2.0g	18.0g	13.0g	1.0g	0.1g
LOW-FAT CARROT CAKE SLICE	470	3.2g	0.9g	19.2g	11.8g	2.2g	0.2g
CEREAL BAR, CRUNCHY GRANOLA	420	8.0g	1.0g	15.0g	5.6g	1.3g	0.1g
CEREAL BAR (LIGHT)	370	1.5g	0.9g	17.0g	9.0g	*0.6–2g	0.1g
CRISPS (25g BAG)	585	9.1g	0.9g	12.3g	0.1g	0.9g	0.3g
CRISPS (LIGHT, 28g BAG)	480	5.0g	0.5g	15.0g	0.1g	1.0g	0.4g

*There is some variation between items of different flavours.

reassure the kilojoule-conscious treat-seeker. These treat foods tend to be small, with a kilojoule content of around 400kJ. The packaging is part of the attraction: it provides an apparent physical barrier to consuming more than the prescribed portion, creating the impression that the treat food can be eaten as part of a kilojoule-controlled plan. It's sold to us as a win-win situation: we get the treat and successfully restrict our energy intake – we 'have our cake and eat it'. But is this really true?

Don't be fooled

Such packaged treats are seldom healthy snacks; they are often high in sugar and salt. They may help people to achieve success as part of a weight-reduction plan by allowing indulgent food items to remain on the menu in a controlled way. But the energy content of little treats is often not much less than a portion of the regular treat. The twin dangers of all these cleverly marketed snacks is that they often fail to fill the hunger gap and, if seduced by their 'slimming' appeal, we eat more of them, jeopardising any kilojoule-controlled regime. A naturally healthy snack is almost always the better choice.

6 Your midday meal

All too often lunch is hurried or skipped as we fill up on whatever is available without caring enough about what we are eating. Wrong, say the experts. Nutritionally, lunch – rather than dinner – should be the most important meal of the day.

Lunch was once the main meal, but for many working people today it is small or sometimes non-existent. The tough 'lunch is for wimps' office mentality frowns on a midday break, concerned that food wastes time or slows you down. This is wrong and unhealthy for the following reasons:

➡ **A balanced midday meal keeps your metabolism active**, supplying the energy to keep you going physically and mentally.

➡ **The right foods help to regulate blood-glucose levels** so you may avoid the highs and lows that create tiredness and mood swings.

➡ **If you don't eat properly at lunchtime**, you're more likely to overeat in the evening, when you are much less likely to be active.

What we eat can determine the degree of post-lunch drowsiness we experience. High-GI carbohydrates such as sugar, white bread and white rice produce a rapid rise in blood glucose. As the body releases insulin to control the levels, the liver and muscles extract glucose from the blood and store it, making us feel tired. The release of insulin also prompts the brain to produce the chemicals serotonin and melatonin, which encourage sleep.

By contrast, wholegrain starchy foods have a lower GI, which causes blood-glucose levels to rise more gradually, avoiding energy peaks and troughs. Combining protein foods with complex carbohydrates tends to lower the GI of the meal overall. Result – less post-prandial sleepiness.

DRIVERS who

eat a large lunch are much more in danger of 'lane drifting' than those who have a light meal, according to research at the University of Loughborough in the UK. Before a long afternoon drive, one group of drivers was given a 1200kJ lunch while the others consumed three times as much fat and twice as much carbohydrate in a 3900kJ meal. After half an hour of driving, those who had eaten the larger lunch felt sleepier and were more likely to drift between lanes.

Lunching at home

As more of us work from home and others live longer in retirement, we could prepare a delicious hot or cold midday meal. But do we? Many of us simply grab what's there, barely pausing to enjoy it. Why not savour good, healthy food instead? The following ideas can be whipped up in 10–15 minutes:

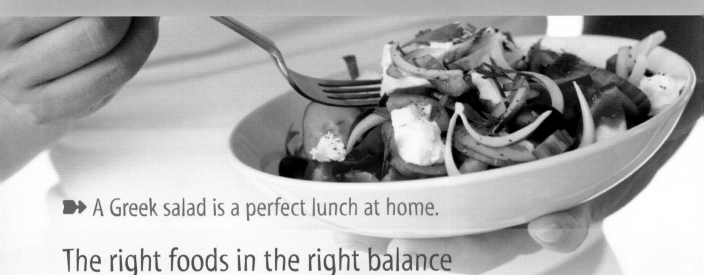

➡ A Greek salad is a perfect lunch at home.

The right foods in the right balance

A light meal based around lean protein and vegetables,
with a small to medium portion of starchy whole grains such as brown rice or grainy bread will
help you avoid post-meal drowsiness and keep up your energy levels throughout the afternoon.

A BALANCED HEALTHY LUNCH MIGHT INCLUDE:

- **A small portion of lean protein** – fish, meat or beans
- **At least one portion of fruit and one of vegetables**
- **Some wholegrain carbohydrates**, such as brown rice or wholegrain bread
- **A serving of dairy food**, such as ricotta cheese or yogurt
- **A small amount of 'good' fat**, such as the omega-3 fats in oily fish, olive oil, nuts or avocado

For women on a diet of 8,000kJ per day, a lunch that delivers around 2000–2500kJ should feel about right. On a
weight-loss diet of 6000kJ a day, lunch would be around 1500kJ. For men consuming the average daily amount of
10,000kJ, a healthy lunch would be 2500–3000kJ.

● SPEEDY MEDITERRANEAN-STYLE SALADS

Start with whatever vegetables and salad you have to hand and add leftover
cold meat, a hard-boiled egg or a can of tuna. Finish with a drizzle of olive
oil and balsamic vinegar, a sprinkling of sesame seeds, pine nuts or poppy
seeds, and serve with a slice of wholemeal bread. For variations, try:

➡ **Greek** chop up tomatoes, fetta, cucumber and red onion. Stir in a
splash of olive oil and a shake of dried oregano.

➡ **Italian** leave out the fetta, add mozzarella, some fresh basil and a small
amount of crushed garlic.

➡ **Spanish** use a little tasty manchego cheese and some grilled capsicum,
then top with a few olives.

Five rules for safe leftovers

Leftovers from the previous night's dinner can easily be reheated as they are or jazzed up with extra ingredients to make a tasty, nutritious and easy lunch.

1 Cover and cool them as quickly as you can, ideally within 90 minutes. If there's a large amount, separate into smaller portions. Once the food is cool, refrigerate immediately.

2 Use refrigerated leftovers within two days. Check your fridge is operating at the right temperature – below 5°C. If reheating leftovers, make sure they're piping hot all through.

3 Don't reheat leftovers more than once. Repeatedly warming food increases the amount of time it spends at the ideal temperature for bacterial growth. The longer the food is warm, the more bacteria are able to multiply.

4 Cool leftovers completely before freezing. For flavour they are best eaten within three months, but can safely be kept frozen longer.

5 Defrost leftovers completely either in the fridge or in a microwave. Frozen leftovers should be defrosted thoroughly before they are reheated. Defrost in the microwave or take them out the night before and let them defrost slowly in the fridge.

WE WASTE

an estimated 20 per cent of the food we buy – either on the plate from serving portions that are too large, from the pan by throwing out that 'last bit left', or directly from the fridge by throwing away out-of-date foods we haven't got around to eating.

● **FRITTATAS AND OMELETTES**

First whisk up the eggs and while they are cooking prepare your filling. Serve with crispy salad leaves and a squeeze of lemon juice.
● Fill an omelette with chopped ripe avocado and a small handful of grated mature cheddar. Or try crumbled fetta and sun-dried tomatoes.
● Fry sliced zucchini in a little olive oil and add to a frittata with leftover cooked vegetables and chopped mint.

● **QUICK SOUP**

It takes about ten minutes to steam vegetables, such as pumpkin, cauliflower or broccoli, then whizz them up in a blender with a dash of milk and some fresh herbs. Finish with a spoonful of low-fat crème fraîche or yogurt and a few grinds of black pepper. Try butternut pumpkin with sage; cauliflower with nutmeg; or classic pea and mint. When you have time, cook batches of soup and freeze in individual portions that can be quickly defrosted. You can avoid the salt and processing of canned varieties, and save money.

● **PANTRY STANDBYS**

Using pantry ingredients (*see* page 153) make a quick fish stew with canned tuna or salmon plus canned beans and tomatoes, or make a carton of soup healthier and heartier by adding leftover vegetables.

Lunch at work

Legally, Australian workers are entitled to a minimum 30-minute break for every five continuous hours worked. In practice most employers offer longer, so why are so many of us skipping lunch? Recent research has shown that only 30 per cent of Australian workers now take a lunch break and more than four million regularly miss lunch altogether. Increasingly, it seems, hectic schedules have pushed lunch to a back seat.

If your workplace provides a fridge and microwave, make use of them. Taking leftovers or home-made soup to reheat at work is an economical way to get a quick, warm and nourishing meal in the middle of the day. On days when you have nothing suitable, many supermarket convenience items, such as noodles and fresh or dried soups, are designed for people with busy lunchtimes. These may be useful if you're pushed for time, but check the labels carefully to avoid high levels of salt and fat.

Luscious lunch boxes

While leftovers can make a delicious and economical lunch, they won't always be available. When choosing other lunch-box foods, the challenge is to keep them healthy and interesting. Try out the 'speedy salads' from the 'Lunching at home' section on page 181 (taking dressing in a separate container so your salad stays crisp), or experiment with the following:

- Swap ordinary bread sandwiches for a tasty wrap or lightly toasted and filled pita bread.
- Prepare a mini buffet in separate small containers: slice a selection of carrots, capsicum, cucumber and celery to dip in hummus, plus a handful of grapes and another of nuts for dessert.
- Make a healthy vegetable pâté – mushrooms and lentils work especially well – and eat with breadsticks or carrot and red capsicum batons.
- Skinned roast chicken drumsticks in olive oil, lemon juice and chopped coriander; make enough for a couple of days and keep refrigerated. Eat with a small prepared salad.
- For a quick and easy dessert, chop fresh fruit into a container and top with low-fat yogurt.
- If you're making dessert the night before that can be eaten cold, make enough for lunch, too – a poached pear, for example, gently cooked in white wine and orange juice flavoured with star anise, or a baked apple, cored and filled with raisins, nuts and honey.

GET THE RIGHT GEAR

to keep food safe and whole until it is eaten – especially when no kitchen facilities are available. Invest in good-quality items, such as:

- Reusable plastic containers in different shapes and sizes for sandwiches, salads, nuts and fruit. Inflatable fruit carriers help to prevent bruising.
- Mini icepacks to keep yogurts and other foods cool.
- A reusable drinks bottle; some have a freezable central core to keep drinks cool.
- A vacuum flask for hot drinks or soup.
- A shorter, fatter food flask to carry hot food, such as pasta or soup, which can be eaten straight from the pot.
- A sturdy cool bag or cool box; buy this last so you can check it's big enough to take the other items.

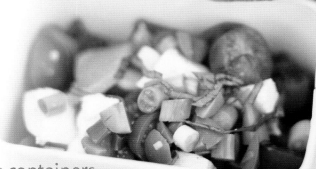

➤➤ It pays to invest in good-quality containers.

Try something different

TRY	WHY?	HOW?
Quinoa – a grain-like crop that looks a bit like couscous	It's a good source of protein and cooks in just 10 minutes.	Cook according to packet instructions and use in salads, in the same way you would rice or pasta. Try it with zucchini, fetta and red onion.
Walnuts and brazil nuts	Walnuts have been shown to help maintain flexible blood vessels. Just three brazil nuts provide your daily selenium requirement, boosting your immune system.	Chop and add to salads or yogurt. Or bake them into a cake, such as a carrot cake.
Sweet potatoes	Orange-fleshed varieties are rich in beta-carotene and are delicious roasted.	Chop into chunks and roast together with capsicum in olive oil. Add a little vinegar and toss with salad leaves.
Linseeds	A vegetarian source of omega-3 fatty acids.	Take a small container of seeds to sprinkle on top of yogurts and salads just before serving.

Spice them up – healthy, delicious sandwiches

Although variety is important at lunchtime, don't ignore the traditional sandwich – named after an 18th-century English aristocrat, John Montague, 4th Earl of Sandwich, a keen gambler who apparently ate meat between two slices of bread rather than tear himself away from the card table for a meal. Here are some tips on refreshing this lunchtime favourite:

- Try artisan breads – a seeded wholemeal loaf, or one with added nuts and cheese, or garlic and olives, or sun-dried tomatoes. The more nutritious your bread, the more nutritious your lunch will be.
- Branch out from the usual mayonnaise and mustard – use a chutney, relish or sauce. Try pesto with mozzarella and tomato, or pickled red cabbage with cold roast beef.
- Pack in more flavour by using strong cheeses such as stilton or gorgonzola, tasty vegetables such as sun-dried tomatoes, and peppery leaves such as rocket and watercress.
- Instead of tuna, try canned crab; it adds immunity-boosting zinc to your diet. Mix it with some chopped spring onions, a small amount of mayonnaise and a dab of Dijon mustard.
- Go 'light' with a carrot and raisin sandwich – peel and grate a carrot, add a few raisins, chopped mint and black pepper, and bind together with a dollop of hummus.

➡ Try pesto with mozzarella and tomato.

as good a source of omega-3 fats as fresh tuna.

Feeding children and teenagers

Coming up with healthy lunch boxes for children can be a challenge; their fussy eating habits combined with peer pressure from schoolmates to choose this or reject that food can make it hard to know what to provide. Most children don't eat healthily enough. One UK survey of children's lunch boxes showed that more than half contained sweets or chocolate and nearly half included a salty snack such as crisps.

While the quality of food in lunches provided by schools has been highlighted by campaigners such as TV chef Jamie Oliver, lunch boxes tend to slip under the quality-control radar. Some schools have adopted special policies aimed at encouraging parents to provide a nutritious packed lunch; these may include a ban on crisps, sweets or chocolate. Even schools without a specific policy often offer guideline recommendations. For a healthy everyday lunch box for your child, try to include:

- At least one portion of fruit and one portion of vegetables.
- Some meat, fish or other source of non-dairy protein such as lentils, kidney beans, chickpeas, or peanut butter (limit processed meats).
- A starchy food such as wholemeal bread, pasta, rice, couscous or potatoes.
- Dairy foods such as milk, cheese, yogurt or fromage frais.
- A drink, which could be low-fat milk or a yogurt drink, a smoothie or simply water.
- At least once a week try to include oily fish, such as salmon.

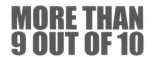

MORE THAN 9 OUT OF 10

Australian children consume too much saturated fat, 70 per cent have too much sugar, 90 per cent do not get enough vegetables, and nearly all eat too much salt, according to the Australian National Children's Nutrition and Physical Activity Survey. Similar results were found in a 2009 New Zealand survey.

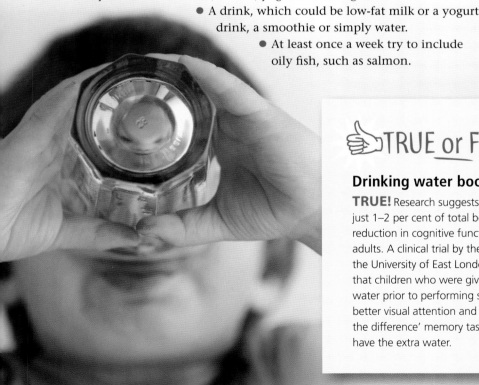

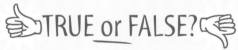

TRUE or FALSE?

Drinking water boosts concentration

TRUE! Research suggests that mild dehydration of just 1–2 per cent of total body weight can lead to a reduction in cognitive function in children and young adults. A clinical trial by the School of Psychology at the University of East London in the UK in 2009 showed that children who were given an additional drink of water prior to performing some tests had significantly better visual attention and ability to perform 'spot the difference' memory tasks than those who did not have the extra water.

Talk to them about good nutrition

As children reach their teens and become more independent, they want more control over what and where they eat. Nutritionally, this is an important time as the body is developing and maturing, so you have to give consistent, positive messages about food to help keep them on track.

If your teenager's school offers lunches, check the menu and encourage healthy choices. If you have to prepare packed lunches, find time to discuss what food is going into their lunch and why you don't want to include crisps, chocolate bars or sweet drinks. You may find you need to compromise between what you would ideally like them to have, and what they feel is 'cool' to eat in front of friends.

Many older teenagers are allowed to eat out of school at lunchtime. It may not be easy, but try to discuss what they are eating in cafés and fast-food restaurants and encourage them to make healthy choices. Make sure they have snacks containing fruits, vegetables and whole grains with them for breaks and after school.

Healthy lunch box swaps for kids (and great for grown-ups, too!)

INSTEAD OF ...	SWITCH TO ...
White bread and rolls	**Seeded bread, wholegrain mini rolls, wholegrain pita bread and wraps, oat-based breads and rolls.** If your children really don't like brown bread, try some of the 50:50 breads available – they are made with 50 per cent wholemeal flour but the taste and texture is more like white.
Fizzy drinks or juice	**Water, milk, smoothies yogurt drinks.**
Cakes	**Malt loaf or home-made muffins** with added fruit and seeds.
Chocolate mousse	**Live yogurt with chopped fruit** such as strawberries or grapes.
Biscuits and confectionery	**Nuts** (if allowed at school), **dried fruit, muesli bars** (but check that sugar content is not too high).
Crisps	**Plain popcorn** or, as an occasional treat, unsalted crisps.
No vegetables	**Some vegetables** – either in the sandwiches or in separate containers. Try sticks of bright red and orange capsicum, raw carrot, cucumber or crisp celery, with a little container of hummus as a dip.

    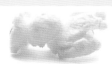

➡ Plain popcorn is a good substitute for crisps.

Eating out and about

Whether you're at work or shopping with friends, the options for eating out at lunchtime, particularly in a city centre, are more varied than ever. Upmarket sandwich shops, and sushi and noodle bars sit alongside the more familiar burger fast-food chains and traditional pubs or cafés. Yet it can be surprisingly difficult to find a lunch that is both healthy and tasty.

Head for somewhere that makes it easy for you to control your choices. A sandwich, sushi or noodle bar may be a better bet than a pizza or burger outlet. But if your willpower can resist the pull of French fries, fast-food outlets are increasingly offering healthier options, such as salads or baguette sandwiches. If you know in advance where you are going, look online; outlets often give nutritional information on their websites.

Whether or not you have nutritional information to guide you, try to stick to healthy food choices from the menu, such as:

- Sandwiches with fillings based on vegetables and lean protein, rather than fillings higher in saturated fats and mayonnaise.
- A salad on the side, rather than chips.
- Meats that are grilled, rather than deep-fried in crispy coatings.
- Tomato- and vegetable-based sauces, rather than creamy and cheese-based ones.
- Extra portions of fruit and vegetables in side dishes and salads.
- Wholegrain varieties of breads, rice and pasta whenever possible.
- The 'daily specials' – often freshly made from whatever is in season, and can make a tasty change from restaurant staples.
- If you are having a dessert, opt for fruit salad or sorbet.

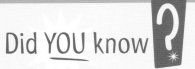

Did YOU know ?

New menu info could save you kilos

Restaurants in New York, USA, already have kilojoule information on display. A survey of more than 15,000 New Yorkers published in the *British Medical Journal* showed that while only 15 per cent of restaurant-goers actually read the kilojoule information, these diners ate around 400kJ fewer than their less observant counterparts. If you like to lunch out once a week, every Friday from work for example, that could save you more than 20,000kJ over the year.

➡ **Choose tomato-based sauces, rather than creamy or cheese ones.**

TRY TO AVOID:
- Processed meats such as sausages, burgers and meat pies.
- Lunchtime drinking, which can make you drowsy. Or minimise the effect by adding sparkling or soda water, or a low-kilojoule mixer.
- Creamy desserts and cheesecakes.

Putting healthy lunch swaps into practice

INSTEAD OF ...	CHOOSE ...	BECAUSE ...
BLT sandwich	Salmon and watercress sandwich	The unhealthy saturated fats in the bacon are replaced by healthy omega-3 fats in the salmon. Watercress provides vitamin C and calcium, and research suggests it may help reduce cancer risk.
Meatball panini	Roast chicken and tomato panini	Saturated fat is reduced by 7g per portion.
Standard salad mains	Order the same salad but with a dressing of lemon juice and no croutons	Adding lemon juice or balsamic vinegar to a salad instead of a cream- or oil-based dressing saves about 800kJ – and removing the croutons saves another 800kJ. Don't be afraid to ask: most good restaurants are more than willing to oblige.
Spaghetti carbonara	Seafood linguine	Switching from the creamy sauce can save 1200kJ a portion; a further benefit is extra zinc and iodine in the seafood.

➡ A salmon sandwich is a good alternative to a BLT.

It's only a bargain if it's something you want

Many lunch venues now offer meal deals, from 'go large' options to 'eat as much as you like' buffets. What might seem like a good deal for your wallet might not be such a good deal for your health. Before buying or refilling your plate, stop to consider whether you would order or eat that amount of food if you had to pay for it. Opting to 'size-up' for just a dollar might sound like a bargain, but if you don't need a soft drink equivalent to two cans of cola or an extra-large portion of fries (and let's face it, not many of us do), then you're wasting that dollar as well as risking your health.

In contrast, some stores offer healthy meal deals that can include sushi, smoothies, salads and fresh fruit. These are worth seeking out if you're satisfied with the quality of the food.

Perfect picnics

Sunny days and warm weather tempt us outdoors for a different kind of lunch, but traditional picnic foods, such as sausage rolls and meat pies, are often laden with fat and salt. Instead, why not take a little time to put together some healthy picnic treats using the vibrant array of fresh summer produce?

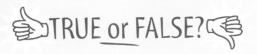

TRUE or FALSE?

Most food poisoning occurs in summer

TRUE! Just under half of reported cases of food poisoning caused by salmonella or campylobacter occur between in the summer months. So be extra careful with food hygiene as the weather warms up.

HERE ARE SOME IDEAS:

- Pull out the soft centre of a large ciabatta loaf and stuff it with roasted capsicum, zucchini and eggplants with a dash of olive oil and a few chopped fresh herbs.
- Quiches don't have to be stodgy. Make your own using 50:50 wholemeal and plain white flour for the pastry. Fill with plenty of vegetables.
- Tabbouleh makes a delicious, healthy picnic salad. Place the burghul in a small pan, cover with water and boil for 10 minutes or as directed on the packet. Add chopped parsley, mint, tomatoes and red onion, and flavour with lemon juice and olive oil.
- Make a salsa. Mix diced tomatoes, avocado, red onion, a little finely chopped garlic and chilli (fresh, dried or ground), then add a sprinkle of ground coriander or cumin, chopped fresh coriander, some diced mango or red capsicums and some cooked black-eyed beans for extra protein.

Keep it safe

Just like everyday packed lunches, picnics need to be kept cool to ensure the ingredients are fresh and safe to eat. Use a purpose-made cool box with freezer packs or frozen juice cartons. Add ice to flasks of cold drinks and avoid leaving your picnic in a hot car for too long.

Once outdoors, keep the food in the shade and covered until you are ready to eat. Take an antibacterial gel or hand wipes, and at the end of the day dispose of any leftover perishable food which has warmed up.

For more advice on eating out and takeaways, see Part 5, pages 300–307.

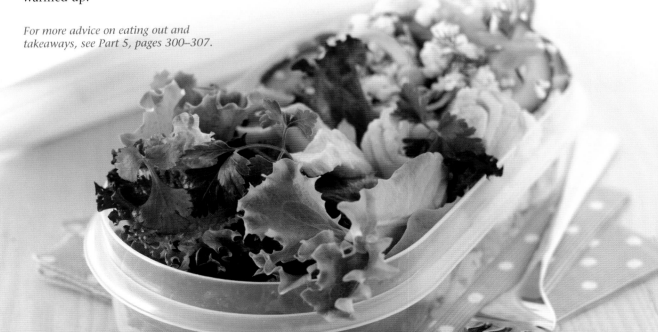

7 Dinner time

For most of us dinner is the key meal of the day. It's usually the one we spend most time preparing, whether eating alone or sharing with family or friends. Make it nutritious but — for your health's sake — not the most high-joule meal of the day.

Whatever time we eat it, our last meal is often the one we enjoy most as we relax in the evening after work or play. It can be a stimulating social and family meal although we may be so tired we simply eat and slump in an armchair and watch TV. Tempting as that can be, it's not a recipe for good health. Nor is regularly eating a large meal late at night when there's little time to digest it or burn off the energy consumed.

3–4 HOURS

before bedtime is the best time to eat your evening meal to avoid digestive problems that can keep you awake. If you are hungry at bedtime, a small snack combining carbohydrates and protein, such as a glass of milk with a banana or an oatmeal cracker can encourage sleep.

Planning ahead

It takes a little effort to eat healthily every evening but planning menus and shopping is time well spent. It gives an opportunity to think about the variety of foods and nutrients in your diet overall. It helps you avoid buying more food than you need, saving you money and cutting out waste. Perhaps the greatest benefit of all is it helps the week run more smoothly, reducing at least one area of potential daily stress.

First, find a system that works best for you. Some people like to plan in advance precisely what they will eat each day of the week and follow set recipes; others prefer a more free-flowing approach depending on what is in the fridge and how much time they have available. If you're cooking for a family on a busy schedule and depend on one big weekly shop, the more structured approach can be the easiest.

You may need to ask yourself the following sort of questions:
➡ **What's already in the fridge that needs using up?**
➡ **What's in the freezer?** If there are key staples in there, such as chicken or salmon, work them into your menu plan.
➡ **Where is everyone this week?** When will the family be home together, and when will you need food ready at different times?
➡ **Which days are you going to be most pressed for time?**
➡ **Who can help cook and take charge on certain days?**

As you plan, try to keep in mind the balance of foods on the Healthy-Eating Plate (*see* page 120) and at each meal include:

- **Good-quality lean protein** – such as fish, turkey, lamb, beef, pork, eggs and legumes.
- **Plenty of vegetables** – fresh, frozen and occasionally canned – for their fibre, vitamins, minerals and other plant nutrients.
- **Starchy carbohydrates** – potatoes, sweet potatoes, pasta, rice and noodles. Use wholegrain products wherever possible.

Dessert is not essential every night, but it is an opportunity to increase the amount of fruit in the diet and to include a portion of dairy foods (check the sugar content of low-fat products). At dinner, you should also:

- **Eat fish** – have at least one portion a week of oily fish such as salmon, sardines, trout or tuna.
- **Eat regular portions of nuts and seeds**.
- **Experiment with new recipes** – it doesn't need to take hours or be overly complicated, but trying something new one night a week will help fend off menu fatigue. It can also help you to build up a repertoire of quick, tasty, easy-to-cook meals.
- **Avoid eating processed meats too frequently** – bacon or chorizo are best used occasionally in small amounts to add flavour to other dishes, such as beany stews and soups.

Did YOU know ?

Most of us still eat together

Despite widespread impressions of isolated eating habits due to social changes, such as long working hours, afterschool activities and computers and TVs in bedrooms, the fact is that most people in Australia and New Zealand still eat dinner with other members of the household. A 2008 survey by the Future Foundation for Kellogg's found that 58 per cent of those questioned ate their evening meal with other members of the household, while in households with children 82 per cent ate dinner together most of the time.

$1.3 BILLION

is what Australians spend each year on ready-made meals, according to food industry figures. That's 65,000 tonnes of food! The market for ready meals is growing, as advertising convinces consumers that they don't have time to cook healthy meals for themselves.

Mapping out your menu

Jot down ideas for the main meal each day. Remember to include vegetables and serving ideas, or you may forget them on your shopping list. Then cross-check your plan with the list on page 191.

To avoid waste, leave at least one meal 'free flow' to use up leftovers or food from the freezer or pantry. Cook double the amount of a dish when you have the time, freezing what you don't need immediately.

Healthy meals in minutes

Some days, time pressures make it harder than usual to provide a healthy evening meal. Try these time-saving ideas for super-fast dinners:

● **Stir-fry saviours** – anything goes. Stir-fry thin strips of meat or fish and set aside. Finely chop some vegetables, garlic and ginger and cook in the same pan for a couple of minutes, then tip the meat or fish back in for a final warm through. Season and serve with egg or rice noodles, which cook in 5 minutes or less.

● **Fish dinners** – soft white fish such as ling and snapper can be grilled in minutes. Add toppings or extra flavour such as lemon and parsley or pesto.

● **'No-cook' dinners** – with cooked chicken from the deli you can whip up a quick Caesar salad. Put crispy iceberg or cos lettuce in a bowl, cut the chicken into bite-sized pieces and toss onto the lettuce with ready-made croutons, plus a few anchovies if you like. Top with parmesan shavings and a drizzle of low-fat Caesar dressing, and serve with fresh wholemeal bread. Experiment with different ingredients and recipes.

● **Dress up a ready meal** – don't do this often, but ready meals can help when things get hectic. Use them as a base, but reduce their total salt and fat and add nutrients by adding, for instance, extra steamed broccoli to broccoli and stilton soup, more kidney beans and chopped tomatoes to a ready-made chilli con carne, or extra toppings to a pizza, such as sun-dried tomatoes, mushrooms or artichoke hearts, all served with a large, colourful side salad.

➠ Nutritious stir-fries make super-quick dinners.

Dinner for one

Across the world, people are living alone in ever-increasing numbers, which means that many of us are cooking for one. It has advantages – you can eat what and when you like, regardless of other people's preferences or routines. On the other hand, it can be hard to drum up the motivation to cook a nutritious meal.

There can be practical difficulties, too. Most recipes are designed to serve four so must be cut down, although you may be able to save some for the next day or freeze it for a later date. Some recipe books specialise in single servings, so it's worth seeking these out or looking online.

Many supermarkets now stock single pre-wrapped portions of meat and fish, plus ready meals and soups in smaller sizes. Better still, buy loose fresh food, so you can have any size or quantity you like. A local butcher will be happy to provide single servings and you can usually select how much fresh produce you need. Here are some easy and delicious ideas for main courses and desserts for one:

➧ **Grilled lamb chops with baba ganoush** – cut an eggplant in half lengthwise, sprinkle with olive oil and black pepper, and roast it. Then scoop out the soft flesh and mash it with a teaspoon of tahini, crushed garlic and juice of half a lemon. Grill two lamb chops under a hot grill then squeeze over the juice from the other half of lemon and serve. Any leftover baba ganoush makes a tasty lunch with toasted pita bread.

➧ **Roasted fillet of trout and new potatoes** – put baby new potatoes in a dish with a little olive oil and roast for 15–20 minutes. Add cherry tomatoes, artichokes and the trout fillet and roast for a further 15 minutes. Sprinkle with shredded basil and balsamic vinegar to serve.

➧ **Baked figs** – set fresh figs in a small ovenproof dish, cut a cross into the top of each and drizzle with honey. Just before they're done, sprinkle a crushed amaretto biscuit on top.

Pantry main courses:

Using some of your pantry stocks and home-grown herbs (*see* pages 152–153), you can also whip up delicious dishes such as the following:

● **Tomato-poached fish with basil** – lightly fry chopped onion and garlic in olive oil. Add a can of chopped tomatoes, black olives and your choice of fish – white fish or canned tuna both work well. Season with black pepper and a little tabasco or paprika and simmer until the fish is cooked. Serve with baby potatoes (these can be added to the simmering mixture to cook before the fish if you like) or pasta, plus a vegetable or salad.

● **Risotto** – soften onions, leeks or spring onions with finely chopped garlic in a little olive oil. Put stock in a pan to heat through. Add risotto rice to onions or leeks and stir to coat the grains. Add the hot stock a ladle at a time, allowing it to be absorbed before adding the next. Leftover cold meat or ham can be cut into small pieces and stirred into the rice towards the end of cooking, together with frozen peas or corn. Heat through and serve with grated parmesan, fresh parsley and a side salad.

Family favourites the healthy way

Traditional favourite ...

... with a healthy twist

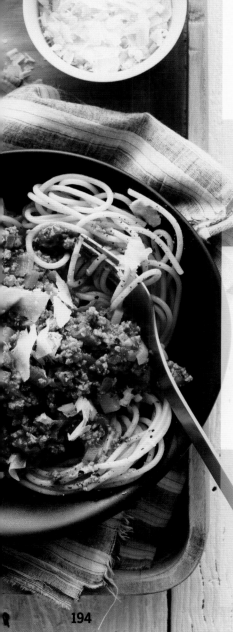

➡ SPAGHETTI BOLOGNESE

Sneaking in some extra vegetables to your Bolognese boosts nutrients and helps your money go further. Use good-quality lean minced beef to reduce the saturated fat. At the end of cooking leave to settle for a few minutes and skim off any excess fat with a spoon.

Fry chopped onion, garlic, minced beef and chopped mushrooms in a little olive oil. Add a couple of cans of tomatoes and tomato puree, and 3–4 large peeled and grated carrots (they won't be noticed once it's cooked). Season with black pepper, dried oregano and a couple of bay leaves, and simmer until cooked. Remove the bay leaves and serve with wholemeal spaghetti.

➡ FRIED CHICKEN & CHIPS

Simply removing the skin from chicken and baking, rather than frying, halves the kilojoules. Chips made with sweet potatoes add beta-carotene, vitamins C and E, plus minerals – potassium, manganese and iron.

Skin the chicken, top with lemon, garlic and a little olive oil, then bake in the oven. Cut sweet potatoes into wedges, coat with olive oil and roast for 30–40 minutes. Serve with a vegetable such as peas, beans or broccoli, or with a side salad.

➡ SHEPHERD'S PIE

Onions, diced carrots and peas are traditional in shepherd's pie, but mushrooms also work well. For extra nutrition and bulk, add a can of black-eyed beans – or put dried beans or lentils to soak the night before and cook them while preparing the rest of the dish.

Brown lean minced lamb and onions, then add diced carrots, peas and mushrooms. Add a little lamb stock and flour to thicken, and season with black pepper. Stir in the cooked black-eyed beans. Put into an ovenproof dish and top with mashed potato – use a dash of olive oil instead of butter and wholegrain mustard rather than salt. Cook in a warm oven for 40 minutes until golden-brown on top.

➡ BEEF IN RED WINE

Traditionally, this rich French dish is made with onions, garlic, red wine, beef and mushrooms. You can make it healthier by adding more vegetables; the added bulk means you can use a little less meat.

Prepare in the usual way but, for four people, add around 250g each of baby carrots, diced parsnips and mushrooms with the wine and bouquet garni. About 30 minutes before the casserole is ready, stir in 200g fresh or frozen broad beans. Serve with a sprinkling of fresh chopped parsley.

Creative carbohydrates

Stuck in a rut with baked potatoes and pasta? Try some of these alternatives for a tasty change:

- **Sweet potatoes** – scrub and bake whole as an alternative to regular baked potatoes. Delicious with vegetable ratatouille.
- **Burghul or quinoa** – these protein-boosting grains are great alternatives to rice or couscous. Boil according to packet instructions and use in salads, soups and casseroles.
- **Brown rice, wild rice and pearl barley** – both brown and wild rice have a nuttier flavour, are more nutritious than white rice and provide extra fibre. Brown takes longer to cook but can be used in most rice dishes. Wild rice (technically a grass) can be added to white or brown rice or used in salads. Pearl barley helps to thicken a soup and makes it healthier and heartier.
- **Beans and peas** – canned are convenient, but dried are cheaper. Both are good value and a nutritious way to bulk out meals. Try out recipes using chickpeas, butter beans, black-eyed beans, borlotti, haricot and kidney beans, edamame (young soybeans), lentils and split peas. Most dried beans need soaking overnight and pre-cooking before adding to stews. Some, such as kidney beans, must be boiled for the first 10 minutes of cooking to neutralise toxins. Check instructions on the packet. Red lentils cook quickly without soaking. Here are two quick bean ideas:

- Try edamame and borlotti beans in a salad with steamed green beans. Crumble over fetta cheese, drizzle with lemon juice and honey and finish with a sprinkling of poppy seeds.
- Make your own super-quick hummus. With a hand blender whizz up a can of chickpeas with a teaspoon of tahini paste, a drizzle of extra-virgin olive oil, a clove of garlic and a squeeze of lemon juice.

Pepping up vegetables

In the Western diet vegetables are often an afterthought. With such a variety of delicious tastes to enjoy and so many vital nutrients, they are far too important to be ignored. If you think vegetables are boring, try pepping them up in one of the following ways:

- Squeeze a little lemon juice over spinach or zucchini – a quick, simple way to enhance their flavour.
- Drizzle steamed broccoli with a little toasted sesame oil, a shake of soy sauce and a sprinkling of sesame seeds.
- Add softly fried spring onions to carrots. Or stir-fry thin sticks of carrot in a little oil, add a teaspoon of lemon juice and garnish with mint or dill.
- Stir-fry quartered brussels sprouts with pine nuts.

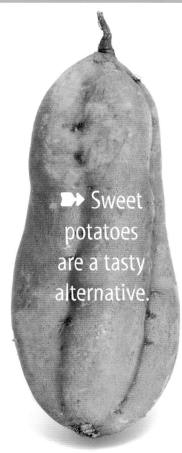

➡ Sweet potatoes are a tasty alternative.

FIBRE IS A VITAL part of our diets that may help to regulate cholesterol levels, prevent constipation and protect against bowel cancer. Most people don't eat enough of it. In Australia and New Zealand, average fibre consumption is 18–25g a day, which falls short of the recommended 30g.

Perfect everyday desserts

If you're catering for someone's sweet tooth, chocolate mousse isn't the answer. Nor is cheesecake; a typical serving of a supermarket product contains around half the recommended maximum daily intake of saturated fat. Try these quick and easy healthy options instead.

● DAIRY DELIGHTS

Low-fat dairy products, such as yogurt or fromage frais, have more bone-building calcium than full-fat versions.

➡ **Put some berries** such as raspberries or blueberries in the bottom of a small dish, add creamy plain yogurt and top with roasted almonds.

➡ **Try frozen yogurt** – a good low-fat, tasty alternative to ice cream. But supermarket products are often high in sugar. To make your own: tip a large 500ml tub of yogurt into a freezer-proof container and freeze for an hour. Remove and whip with a fork to break up the developing ice crystals, then put back in the freezer. Repeat two or three times until frozen.

➡ **Make a healthy rice pudding** – many recipes use cream but you can make tasty rice pudding using low-fat milk (or soy milk), lemon and a little sugar. Top with a spoonful of fruit compote.

A fruity end

Experiment with the many types of fruit available. All contain important micronutrients that boost the immune system. Try these:

● **Roast autumn fruits**, such as pears, plums and apples, with a splash of apple juice, a sprinkling of brown sugar and chopped dried apricots and walnuts. Serve with a small dollop of whipped ricotta or low-fat fromage frais.

● **Roasted pineapple** Peel a fresh pineapple with a sharp knife. Cut into wedges and remove the woody core. Arrange on a baking tin, drizzle with honey and a grated star anise, then roast until bronzed and slightly caramelised at the edges.

● **Fresh mango or red papaya**, sliced and served with a squeeze of lime juice.

● **Fruit crumbles and pies** – make them 'deep fill' to get in extra fruit and omit a pie's pastry base to reduce kilojoules and fat. Add oats and chopped walnuts to your crumble toppings.

30g OF WALNUTS

a day can improve 'endothelium-dependent vasodilation', according to the European Food Safety Authority. In lay terms, this means that eating walnuts helps to keep blood vessels 'stretchy', which is important for good circulation.

Did YOU know ?

A single meringue nest has only 250kJ

Meringues may look and taste indulgent, but being made of whisked-up eggwhites they are light for their size. Sweetened with a little sugar, then baked very slowly until crisp and golden on the outside, they store well in an airtight tin. With a little artistic use of yogurt and fruit for toppings, they make a great sweet treat.

Easy pantry sweets

- **Mini pavlovas** – top ready-made meringues with a scoop of sorbet or frozen yogurt and a few part-defrosted berries.
- **Smoothie sundae** – whizz frozen yogurt and berries together, then pour into a tall glass and top with crushed meringue or chopped toasted almonds.

Cooking for kids

If you are feeding children every day, you want them to eat the same foods as everyone else. To encourage them to try new flavours, the best approach is to offer a few different foods on the plate so they can leave some without a battle. The balance of foods and nutrients on the Healthy-Eating Plate (*see* page 120) is suitable for children from the age of about two years, although portions will be smaller than for adults. Before the age of five, children may need a slightly different diet. This should include:

- Whole milk between the ages of one and two years, then low-fat milk from two years. Skim milk does not provide as much vitamin A, which is important for the developing immune system.
- Small portions of energy-dense foods, as children need more energy for growth but only have small stomachs. Nuts, seeds, eggs and sardines are better options as they supply healthy fats, rather than salty crisps or chips and sugary cakes and biscuits. (Whole nuts should not be given to children aged under five because of the danger of choking.)
- Plenty of fruit and vegetables as snacks, as well as with meals. A portion for a child is about the size of their fist.

If you want to cook something special, make it colourful and fun. Here are a few ideas:

- **Macaroni cheese faces** – make a simple macaroni cheese more enticing and healthy by adding green broccoli hair, cucumber eyes and a smiley tomato mouth.
- **Pick-and-mix plates** – on a pretty plate set out small portions of diced cheese, sliced cucumber, chopped tomato and avocado, wholegrain crackers spread with cream cheese, a little pile of grapes or strawberries, some dried apple and other tasty ingredients. It's a good way to use up leftovers and the kids will feel they are getting a treat.
- **Invisible vegetables** – it's important to offer vegetables on the plate so children get used to having them, but if your child is picky about vegetables, take the pressure off by whizzing vegetables into pasta sauces and adding extra toppings to pizza.

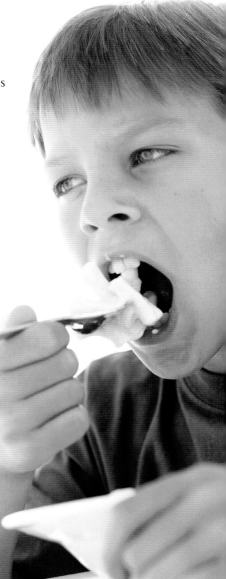

- **Melon boats** – cut ripe rockmelon or honeydew melon into wedges and remove the seeds; slice the fruit away from the skin and cut it into chunks, leaving in its skin 'boat'. Orange slices on toothpicks can make sails, topped with a grape or half a strawberry for the crow's nest. Younger children will need supervising when they dismantle it.

Home entertaining

Inviting guests for dinner doesn't have to mean hours of stressful slaving in the kitchen producing soufflés, complicated mains and rich sauces. Don't be afraid to serve up simple, healthy dishes made with good-quality ingredients and bold flavours. You'll find your guests enjoy this just as much as fancy finishes. As always, planning ahead is crucial:

- Find out in advance if any of your guests are vegetarian or have a food intolerance or allergy. *See* Special diets, page 200, for ideas on how best to cater for special requests.
- When and where can you shop? If possible make time to visit a good market, butcher or fishmonger to get the best, freshest main ingredients.
- Plan courses that complement each other and the season. If you have a creamy curry or rich casserole, for example, cheesecake is too heavy for dessert. A rich main course requires only a light starter and dessert. Use fresh seasonal produce when you can and see if your guests can taste the difference.
- Get your timing right – simpler food ready at a reasonable hour will go down far better than a flustered you serving elaborate dishes hours late.
- Don't panic if you get a bit behind. Set the table, light some candles, have some healthy nibbles (*see* page 174) and drinks ready and no one will notice if it takes a little bit longer for dinner to arrive.

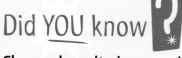

Did YOU know

Cheese doesn't give you nightmares

Perhaps the first and only research to test the old myth found that no study subjects suffered bad dreams after eating a small portion of cheese 30 minutes before bed. The British Cheese Board study involved 200 volunteers, 72 per cent of whom said they slept very well, after eating 20g of one of a variety of British cheeses. The dreams of the 67 per cent who could recall them, differed according to the cheese consumed. Stilton blue cheese eaters had the strangest dreams, ranging from talking soft toys to dinner party guests being traded for camels. Despite these findings, health professionals point out that too much cheese late at night may upset your digestion and make it difficult to go to sleep.

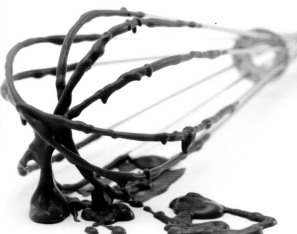

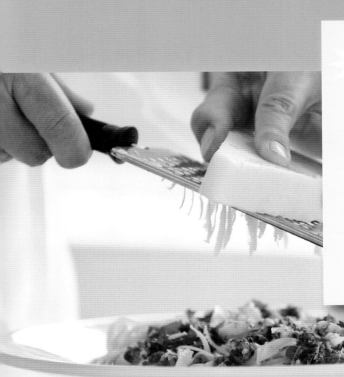

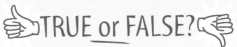

👍 TRUE or FALSE? 👎

The vegetarian option is always the healthiest

FALSE! You might think the vegetarian option will be healthier or lower in energy than the meat on the menu, but this isn't necessarily the case. Vegetarian restaurant meals normally contain more vegetables – so far so good – but they often also contain a lot of cheese, which pushes up the fat and kilojoule count. Think what the key ingredients in the dish might be before you order it. If you are not actually vegetarian, you might be better off with a meat option or grilled fish with new potatoes and a side order of vegetables.

Making healthy restaurant choices

In many ways, a healthy choice in a restaurant is much the same as a healthy choice at home: steamed or grilled rather than fried, especially deep-fried; boiled potatoes rather than chips or sautéed; tomato- or vegetable-based sauces rather than cheese or cream ones. The difference is that at home you control the amount of ingredients such as salt, cream, butter and oil, whereas chefs often use these liberally. Their primary concern is not health but flavour.

Whether you need to worry about this really depends on how often you eat out. If, like many of us, you dine out only occasionally for a celebration or special treat, don't worry – your meal is meant to be enjoyable, not a source of anxiety. Go ahead and have a main course with a cream sauce; just have a fruit dessert or a sorbet instead of a rich cream dessert. If you eat out regularly, you should try to choose the healthier options.

Always be wary of the extras: the nibbles to start, the bread rolls with butter, the side order of chips, coffee with cream, the cheeseboard, the after-dinner mints. Taken together, these can add up to almost a meal in themselves. Concentrate on your favourite courses. If you love savoury foods, have a starter and main course but skip dessert. If you have a sweet tooth, leave out the starter. If you like all the courses, choose lighter options, or go for a second starter as your main with a side of vegetables. You'll still enjoy all the different flavours and leave room for dessert.

SALT is used liberally in most restaurants, with one survey finding that some single dishes were providing more than 6g salt (the safe limit for a whole day). Nearly half of the surveyed meals were too salty, providing over fifty per cent of this safe limit.

For more cooking ideas, see Home-made is best, page 148. For further information about restaurant meals and takeaways, see Part 5, pages 300–307.

8 Special diets

For many people, adopting a particular diet is a lifestyle choice; for others it is a crucial matter of health. In every case, special diets can and must supply all the nutrients you need.

Your teenage daughter announces, out of the blue, that she is now a vegetarian. Or your young son has been diagnosed as lactose intolerant and can't drink milk, which you know is so important for bone development. Or your mother who'd complained of thirst and tiredness has been told she has type 2 diabetes. Problems like this confront someone every day and require rethinking and changing normal everyday meals.

Special diets mean different food choices for medical and ethical reasons. They may mean avoiding particular foods, or eating more of one type of food but should always supply all the nutrients required for good health.

Getting help for food-related problems

If you have symptoms that you think may be linked to what you eat, it is worth consulting reliable internet websites, but make sure you take advice from a health professional. An immediate diagnosis may not be possible, but an initial discussion of symptoms with a qualified expert can indicate a sensible way to investigate possible food links to feeling unwell. In some cases, short-term trial-and-error diets can help confirm a diagnosis.

Seeking professional dietary advice is especially important for people who are more vulnerable to deficiencies such as fast-growing young children, teenagers and the elderly. Pregnant women and people who are unwell or recovering from illness also need expert nutritional guidance.

Once there is a clear diagnosis, a registered dietitian can suggest a suitable special diet. Voluntary patient associations and appropriate charities can often supply additional advice and support.

➡ Lactose intolerance is just one of the problems that requires rethinking and changing normal everyday meals.

Not eating 'food with a face'

Even among those who still eat meat, an increasing number are choosing to eat less or have more meat-free meals. In the Western world, going one step further and becoming vegetarian is usually a health or ethical choice. By contrast, in countries such as India, millions of people are vegetarian for cultural and religious reasons dating back to ancient times. In the West, most vegetarians follow a lacto-ovo vegetarian diet, not eating any kind of meat, poultry, fish or shellfish, or products made from them (such as foods containing gelatine), while still eating eggs and dairy products. In India, eggs are often excluded, too.

Being vegan is a far more challenging and less common dietary choice, currently made by fewer than one per cent of adults in the West. As it cuts out all animal products from the diet – eggs, milk and all dairy products, not just meat – it demands more radical changes to a typical Western diet in order to maintain a healthy balance of nutrients.

Is being vegetarian healthy?

Provided that you eat a variety of foods that are good sources of particular nutrients, a vegetarian diet is perfectly healthy. In fact, it actually seems to offer health benefits. Many large surveys confirm that, compared to meat-eaters, vegetarians are less likely to be obese and also seem to be better protected from heart disease and the risk of certain kinds of cancer. Almost by definition vegetarians eat more plant-based foods,

ANIMAL-BASED FOODS are known as 'perfect' proteins because they supply all the 'essential' amino acids our bodies need, which many vegetable protein sources do not. But different vegetarian ingredients can be combined to make up a complete protein. Some traditional combinations from around the world do just that, such as rice and dhal from Indian cuisine, or beans and tortillas from Mexico.

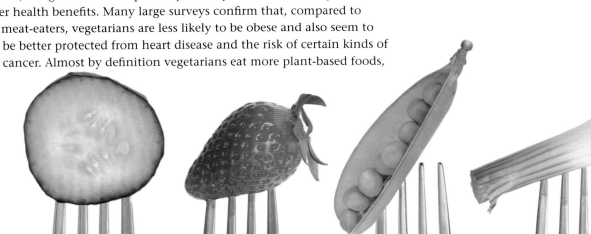

Different kinds of vegetarians

Semi-vegetarians ('meat avoiders') eat little or no red meat, but eat fish and poultry occasionally

Vegetarians (lacto-ovo) eat dairy products and eggs, but no meat, fish or poultry

Vegans eat no foods derived from animal sources. This means no meat, fish, poultry, dairy, eggs, honey, gelatine or any foods containing such ingredients

Fruitarians – raw food diet eat only raw and dried fruits, nuts and seeds and this is linked to having higher intakes of fibre, antioxidants and some vitamins and minerals. Also, vegetarian diets are usually lower in saturated fats, which are a risk factor for raised blood cholesterol levels.

But these health benefits depend on vegetarians knowing what nutrients are essential for health and what foods provide them, then making sure that these are included in their everyday diet. A diet based principally on pasta-and-tomato sauce, for example, or on other starchy foods that are low in nutrients and high in sugars and salt, is not a healthy way to be vegetarian. If a restaurant or supermarket food is labelled 'suitable for vegetarians', always check that it also supplies the nutrients – especially protein – that you need.

Getting enough protein, vitamins and minerals

In the past nutritionists were concerned that vegetarian diets might not contain enough protein. In most cases they contain enough for good health (about 10 per cent of energy) but tend to be lower in protein than the diets of meat-eaters. Lacto-ovo vegetarians get protein from eggs and

➡ A diet based principally on pasta and tomato sauce is not a healthy way to be vegetarian.

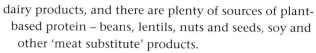

dairy products, and there are plenty of sources of plant-based protein – beans, lentils, nuts and seeds, soy and other 'meat substitute' products.

Vegetarians must also ensure they get adequate levels of all the necessary minerals and vitamins. Lower total intakes of iron, and the fact that iron is less well absorbed from plant foods, mean that vegans may not get enough. Adequate intake of calcium can also be a challenge for vegans.

Of the vitamins, B_{12} can only be found in animal-sourced foods, so vegans have to make sure that they eat products such as breakfast cereals that are fortified with this vitamin (or take supplements); vegetarians usually get their quota of B_{12} from dairy foods and eggs. Although vitamin D comes mainly from the action of sunlight on skin, vegetarians, especially vegans, may not get enough from food. Again, vitamin D–fortified foods and supplements are helpful.

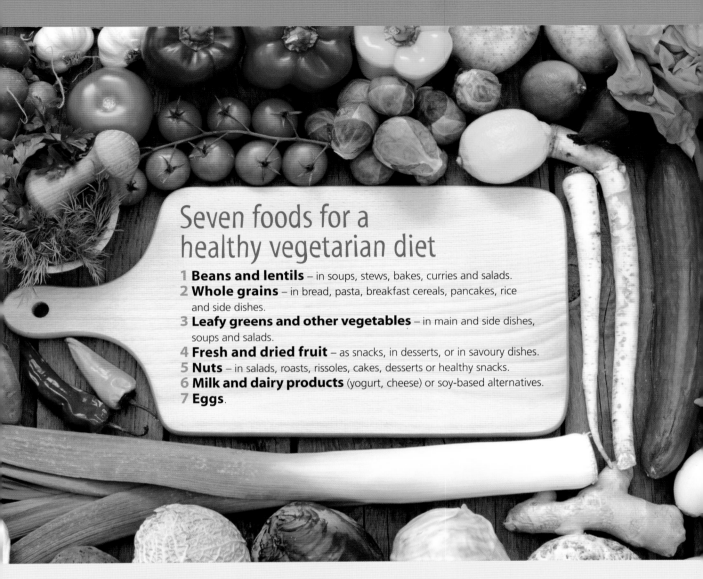

Seven foods for a healthy vegetarian diet

1 **Beans and lentils** – in soups, stews, bakes, curries and salads.
2 **Whole grains** – in bread, pasta, breakfast cereals, pancakes, rice and side dishes.
3 **Leafy greens and other vegetables** – in main and side dishes, soups and salads.
4 **Fresh and dried fruit** – as snacks, in desserts, or in savoury dishes.
5 **Nuts** – in salads, roasts, rissoles, cakes, desserts or healthy snacks.
6 **Milk and dairy products** (yogurt, cheese) or soy-based alternatives.
7 **Eggs**.

Vegan food sources of vital nutrients

Iron	Beans, peas, green leafy vegetables, dried fruit; fortified foods: breakfast cereals and bread.
Calcium	Beans, almonds, green vegetables such as kale and cabbage; fortified foods: soy milk, tofu and bread.
Vitamin B$_{12}$	Fortified foods: breakfast cereals, soy milk, rice milk and yeast extract (e.g. Marmite™).
Vitamin D	Fortified foods: breakfast cereals, soy milk, soy cheese and margarine.
Protein	Beans and lentils, nuts and seeds, soy products, cereals and meat 'substitutes' (e.g. Quorn™).

See also What if I'm vegetarian?, page 113.

Diet for diabetes: not so sweet

Diabetes is a major health concern in the world today. Some health experts already describe it as having reached epidemic proportions. At the end of 2012 there were almost 370 million people around the world with diabetes – by 2030 it is estimated that the number could exceed 500 million.

Having diabetes means your body doesn't produce enough insulin or cannot use it effectively; insulin is the hormone needed to transfer glucose from the blood to the muscles, liver and other tissues. If your diabetes is not identified and treated, carbohydrate foods in the diet cause glucose to build up to very high levels in the blood, which will make you excessively thirsty.

The condition also means that too little glucose gets transferred to the muscles, making you feel tired and weak. The aim of treatment, whether through diet, insulin or drugs, is to keep blood-glucose levels within a narrow normal range, avoiding both hyperglycaemia (high levels of blood glucose) and hypoglycaemia (low blood glucose).

➡ There are two types of diabetes:
- **Type 1 diabetes**, which used to be known as insulin-dependent diabetes, occurs when the body cannot produce insulin and requires life-long insulin injections to match the amounts of carbohydrate foods eaten.
- **Type 2 used to be known as adult-onset diabetes**, but today many young people are also developing the disease. It is caused by an insulin deficiency or insensitivity to the insulin made by the body and is often linked with being overweight. Drug treatments can either increase the production of insulin or enhance its effectiveness, but weight reduction and control of carbohydrates are central to managing the disease.

The 'what' and 'when' of eating carbohydrates

While people with diabetes should eat a normal balanced diet, the extra hurdle is learning 'glycaemic control' – how to balance the glucose-raising effects of eating carbohydrate foods with the glucose-lowering effects of insulin injections or hypoglycaemic drugs. Foods high in protein or fat have little effect on blood-glucose levels, but eating too much can lead to becoming overweight, which is a high risk factor for type 2 diabetes. Too much saturated fat also increases the risk of raised blood cholesterol levels, which are linked to cardiovascular disease.

However, when planning daily meals and snacks, if you have either type of diabetes, you'll need to be especially aware of what carbohydrates you are eating and when.

You should be able to achieve normal glucose levels with carbohydrate intakes ranging from 45 per cent to 60 per cent of total energy. Here's how to work it out:

1g carbohydrate = 16kJ
45–60 per cent of kilojoules = 3600–4800 kJ
(in a daily diet of 8,000kJ)

Within this range, individual fine-tuning depends on the type and timing of insulin or medication, and on factors such as levels of activity and the type of carbohydrate.

If you are on fixed dosages of insulin at specific times of the day you'll need a daily plan of carbohydrate intake timed to match the action of the insulin. If not, monitor your blood glucose and adjust your insulin intake to match the variations you find. It may take a while to balance insulin and carbohydrate to achieve long-term blood-glucose control; your dietitian will be able to help. If you're using insulin, make sure you have access to 'emergency' carbohydrate snacks to counter possible episodes of feeling weak and shaky due to very low levels of blood glucose (hypoglycaemia).

You'll need to learn about the glycaemic effect of foods – that is, the rate at which they increase blood-glucose levels measured by the glycaemic index (GI). Some carbohydrate foods, such as wholegrain cereals, beans and many vegetables, are described as low GI because they cause blood glucose to increase only slowly after eating. Others, such as potatoes, white bread, fruit juices and sweets, are high GI because they cause a rapid rise in blood glucose; sweet foods are not always higher GI than starchy foods.

Can diabetics eat sweet foods?

The short answer to this is yes, in moderation. If you're diabetic, you can consume some sugar-containing foods, as long as most carbohydrates in the diet comes from starchy, preferably high-fibre foods. The use of kilojoule-free sweeteners does not affect blood glucose levels. Nutritive sweeteners (such as fructose or sorbitol) have some effect and consuming too much of them can also cause diarrhoea or flatulence.

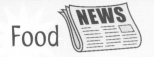

Food NEWS

A restricted diet offers hope

In a 2011 UK study, 11 volunteers with type 2 diabetes followed a diet of just 2500kJ a day, made up of diet drinks and non-starchy vegetables. After eight weeks, the group had lost an average 15.3kg each and all had recovered a normal ability to make insulin; seven retained this ability three months later after returning to a regular healthy diet. 'This is a radical change in understanding type 2 diabetes ... we have shown that we can reverse the condition,' said Professor Rod Taylor of Newcastle University, who led the trial. But such an extreme diet should only ever be undertaken under medical supervision.

TEA-DRINKERS
may have some protection against type 2 diabetes. Studies comparing rates of diabetes in different countries report a correlation between drinking lots of black tea and a lowered risk of type 2. Data analysis seems to show that three or more cups of tea a day provides some protection, but a causal link has not yet been established and more research is required.

No gluten for one-in-a-hundred

Around one per cent of adults in industrialised countries have coeliac (pronounced SEE-lee-ak) disease, meaning they have to avoid gluten, a protein found in wheat, barley and rye. For people affected, eating foods containing gluten provokes an autoimmune reaction in which the body's immune system attacks its own tissues. The damage is done to the lining of the gut, so food is poorly digested, reducing nutrient absorption. Untreated, the disease can lead to malnutrition and sometimes intestinal cancer.

The symptoms of coeliac disease can vary widely between people, but the usual problems are indigestion, bloating and diarrhoea. Sufferers often feel unwell or lethargic after eating and may experience unintended weight loss. There are many possible diagnoses for these general symptoms, so confirmation tests are needed to be sure that the trigger is gluten. Blood tests to identify heightened levels of tTGA (tissue transglutaminase), an enzyme produced by damaged gut cells, is a reliable predictor of coeliac disease. A biopsy showing damage to the gut is the 'gold standard' method of diagnosis.

Treatment for coeliac disease is effective and simple: eat no gluten. But if you are diagnosed, you'll soon discover that what is simple in theory can prove difficult in the real world of restaurants, canteens and everyday life. Foods may not be clearly labelled, and family and friends who cook for you may not be completely aware of what 'gluten-free' implies. Treatment must also be life-long, so that means saying goodbye to wheat- or rye-based bread – although gluten-free pastas and pizzas can now be found.

A gluten-free life

When planning a gluten-free diet, you must first become familiar with the huge variety of healthy, nutrient-rich foods that can be eaten. The good news is that most fresh foods are fine – fresh fruit and vegetables, meat and fish, beans and lentils, nuts and seeds. Just make sure they have not been battered, sauced or otherwise prepared with ingredients containing gluten. Rice and potatoes are gluten-free and can fill the gap in starchy foods, or try buckwheat or millet for a change. Cornflour, rice flour, potato flour or chickpea flour can take the place of staple wheat flour.

Processed foods present more of a challenge. Some of the 'do-not-eats' are fairly obvious: no bread, biscuits, doughnuts, scones, cakes, pasta, pizza or most breakfast cereals. Avoiding these is a start but it's not enough, as very small quantities of wheat, barley or rye are in many foods, often as components of other ingredients. Studying food labels will reveal surprising examples of 'hidden' gluten ingredients, so label-reading is an essential skill that must be mastered.

MOST BEERS are not gluten-free because of residues of barley from the brewing process, but if a beer contains fewer than 20ppm (parts per million) gluten, it may be described as gluten-free. A few gluten-free beers are labelled in this way, so a visit to the pub may now allow coeliacs a wider choice of drinks.

Is a food suitable for my gluten-free diet?

- The first thing to look for is a gluten-free logo or statement on the label. The 'crossed grain' logo of the various national coeliac support societies indicates foods are safe for coeliacs, and some retailers have their own symbols. The health foods aisle in large supermarkets almost always include gluten-free items, often labelled 'gluten-free' or 'very low gluten'. In Australia and New Zealand, this is defined as 'no detectable gluten', whilst overseas the definition is 'less than 20ppm' (parts per million). To simplify labelling and reduce confusion, coeliac societies have been campaigning FSANZ to change local standards in line with the international definition.
- The next check is the ingredient list – is there any hint of a wheat, barley or rye component in the food? Sometimes it is difficult to decide, because components of an ingredient such as 'spice mix' may contain small quantities of wheat flour.
- The final check is for 'allergen alert' boxes. The presence of an ingredient containing gluten is one of 14 food categories that most manufacturers now declare outside the ingredient list. Allergy-alert information is not a legal requirement, but it is quite common on food labels today.

Recent years have seen a dramatic increase in the number of products labelled fully and often specifically as gluten-free, so being diagnosed as coeliac is less of a burden today than in the past. And you can always ensure that food is gluten-free when you buy and cook your own fresh ingredients. If you are a diagnosed coeliac you might also be advised to take multi-vitamin supplements because at times you may not be absorbing enough of certain nutrients.

COELIACS CAN EAT OATS

– that's usually TRUE. Oats do contain gluten, but of a kind called avenin that appears to be well tolerated by nearly all coeliacs, showing no evidence of causing damage to cells in the gut wall. But because oats are often milled in plants that handle other grains and cereals, they carry a high risk of 'contamination' with gluten from other ingredients. Advice is to avoid oats immediately after diagnosis, then ensure that any oats consumed are labelled 'gluten-free'.

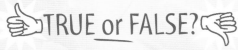

➡ Many gluten-free products such as rice pasta can now be found.

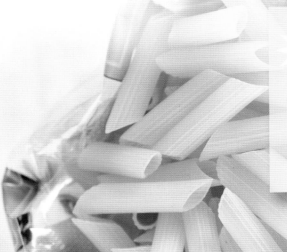

👍 TRUE or FALSE? 👎

'Wheat-free' means the same as 'gluten-free'

FALSE! Some wheat-free products are gluten-free, but others might contain components of rye, barley or spelt, all of which contain gluten. Always double-check items labelled wheat-free and if in doubt, leave them out.

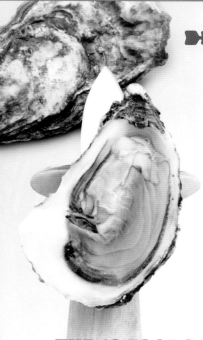

Adverse reactions to food

Sometimes, however much you like a food, when you eat it you experience a range of unpleasant symptoms. It may be difficult to establish if a food reaction is to blame and if so, which food is the culprit.

Adverse reactions to food are labelled as either a food intolerance or a food allergy. An intolerance is not a dislike; generally it means a physical adverse reaction to one of the natural or added chemicals in the food. Surveys indicate that up to 25 per cent of people in Australia and New Zealand believe they have some kind of food intolerance. Food allergy is a specific kind of food intolerance where a food protein sparks an abnormal, sometimes dangerous, immune response in the body. It is estimated that allergies occur in one to two per cent of adults, and four to six per cent of children in Australia and New Zealand.

THE 10 FOODS

known to cause allergic or intolerant reactions that must be listed on ingredient labels in Australia and New Zealand are, in alphabetical order:

- Eggs
- Fish
- Milk
- Peanuts
- Royal jelly
- Sesame seeds
- Shellfish
- Soybeans
- Tree nuts (including almonds, cashews, walnuts)
- Wheat and any other cereals containing gluten

When milk isn't good for you

The most common form of adverse reaction to milk and other dairy foods is lactose intolerance. To digest milk the gut must break down milk sugar (lactose), and to do that an enzyme known as lactase is required. Levels of lactase are high in the guts of infants, for whom milk is the only food, but in most adults levels of this enzyme are much lower. When large amounts of milk are consumed, the lactose cannot be absorbed and passes undigested into the colon. Here it gets fermented by gut bacteria producing symptoms of bloating, gut pain and diarrhoea.

Lactose intolerance can be diagnosed with a hydrogen breath test. As symptoms depend on the amount of lactose consumed, you will usually be advised simply to reduce the amount of milk and fresh dairy foods you consume, although it may be necessary to exclude them. The tiny amounts present in hard cheese do not seem to cause adverse reactions.

Infants and very young children can also be allergic to the protein in cow's, goat's or sheep's milk. This can affect the gut (producing symptoms such as vomiting and diarrhoea), the skin (atopic eczema, dermatitis) and the respiratory system (wheezing, rhinitis). Once the allergy is diagnosed, all dairy products must be avoided. For infants, there are suitable replacement formula milks made with soy protein or casein/whey hydrolysate. Some children 'outgrow' the allergy and, by the time they reach school age, milk may no longer produce the adverse symptoms.

Problems with nuts

Peanut and nut allergies are less common, but reactions to even the smallest amount of nut can be severe. Symptoms can include urticaria (skin rash) and asthma. Extreme reactions can be life-threatening, causing shock and swelling of the tongue and throat. People diagnosed with these allergies must ensure that they eat nothing containing peanuts or nuts. Although they may be allergic to one or the other, the advice is often to avoid both.

One ingredient to look out for is peanut oil, sometimes called groundnut oil, in cakes and sauces. Check food labels carefully. The oil is also used in many Chinese, Thai and Indonesian, and some West African meals, so these are 'high risk' areas where you must make sure that dishes are peanut-free. Research suggests that peanut allergies, which are commoner, occur more often in children and tree nut allergies occur more often in adults.

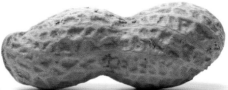

Did YOU know ?

We couldn't always digest milk

Prehistoric Europeans couldn't drink milk, according to UK archaeologists. The gene which helps to break it down developed in the population with the advent of dairy farming. Today more than 90 per cent of Europeans have the gene. Yet, the Western life-long love of milk is an exception rather than the rule. In most parts of the world children stop drinking milk when weaned, just like the young of other mammals.

Detox diets

The gossip magazines frequently report that celebrities attribute their good looks and 'glowing' health to detox (detoxification) diets. These diets are very restrictive, with unusual food combinations. Most involve a fast or semi-fast for the body and the 'flushing out' of toxins by drinking lots of water and herbal teas. Detox diets contain no protein foods nor processed 'junk' foods; the menu is made up of mainly salads and raw vegetables. Short-term 'purification' programs can also include saunas, laxatives or colon cleansing.

Do they work?

The difficulty in assessing such diets is that there is no real definition of 'detoxification'. It's true that if some substances we consume or produce accumulated to elevated levels, they could indeed make us feel very ill. But we have certain body organs, especially the liver, kidneys and colon, whose day-to-day job is to keep toxin levels within a normal range. So, are these diets in any way more effective? Beyond excluding alcohol – one of the most commonly consumed 'toxins' – and supplying plenty of fibre to stop you feeling congested and constipated, they don't seem to have any special powers to boost the rate of elimination of adverse substances.

A few days of detox dieting can certainly produce temporary weight loss, but whether the body is less 'toxic' as a result of following them has not been proven. They are not advised for more than a few days because they are restricted and contribute little energy, and so can make you feel weak and tired.

9 Effective weight control

As obesity rates soar, diets have become big business. But weight control isn't just about dieting. It's about finding a healthy eating and activity regime that works for you long term, keeping you trim, feeling well and full of zest for life.

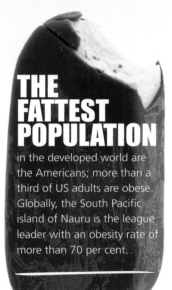

THE FATTEST POPULATION in the developed world are the Americans; more than a third of US adults are obese. Globally, the South Pacific island of Nauru is the league leader with an obesity rate of more than 70 per cent.

More of us are getting fatter year on year. At its simplest, extra weight places greater strain on your joints, heart and lungs. At a more complex level, excess fat can cause an imbalance in your body's biochemistry, now linked to a number of serious disorders including type 2 diabetes, high blood pressure, heart disease, stroke and certain cancers. As national weight figures go up, so does the incidence of these disorders.

With weight gain your risk of psychological issues such as poor self-esteem and depression increases, as does infertility and impotence, and problems sleeping, breathing and moving. Exercise becomes more difficult and the sheer pleasure of physical activity is often lost.

The bottom line: being overweight increases the chances of suffering poor health and having a lower quality of life. But it doesn't have to be that way. If you're determined, weight – however great – can be controlled.

How did we get here – what's changed?

So what's gone wrong?

- **Sedentary lives and fatty, sugary foods** We are all sitting more. Surveys in 2012 found that 67 per cent of Australian adults, and nearly 50 per cent of New Zealanders, were sedentary or had inadequate levels of exercise. At the same time we are eating far more sugary snacks and high-fat takeaways, ready meals and convenience foods.
- **Haywire hormones** Excess weight can affect sleep; poor sleep may then lead to further weight gain as it interferes with the production of two key hormones, ghrelin and leptin, which have roles in triggering the urge to eat and controlling how much we eat before feeling full.
- **Large friends** As we've all got fatter, another factor may be our nearest and dearest. A 30-year US study suggests that having family and especially

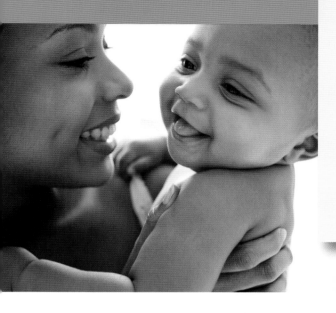

Did YOU know ?

Obesity can be triggered before birth

If a mother has a poor diet during pregnancy, her child is 25 per cent more likely to become obese, according to Professor Keith Godfrey of the MRC Lifecourse Epidemiology Unit at Southampton University, UK. Undernourishment in the uterus can set the unborn child's metabolism to conserve fat against poor food supplies in future, which can lead to adult obesity when food turns out to be plentiful. Exposure to junk food before birth also predisposes a child to obesity.

close friends who are overweight can triple your own chances of becoming overweight. This is probably because friends and family influence our food intake; there may also be little incentive to diet if overweight is the norm in our social group.

● **Fat-disposing gene** British scientists have discovered a gene that regulates the amount of fat in the body: a variant in this gene could explain why some people seem to retain more fat than others. As Professor Andrew Hattersley of the Peninsula Medical School in Exeter put it, this gene might answer the question: 'I eat the same and do as much exercise as my friend next door, so why am I fatter?'

Identifying a weight problem

A good starting point for assessing your weight is the body mass index, or BMI – a measure of how heavy you are relative to your height, used widely by the medical profession.

▶ **The BMI equation:** Weight in kilos ÷ [height in metres × height in metres]. To take an example of a person 1.7m tall who weighs 68 kilos:
$1.7 \times 1.7 = 2.89$ and $68 \div 2.89 = 23.5$
The BMI of 23.5 lies within the healthy weight range of 18.5–24.9:

▶ **The BMI Adult Weight Guide**
Underweight ▶ Less than 18.5   **Healthy weight** ▶ 18.5–24.9
Overweight ▶ 25–29.9   **Obese I** ▶ 30–34.9
Obese II (severely obese) ▶ 35–39.9
Obese III (morbidly obese) ▶ 40 or more

The BMI is a useful tool, but can be misleading. A rugby player with a lot of muscle could be heavy relative to height without being overweight. Conversely, if you have a small frame your BMI might fall in the healthy weight range while you're actually carrying too much fat.

Some variations come down to ethnicity. People of Asian heritage, for example, tend to be smaller-framed and carry more fat at a lower weight. There are also different BMI values for children because they have not yet fully developed.

How big is your waist?

The next step is to look at where the unwanted fat is going. Fat stored just under the skin, called subcutaneous fat, and fat that accumulates on the thighs and buttocks is not such a health worry as abdominal or visceral fat around the organs. Build-up of visceral fat is linked to an increase in inflammatory chemicals in the body and to metabolic syndrome, a condition marked by high blood pressure and cholesterol – two factors that greatly increase the risk of heart disease and type 2 diabetes.

To check if you have too much fat around your middle, measure your waist 1cm above the navel and look at the list below; the lower measurements are where doctors consider your risk begins. The higher your waist circumference and the higher your BMI, the greater your risk.

- **Men: 94–102cm or more**
- **Women: 80–88cm or more**
- **Asian men: more than 90cm**
- **Asian women: more than 80cm**

Getting ready for change

To achieve lasting weight loss and weight control, you have to really want to and be determined to stick at it. This might sound like stating the obvious, but many people fail because they are not prepared psychologically for the changes and challenges ahead. Thinking in advance about why you want to change, what it will mean and what benefits it will bring can mean the difference between success and failure.

You'll also need to do some research and work out a strategy before you embark on your weight-loss plan. Identify potential difficulties and think of who you can call on for support if necessary. When you start, be aware that some weeks will be harder than others, with less to show for it, and don't be shy of asking for help. To achieve long-term weight control, the changes you make to your diet and lifestyle must be sustainable.

HALF YOUR HEIGHT

or less is the ideal waist measurement. Scientists have found that this simple calculation is just as reliable as the more complicated BMI–waist ratio for predicting future health risk. 'Keeping your waist circumference to less than half your height can help increase life expectancy for every person in the world,' says Dr Margaret Ashwell, former science director of the British Nutrition Foundation.

Know your drivers for eating

Are you someone who eats out of boredom? Or an emotional eater using food to cope with highs or lows? Do you eat from habit, while you watch TV? Or is your overeating social, or related to work and eating out with clients? Analyse where and why you eat to see what the problems are, then think about how you could reduce your energy intake and increase your activity levels.

Different situations require different approaches. If you eat out of habit, find alternatives that do not involve food. Try knitting instead of snacking while watching TV, for instance. If it is social or work eating that is the root cause, make menu choices that fit with the food plan you decide to follow, be aware of portion sizes and skip dessert. If you're an emotional eater seek advice to help tackle more deep-rooted psychological issues.

Getting information

Family doctors may not give diet advice but can help you to work out your best starting point – whether you need specialist help from a dietitian or psychologist, or if there are other medical issues that need investigation, such as diabetes or thyroid problems. If you want advice on food and diet, ask for a referral to a registered dietitian; when seeking nutrition advice, via your doctor or independently, it's important to consult a qualified professional.

Typically dietitians do not give out prescriptive diet plans, but aim to guide you through decisions about food and answer practical questions. Some dietitians may be able to offer a regular point of contact to help keep you motivated, or recommend a weight-loss support group. A private registered dietitian can usually offer individual support.

Overcoming barriers

Is there anything holding you back? For example, is lack of time or cooking skills getting in the way of eating healthily? Is the cost of food an issue? Does shift work dictate the times you can eat? Think of practical solutions.

Finding out about easily prepared healthy foods and learning some simple recipes to cook may be part of the answer. Shopping with friends for bulk bargains can help finances. Getting your partner or children involved can help, too, and lay the foundations for healthy family nutrition.

Did YOU know ?

Central heating can affect your weight

In the days before central heating and air-conditioning, a greater proportion of kilojoules were used up simply to keep warm in winter, while in summer the heat naturally depressed appetite. Our bodies no longer need to burn fat to keep warm in cold weather; central heating does it for us. In summer, with so much time spent in air-conditioned places we've lost another natural factor that once helped to regulate weight.

BP RISK

rises as your waist measurement increases. Men with large waists are twice as likely to have high blood pressure, and women three times as likely.

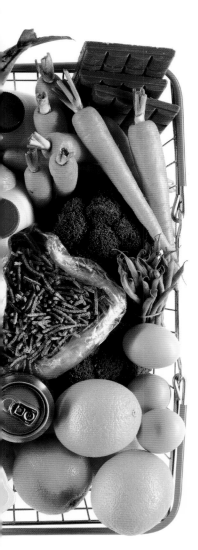

Energy in...

Your weight-loss strategy

There's no magic to weight loss: despite all the different diets and thousands of words devoted to this subject, it comes down to the energy balance equation. If you take in more energy (kilojoules) in food and drink than you use, you'll gain weight; if you consume less than you use, you'll lose weight. So the options are: eat less, get more active or – best of all – do a bit of both.

ENERGY IN – three steps to healthy eating

Before considering more extreme diets or other measures, start with the basics of healthy eating; it may be all you need. The three things to consider are:

- **WHEN YOU EAT**
- **WHAT YOU EAT**
- **HOW MUCH YOU EAT**

• WHEN YOU EAT – meal timings

Meal times are critical to healthy eating. People who 'graze' erratically have been shown to eat more, not burn energy as effectively, have higher cholesterol and produce more insulin than those who eat regular meals.

To balance your energy levels and keep cravings at bay aim to eat every 3 to 5 hours, as this is the time it takes for the stomach to empty after an average balanced meal. Building in mini-meals in the form of healthy snacks helps to keep hunger in check and prevent overeating at the next main meal. Timings for a typical day might be: 7–8am breakfast, 11am snack, 1pm lunch, 4–5pm snack, 7–8pm dinner. No grazing, no sugary drinks, no high-energy snacks – just healthy food keeping you satisfied until the next meal.

• WHAT YOU EAT – the major food groups

To supply all the nutrients you need, your diet must strike the right balance between the three major food groups: protein, carbohydrates, fruit and vegetables, plus some dairy products. You'll need some fat for good health. You don't need sugar, although a little sweetness can help combat food cravings.

- **Protein foods** are essential to fuel growth and maintain, repair and replace tissue in your body. Protein is also digested slowly, keeping you feeling full for longer, so for lasting satisfaction eat some protein with all meals. You can get protein from animal or plant sources, although some non-animal sources may need to be combined – such as rice and beans – to give you a 'complete' protein. (*See* Healthy lean protein, page 106.)

- **Carbohydrates** are an energy store for plant foods and they do the same for us. Eating low-GI carbohydrates such as wholegrain foods keeps energy levels steady for longer as they are digested slowly, and also supplies fibre to boost a sluggish gut and prevent constipation. (*See* Fibre, page 92.)
- **Fruit and vegetables** are perfect for piling on the plate because, with a few exceptions, they are low in energy but packed with protective nutrients – fibre, vitamins, minerals, antioxidants, microchemicals. The World Health Organization (WHO) suggests a daily minimum target of 400g fruit and vegetables, or five portions. One portion of fruit is about the size of a tennis ball, so that's an apple, an orange, a couple of plums, a handful of grapes; a portion of vegetables is 80g, or about 3 to 4 tablespoons. (For more on fresh produce, *see* page 84.)

- **HOW MUCH YOU EAT** – **controlling portion size**

Many of us pile too much food on our plates and too often it's the wrong kind of food. An easy way to portion food for weight loss is to start with a smaller plate – a medium-sized (20cm) plate is ideal. Fill half with salad and vegetables, then split the other half visually with a quarter for your protein choice and a quarter for carbohydrates – about two tablespoons of rice, potato or pasta, or a slice or two of bread. The plate should look full, which is visually satisfying, and the food should take time to chew and eat, which helps you to feel full.

ENERGY OUT – exercise and activity

Diet alone can only take you so far before the body's metabolic rate slows down to compensate for getting less food. To lose weight and keep it off, you've got to get up and move. One US study found that on top of a reduced-energy diet you need an hour's exercise five days a week to lose 10 per cent of weight and keep it off.

To increase your metabolic rate and burn off more energy, you have to get your heart pumping and build up your muscles; muscle is an active tissue, which burns energy even when it's doing nothing. Aerobic activity will raise your heart and lung rate, while weight-bearing or weight-resistance exercise builds and strengthens muscles.

At least 30 minutes of exercise should be a regular part of every day, so find activities you enjoy. Dance, swim, play tennis or walk the dog. Use the stairs rather than the lift at work to strengthen your leg muscles. Never sit still for long periods; get up every half hour. You don't have to go to the gym but structured, guided exercise classes could introduce you to new activities and help you push your fitness to new limits.

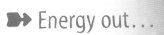 Energy out…

DRINKS DISRUPT

diets; alcohol has 29kJ per gram, almost double the kilojoules in protein and carbohydrate (17kJ per gram). Two 175ml glasses of wine or a pint of beer add up to about 1000kJ. Cocktails could have up to 1500kJ. This energy is quickly absorbed and easily stored as extra weight. Sweet fizzy drinks can be equally fattening and the largest white chocolate mocha can have 2500kJ – similar to a plate of spaghetti bolognese.

Diets, diets – find one that works for you

Although the same principles run through all diet plans, you may well find that some work better for your personality and lifestyle than others. Look for the one you are most likely to enjoy, because that's the one you will be able to follow for longer. If something isn't working, go back to the basics of healthy eating – you may be surprised to see how far you have strayed.

Popular diets usually hit the headlines with some catchy angle that makes them sound fresh and new. Here's a closer look at some of them.

'Five and two' fasting
One of the most recently fashionable diets, the 'Five and Two' eating plan involves two days of fasting in a week of otherwise normal eating. One 2011 study compared a regular weight-loss diet that reduced daily energy by 25 per cent with the weight-loss results achieved by following a normal healthy diet five days a week, then a very low energy diet of just 2500kJ on the other two days. The 2500kJ was made up of 1200ml of low-fat milk, 320g of vegetables, a piece of fruit, a low-joule salty drink and a multivitamin. Although some participants reported low energy, headaches and constipation, those who stuck to the plan without bingeing on normal days lost as much weight as people on the daily diet. If this pattern suits you, rather than restricting energy every day, this could be a useful way to lose weight.

Low-carbohydrate plans
These restrict carbohydrates (rice, pasta, grains, fruits and some vegetables) to unnaturally low levels. The main food supply is protein (meats, fish, poultry, eggs) and fats. Treat foods (cakes, biscuits, chips, crisps) are strictly off limits – a key reason why the plans work; those on them eat fewer kilojoules. The diets all produce rapid initial weight loss, in part from water, so are effective in the short term. Protein is good for keeping you feeling full, so if plenty of meat with salad on the side is to your taste, this may be an easy type of diet to follow. No problems have been reported but concerns have been raised about potential future effects on health.

➡ **The Atkins diet** is the oldest and most basic. It puts strict limits on carbohydrates in the first phase, but no limits on fatty or fried foods. It puts the body into a state of ketosis, which means the body burns fat instead of carbohydrates as fuel; side effects are bad breath and constipation as no fibre foods are allowed.

➡ **The Dukan diet** offers a healthier choice of foods than Atkins. It is still very low carbohydrate, but fat is also kept at very low levels. Stage one is protein only, plus some oat bran to help with constipation, and daily exercise. The next stages allow increasing amounts of carbohydrate, but at least one protein-only day is retained. It should not be followed long term.

➡ **The Zone diet** works on a 40:30:30 ratio of carbohydrate, protein and fat, so is not as extreme. But it is a fussy diet to follow as the ratios must be

Did YOU know

Overweight children
Your slimming plan may not suit a young child. Children have different nutritional requirements as their bodies need to fuel growth. They also have a smaller stomach capacity, so filling them up with high-fibre foods may not give them all the nutrients and energy they need. Seek professional advice if your child is overweight.

converted to real food by following pre-calculated recipes or else by calculating and weighing everything you eat. Overall, kilojoules come down quite drastically on the plan, and people report finding the food enjoyable and satisfying. It has been used to help reduce blood glucose levels in cases of type 2 diabetes, as well as for weight loss.

Low-GI diets

These diets cut out carbohydrates with a high GI (white breads, sugary and refined cereals such as cornflakes, potatoes, white rice, sweet confectionery) and replace them with smaller portions of low-GI carbs such as oats, brown basmati rice, wholemeal pasta and noodles, baby new potatoes, wholemeal pita and other breads, lentils and beans. A low-GI diet doesn't produce rapid weight loss, but works for some because it is easy to maintain long term as part of a standard healthy eating-and-exercise plan. Essentially, it's a normal healthy diet, with a few small adjustments.

Kilojoule counting

Just a couple of biscuits extra each day, 650kJ on top of your usual intake, adds up to 240,000kJ in a year. If you don't use up those kilojoules, they will add an extra 6.5kg to your weight by the end of the year. Keeping a food diary, noting everything you eat and drink, has been found to raise awareness of the little things that add up. It's easy to do and worth a go to help you self-diagnose where you could make simple changes. There are mobile phone and online apps designed to help keep a daily log and calculate the details. They can be useful, but there is a danger of users obsessing too much on kilojoule detail while missing the basics of healthy eating.

Food combining

In the 1920s, William Hay, a doctor in New York, USA, said that the human body cannot digest protein and carbohydrates efficiently at the same time, as one needs an acid environment, the other alkaline. He launched a diet for better digestion, in which protein and carbohydrate foods are not eaten together as part of the same meal; vegetables and a certain amount of fat can go with either. So if lunch, for example, is a ham salad, dinner might be vegetable risotto. Food combining still has many fans, but there is little scientific evidence to support the underlying theory: any weight-loss benefit comes from a reduction in energy consumed.

Slimming groups

Commercial slimming groups such as Weight Watchers and Jenny Craig have good success rates. The weekly meetings help to motivate, inform and encourage dieters, and are a place to build community support and learn about healthy eating. The weekly weigh-in provides a timed goal for everyone to work towards.

Very low energy regimes

Lighter Life, Cambridge Diet, Optifast, NG tube. These are the most restrictive of all, based on 3500kJ a day or less made up of shakes or meal replacements. They are very tough to follow, but do produce rapid short-term weight loss. Anyone attempting a very low energy diet must discuss it with their doctor before starting and be monitored throughout. The daily shakes must include a good supply of protein to help limit muscle loss.

These diets have been found to slow the metabolic rate, which eventually slows weight loss. Typically, when the diet is finished weight can pile back on, but a second-stage program to reintroduce healthy eating can help to avoid this. Very restrictive diets are not recommended for everyone and should not be followed for longer than 12 weeks. However, for some they are an effective weight-loss solution.

Extreme measures

If weight has soared out of control, more drastic measures may be needed. Going on an extreme diet is not to be taken lightly: it's important to take medical advice, to understand the limitations and to return to the basics of healthy eating once the diet is complete.

● **Diet pills** These can be prescribed by your doctor and give up to ten per cent weight loss, but if you do not follow a strict low-fat diet they can have the unpleasant side-effects of rapid diarrhoea and anal leakage, making them socially challenging.

● **The nasogastric tube diet** This involves a medical intervention to fit a tube through the nose to the stomach; a tightly controlled, very low energy quantity of liquid protein is then fed through the tube for seven to ten days, with no other food allowed. The patient alternates weeks on a low-energy diet with weeks being fed through the tube. Some spectacular weight losses have been recorded, but some reports suggest that the mental and social challenges of avoiding food altogether can lead to psychological problems. Some doctors express concerns about tube hygiene and whether it is appropriate to use a feeding method devised for sick patients who cannot chew or swallow as a means of inducing weight loss.

● **Bariatric surgery** The most extreme of all measures is reserved for people who have severe health problems as a result of being obese. Surgery can reduce the stomach to the size of an egg; it can bypass the stomach so food is not absorbed properly; or a band can be placed at the top of the stomach to reduce the amount that can be eaten. Patients eat only a meal the size of a yogurt tub three times a day. Surgery can be life-saving with dramatic results reversing diabetes, high blood pressure, sleep problems, breathlessness, depression and mobility problems. In the long term, surgery may also reduce the drive to eat, altering a taste for sweet or fatty foods. It is not an easy option and requires a lot of commitment from the patient. The rapid, extensive weight loss can also lead to unsightly excess skin requiring further surgery. As with all diet procedures, some weight regain can occur over time.

After surgical measures, medical follow-up is important to avoid problems and ensure you do not suffer any nutritional deficiencies.

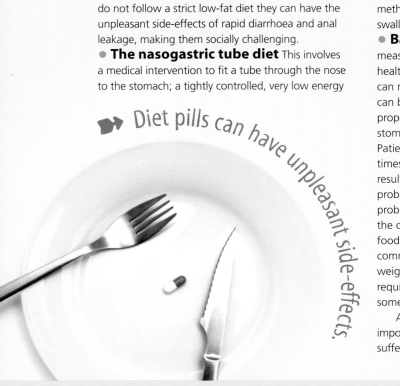

➤ Diet pills can have unpleasant side-effects.

Severe underweight – an equal danger

At the other end of the scale, extreme weight loss, often associated with eating disorders such as anorexia, is equally damaging. Young people are increasingly susceptible and many elderly people are severely underweight, too. Because fat plays an essential role in the body (*see* page 98) health problems arise when there is not enough. The immune system can soon weaken, making the body more susceptible to infections, colds and flu. Recovery is slower, often with complications, and wounds take longer to heal. Nutritional deficiencies contribute to extreme tiredness and can impair heart function. All over the body, muscle tissue is broken down to supply essential energy for heart and lung function; as heart muscle weakens, blood pressure may fall to very low levels and the heart beat becomes irregular.

In younger women it is common for the menstrual cycle to stop, while men often experience impotence. The thyroid function slows in a bid to conserve energy, which affects growth hormones in children and teenagers. Younger people with extended anorexia may suffer osteoporosis in later life.

Monitoring and maintaining weight loss

Weighing yourself regularly – once a week, always at the same time of day – will help you keep track of progress but it only gives you part of the picture. Muscle weighs more than fat, so if you are exercising and shaping up, you may not lose weight as quickly as you expect. Fluid levels may also change your weight significantly from one day to the next.

Well-fitting clothes with a fixed waistband can provide a good reference point: take note of how they loosen or tighten in different places. Once a month measure your mid upper-arm, bust or chest, waist, hips, upper thigh and make a note, so you can compare that with your weight loss and see how your body is changing over time.

What rate should I aim for?

The figures usually quoted for a safe rate of weight loss are about 0.5–1kg a week, but everyone is different. For some, weight loss is faster in the early weeks, then slows down as the body adjusts to changes in the diet. In practice weight loss tends to follow a stepwise pattern, rather than a straight downward line, with plateaus and occasional rises, too. If the overall trend is down, you know you are on the right track.

Set yourself upper and lower boundaries to allow for fluctuations, then adjust downwards as you lose weight. Or use body measurements or clothes as markers.

If you hit a plateau but know you are following a good routine, don't panic. An occasional levelling off is normal and eventually will indicate that you've reached your ideal weight. But if a plateau persists while you're still overweight or if you start to cross an upper boundary, check for bad habits – diet deviations or less exercise, perhaps – and adjust your regime accordingly.

The same upper and lower boundary technique works equally well for maintaining your target weight once you reach it. The key is to monitor yourself regularly: if you notice a weight increase, think about what has changed in your lifestyle to cause it and take small simple actions to get back on track.

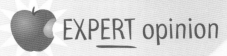 **EXPERT opinion**

Slow, steady weight loss is best

Amanda Genge, an editor at WeightWatchers.com, says the best way to lose weight is slowly. Trying to lose too much too quickly can harm your health, rather than helping it: '… losing weight at a rate greater than an average of 1kg per week (after the first few weeks, when you may lose more because you're shedding water weight) increases your risk of developing health problems like heart-beat irregularities, anaemia, excessive loss of lean body mass (muscle), bowel irregularities and gallstone formation.'

Amanda Genge, *WeightWatchers.com*

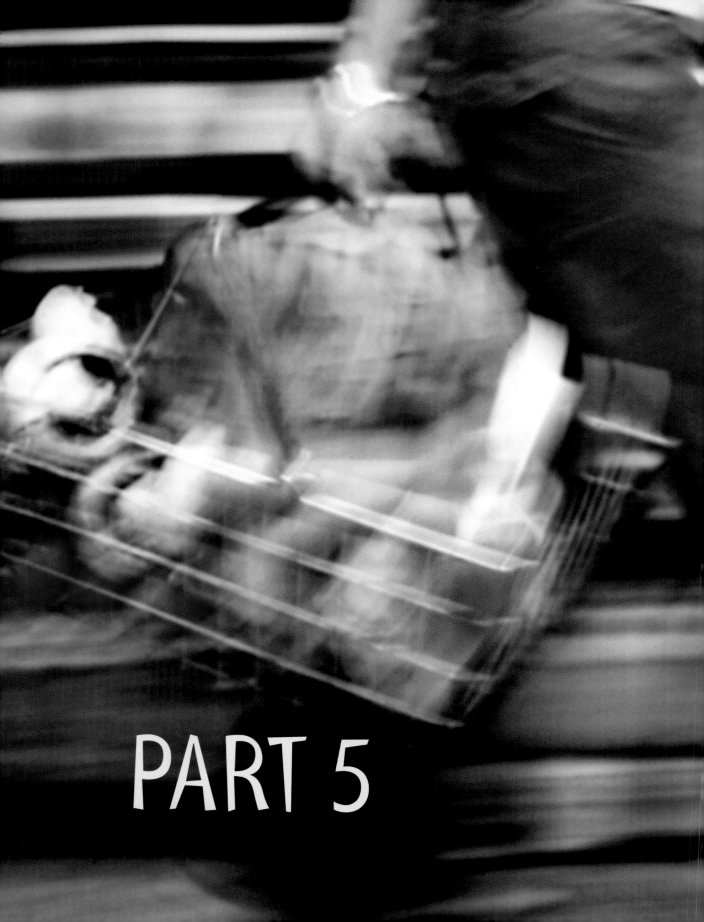

PART 5

Your live-long food guide

Make the right food choices – every day

Wherever and however you buy food, you have to choose – often from dozens of competing brands and types. Knowing what lies behind the packaging and hype will help you make decisions that are crucial to your own and your family's health.

Every day we make lots of food choices – often out of habit or triggered by the sight or smell of a tempting product. It's almost inevitable in a world where drinks or snacks seem omnipresent, ready to catch our eye.

Yet we need to think and know more about what we're buying. As you'll discover again in this section, you can't assume that all food is good for you. From meat, fish and eggs to rice, bread or ice cream, you'll be surprised – perhaps shocked – by what some products can contain. This section points you to the better choices – nutritious foods produced in the most natural way and therefore free of potentially unhealthy added extras.

Buying the best

Your Live-Long Food Guide explains how everyday foods and drinks get to us, the many varieties of each type, how they fit into a healthy diet, cooking methods that retain their nutrients, preparation and storage advice, and more. That knowledge can inform your choices, which, in time could influence manufacturers. If most of us chose to buy only from those who respect their products and value good nutrition, the industry would have to listen – and we would be healthier as a result.

Meat & poultry The top source of protein in our diets, beef, lamb, pork and poultry are widely eaten worldwide. However, the practices of intensive farming – giving hormones to stimulate growth in cattle, mass antibiotics to contain infection in cruel, overcrowded conditions – can affect our health. Find out how to shop for better-quality meats and the pluses and minuses of individual products.

Fish & seafood As protein-rich alternatives to meat, both have much to offer. Oily fish are especially nutritious. Whether wild or farmed, you need to know the source; wild may be overfished or polluted, and farmed can be as intensively reared as livestock, with similar problems. These pages explain what to look for and how to choose the best.

Fruit & vegetables Given the delicious variety and powerful disease-fighting nutrients these foods contain, we should all

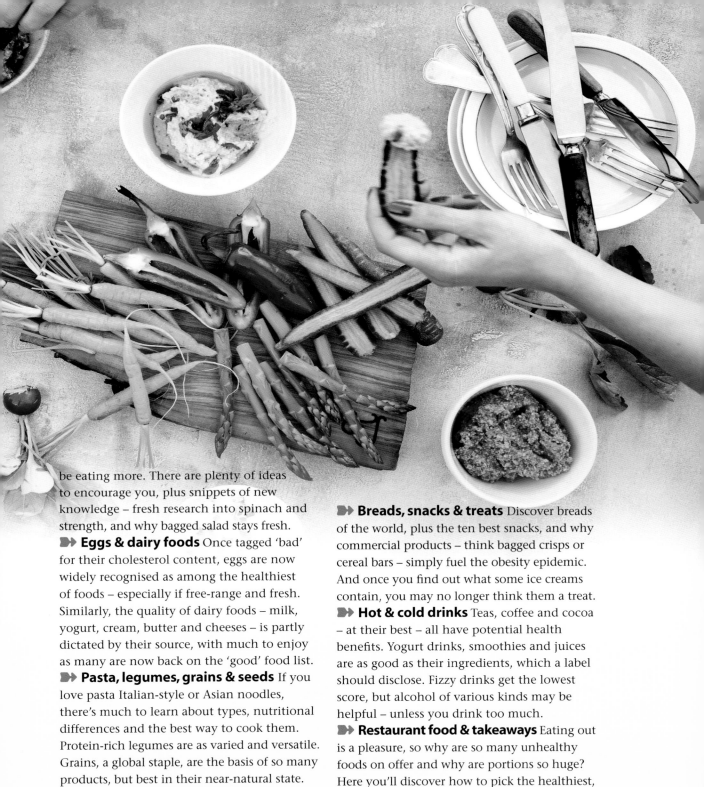

be eating more. There are plenty of ideas to encourage you, plus snippets of new knowledge – fresh research into spinach and strength, and why bagged salad stays fresh.

▶▶ Eggs & dairy foods Once tagged 'bad' for their cholesterol content, eggs are now widely recognised as among the healthiest of foods – especially if free-range and fresh. Similarly, the quality of dairy foods – milk, yogurt, cream, butter and cheeses – is partly dictated by their source, with much to enjoy as many are now back on the 'good' food list.

▶▶ Pasta, legumes, grains & seeds If you love pasta Italian-style or Asian noodles, there's much to learn about types, nutritional differences and the best way to cook them. Protein-rich legumes are as varied and versatile. Grains, a global staple, are the basis of so many products, but best in their near-natural state. Seeds are well worth exploring, too, for their nutty flavours and important nutrients.

▶▶ Breads, snacks & treats Discover breads of the world, plus the ten best snacks, and why commercial products – think bagged crisps or cereal bars – simply fuel the obesity epidemic. And once you find out what some ice creams contain, you may no longer think them a treat.

▶▶ Hot & cold drinks Teas, coffee and cocoa – at their best – all have potential health benefits. Yogurt drinks, smoothies and juices are as good as their ingredients, which a label should disclose. Fizzy drinks get the lowest score, but alcohol of various kinds may be helpful – unless you drink too much.

▶▶ Restaurant food & takeaways Eating out is a pleasure, so why are so many unhealthy foods on offer and why are portions so huge? Here you'll discover how to pick the healthiest, tastiest dishes from ten top world cuisines plus delicious takeaway food to enjoy.

1 Meat & poultry

Across the world, we're eating more meat, often from livestock reared intensively to feed our growing appetite. In the industrialised world we eat an average 1.5kg each per week; it's just over 0.6kg in the developing world. Pork is the most widely consumed, followed by poultry, beef and lamb.

What does it do for me?

There's been so much talk about the 'dangers' of eating too much red meat that it's easy to forget that all meat and poultry is highly nutritious, supplying:

▶▶ **High-quality protein** with the full complement of essential amino acids our bodies need for health. Protein is also the best nutrient for satisfying the appetite for hours at a stretch, making us less likely to snack unhealthily between meals.

▶▶ **Essential minerals**, especially iron and zinc. The **iron** is in a form that is easily absorbed by the body, helping prevent a deficiency that can lead to anaemia, causing fatigue, irritability and difficulty concentrating. **Zinc** is important for growth, a healthy immune system, fertility, wound healing and healthy skin – and meat is the richest dietary source there is.

▶▶ **B-group vitamins** – red meat is one of the very best sources of these, including B_1 (thiamin), B_2 (riboflavin), B_3 (niacin), B_6 and B_{12}. The B vitamins have a role in many vital body functions, including the workings of the brain and nervous system and in generating energy. B vitamin-deficiency is not uncommon, especially among the elderly.

Isn't saturated fat a problem?

If you eat too much red meat, yes; white meats are much lower in saturated fat. Most health experts recommend limiting red meat consumption to reduce the risk of heart disease and other health problems. But in moderation, it makes a valuable contribution to the diet without compromising health.
● **Not all the fat in red meat is saturated**. More than half the fat in leaner cuts is of the healthy monounsaturated or polyunsaturated types. These include omega-3 fatty acids and conjugated linoleic acid, which are thought to reduce the risk of cancer and heart disease.
● **Levels of healthy fats are higher in meat from grass-fed and free-range animals**. Grass-fed animals also contain higher levels of a recently identified protein present in grass, called glutathione, which functions as an antioxidant, protecting cells from DNA damage.
● **Game meats contain very little saturated fat**.

Any other health issues?

Some epidemiological studies have suggested a statistical link between eating large amounts of red meat and increased risk of bowel cancer. The

30 years ago it took nearly 3 months to grow
a broiler chicken to slaughter weight (2 kg) – **today it takes 41 days.**

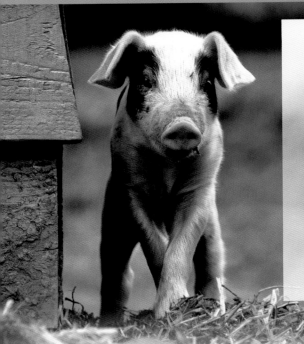

70% of all antibiotics sold in the USA **are fed to cattle, pigs and poultry** on industrial animal farms, for purposes other than treating disease.

Antibiotics in livestock

In factory farming antibiotics are widely used, not just to cure illness but as a routine preventative measure to keep the animals healthy in the crowded, stressful conditions. There are now urgent concerns that the overuse of these vital drugs in intensive farming is compromising their ability to treat illness in humans. As the World Health Organization puts it: 'The widespread use of antimicrobials … in livestock production has intensified the risk for the emergence and spread of resistant micro-organisms. This raises particular concern since the same classes of antimicrobials are used both in humans and animals.' The highest antibiotic usage in European farming occurs in intensive pig and chicken production. In the USA the problem may be greatest in cattle, where antibiotics are also used as growth promoters, a practice banned in Europe. In 2009 alone, US farmers got through 13,620 tonnes of antibiotics.

consensus is that there is a risk when you eat more than 500g per week. But the greatest risk comes from eating a lot of cured and processed meats, which often contain chemical preservatives.

How much can I eat?

70g red meat a day, or up to 500g per week, is the limit suggested by the World Cancer Research Fund. There is no recommended limit for unprocessed white meat, which contains much less saturated fat.

To get its dietary benefits we don't need to eat much meat as it is such a concentrated, high-quality source of protein and other nutrients.
- **Current advice** is to eat red and white processed meats only in small amounts or to avoid them. Most of the meat in a healthy diet should be fresh.
- **The skin of poultry** is best removed before cooking or eating, as it is the fattiest part of the meat.
- **Pregnant women** should avoid liver, including chicken liver and liver pâtés, as it is so rich in vitamin A; an excess of vitamin A has been linked to birth defects.

Six steps to safe eating

Raw meat of all kinds can contain food-poisoning bacteria. Follow these simple steps to ensure your meat is safely stored and prepared:

1 **Wash your hands with soap** before and after handling raw meat and clean any surfaces or equipment in contact with the meat.
2 **Use a separate chopping board** for cutting up meat and do not allow raw meat to come into contact with other foods.
3 **Check your fridge temperature** is no higher than 5°C. Place raw meat in a covered dish on the bottom shelf to avoid drips falling on other food. Keep raw and cooked meats separate.
4 **Put leftovers in the fridge** as soon as possible and eat them within two days. Do not reheat leftover meat more than once.
5 **Freeze meat as quickly as possible**, using 'fast-freeze' if your freezer has the option. Clearly label each package with contents and date.
6 **Defrost meat slowly**, ideally by moving it to the fridge the day before you cook it. Make sure it is completely thawed before cooking, then cook it as soon as possible. After cooking, meat can be re-frozen. **NEVER** re-freeze defrosted raw meat.

Beef

Quality meat from grass-fed cattle is both the healthiest and most delicious.

How does it get to us?

▶▶ Traditional beef comes from outdoor herds of cattle, such as Aberdeen Angus, Hereford and Charolais, selected and bred for their quality of meat and fed on grass. Outdoor-reared, grass-fed beef takes at least two years to produce and is usually more expensive than beef from a commercial herd. Grass-fed beef has been shown to have more vitamins and healthy omega-3 fats than beef from cattle fed on cereals and soybeans.

▶▶ Commercial beef is usually from a mixture of traditional beef breeds cross-bred with faster-growing beef breeds or with dairy breeds. Commercial herds are reared outdoors on grassy pasture for part of their lives, but the animals are usually brought inside into barns as they get older to be fattened up more quickly on a cereal-based diet. They are ready for market between 12 and 18 months of age, so are more commercially viable.

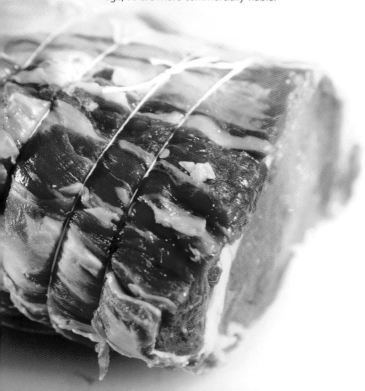

Buy the best

The hallmark of good beef is its rich flavour. Huge portions are not essential – and may be harmful – so it is worth buying the best you can find and afford.

What to look for

There are **three visual characteristics** that reveal the quality of beef:
● **It has quite a dark colour** – wine-red rather than bright red.
● **It does not look wet**, or exude liquid.
● **The fat is creamy in colour** (a sign of grass-fed beef), not white (a sign of cereal-fed). Marbling is when threads of fat run through the meat. From a taste perspective, many cooks think this is desirable as the fat bastes the meat naturally as it cooks. But from a health perspective, experts recommend leaner meat.

Where to shop

▶▶ A local butcher is probably your best bet:
● **Traditional butchers hang beef properly** in a cool, dry atmosphere for two to four weeks. This gives it time to mature, tenderises the meat and allows the flavour to develop.
● **They have the skills to butcher meat correctly** and the knowledge to direct you to the best cuts for your purpose, which are not always the most expensive.
● **A local butcher is often cheaper** than a supermarket, so you win on taste, service and price. Butchers may sell traditional beef alongside more commercially reared beef, so you may want to check which you are getting.

▶▶ Specialist suppliers sell beef from heritage herds or less commonly farmed breeds – such as Dexter, Galloway, South Devon or Red Poll. Heritage beef tends to command a premium price. However, as farmers often sell direct from the farm to the public, cutting out the middlemen, it can work out much the same price as good-quality beef from a butcher's shop. You may also find specialist beef at farmers' markets.

▶▶ What about supermarket beef?
● **Typical supermarket beef is** butchered straight after the animal is slaughtered, wrapped in plastic and delivered direct to stores for sale. Cuts are

A shop-bought burger can be just 59% beef

plus 15 or more other ingredients including fat, additives, water and seasoning.
For quality control, cook your own.

packed on an absorbent mat to soak up the fluid that would evaporate in the air if the meat was hung.
● **It is usually a bright red colour** and soft in consistency, but not reliably tender when cooked.
● **If you buy supermarket beef**, unwrap it, pat it dry with kitchen towel, then leave it to dry at room temperature before cooking. This will help it to brown.

How can I use it?

Beef can be stored in the fridge for up to three days, and in the freezer for nine to 12 months. For mince storage is shorter – just a day in the fridge and up to three months in the freezer. Always serve with vegetables for the complementary vitamins and fibre.

▶▶ Grill it In general, this is a healthier way to cook meat than either frying or barbecuing.

▶▶ Roast it Sirloin, forerib, topside and top rump are the best cuts for traditional roasting.
● **Silverside and brisket** are better in a pot roast, slow cooked in a little liquid.

▶▶ Stew it For a tasty, inexpensive dinner that's especially satisfying in cold weather, brown cubes

of cheaper cuts of beef; add onions and liquid and slowly cook. Add plenty of vegetables such as carrots and mushrooms partway through.

▶▶ Stir-fry it Thin strips of beef are great with thinly sliced onions, mushrooms and Asian greens.

▶▶ Mince it Lean beef mince makes lots of healthy, affordable meals: cottage pie, burgers, chilli con carne, lasagne, spaghetti Bolognese or meatballs.

▶▶ Make stock A few bits of marrow or knuckle bone and a small piece of flank beef, simmered with an onion, carrot, celery stick, bay leaf and black peppercorns, will produce a large pot of stock, giving you the basis for delicious soups, risottos and casseroles.

Why is it important to rest meat before carving?

During cooking, the juices in meat migrate into the middle of the cut. Allowing cooked meat to rest away from the heat before carving or serving lets the juices redistribute throughout so the meat is juicy and tender. To rest meat, place it on a warm plate and cover loosely with foil to keep it warm (covering it tightly will make the hot meat sweat). Rest steaks or chops for at least 3 minutes, and a roast for 10–20 minutes before carving.

Cured beef products

These are high in salt, so should be eaten only in small amounts and infrequently.
● **Bresaola**, an Italian dry-cured delicacy with a 'gamey' flavour, is sold in very thin slices and traditionally eaten as an antipasto.
● **Corned beef** is cured, boiled, compressed, then packed into cans. It is high in both fat and salt, but is a cheap and convenient pantry standby.
● **Pastrami** is beef brisket cured with spices, sugar and garlic, then smoked and steamed.
● **Jerky** is a lean meat, thinly sliced, salted and/or marinated, then dried or smoked at a low temperature.

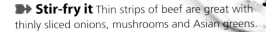

Lamb & mutton

Lamb is a versatile and highly nutritious red meat from grass-fed animals. Around half its fat is monounsaturated or polyunsaturated 'good' fats.

How does it get to us?

Of all of our farm animals, sheep live the most natural life closest to that of a wild animal.
- **Most sheep** spend active lives outdoors, foraging on grass and other plants.
- **Where they graze** may vary from lush pasture to much barer terrain. If the terrain is not fertile enough to fatten them up for market before winter, the farmer will move his flock to better pasture or he will feed the sheep on crops during the winter months to supplement their natural grass diet.

Different types

The flavour of lamb differs according to the age of the animal and also the type of land on which it has grazed.

BY AGE:

➡➡ **Spring or 'new season' lamb** is from lambs that are just a few months old. These may be early maturing breeds or lambs housed indoors and fed cereals and other crops to fatten them up. Available for the first few weeks of spring, this is the mildest-tasting lamb, prized for juicy tenderness rather than flavour.

➡➡ **Lamb** – the most common type – is meat from free-ranging sheep, aged from six months to one year old. Redder than spring lamb, it has a stronger, meatier flavour. At its best in autumn and winter.

➡➡ **Hogget**, usually only on offer direct from farm outlets, is meat from more mature, free-ranging sheep over a year old. The meat is darker than standard lamb, and extremely flavourful. Usually on offer in winter.

➡➡ **Mutton** is from free-ranging sheep or rams that are at least two years old. The meat has more depth and character because older sheep have grazed for longer on a diet of varied plants and grasses. It has a tighter grain, with a marbling of healthy omega-3 rich fat.

BY PASTURE:

➡➡ **Lowland** lamb, farmed in milder, more fertile climes, often tastes relatively sweet because the sheep have fattened up on abundant grass.

➡➡ **Marshy, coastal** lamb reared on Australian outback saltbush, or in marshy, coastal areas, has a richer, slightly saltier flavour.

➡➡ **Rugged upland** lamb from sheep reared in rugged upland areas, on rougher, less hospitable land, often has a deeper, more complex flavour.

Where to buy it

➡➡ **Your local butcher** Lamb becomes more tender and tasty when it is hung for at least a week – longer for hogget and mutton. Traditional butchers have the skills and knowledge to hang and cut lamb so that it is dependably tender, evenly cut and expertly trimmed. Most supermarket lamb is not hung.

➡➡ **Direct from the farmer** – by phone or online. Lamb from rare breeds and more mature hogget, shearling (a sheep that has been sheared once) and mutton is mostly sold this way. Buy mutton from a producer or butcher who takes pride in their produce and knows how to prepare it for the table.

Good to know

- **Lamb freezes well** so if you can make space for half a lamb in your freezer, or can share a bulk order with a friend, you can cut the cost considerably. The lamb can often be supplied ready cut into joints.
- **Buying a whole or half carcass of lamb** means that you get some of the more economical but tasty cuts that can be hard to find such as sweetbreads, scrag end, breast and flank, which can be used in many varied dishes.

● **Lamb keeps for up to three days** in the fridge and for six to nine months in the freezer. Storage for lamb mince is shorter: one day in the fridge and up to three months in the freezer.

How can I use it?

Lamb supplies good flavour, so you don't need a lot. A small amount will flavour a dish that is otherwise mainly vegetables.

▶ **Roast it** Leg is the classic, but for a cheaper roast that many consider tastier try shoulder slowly roasted on a rack to allow the fat to drip out, naturally basting the meat as it cooks. Leftover meat can be used to make shepherd's pie or a quick curry.

▶ **Stew lamb** It makes an economical Irish stew, topped with sliced potatoes; a simple casserole of root vegetables, passata, stock and leftover wine or water; or a sustaining soup with leeks, potatoes, tomatoes and cabbage. Shanks are particularly good for slow-cooking.

▶ **Use lamb mince** It's a handy freezer standby that makes tasty meals, such as Middle Eastern-style dolma or kebabs; lamb and mint burgers served with yogurt; shepherd's pie; moussaka; or stuffed eggplant, capsicums and zucchinis.

▶ **Quickly sear prime cuts** Chops and leg steaks are beautifully tender when quickly seared.

▶ **Grill or fry it** A piece of expensive, quality lamb fillet, leg or neck will go further if you cook it, then slice finely and serve warm on top of hummus with pita bread as a main course with salad.

▶ **Gently boil or slowly roast hoggett**, shearling or mutton. Then serve it with a delicious and highly nutritious Italian salsa verde made with capers, anchovies, olive oil, lemon juice and lots of chopped parsley, basil and mint.

Cured lamb products

These are a rarity compared to other red meats.
● **Merguez** Perhaps the most famous lamb sausages are spicy Merguez from Moroccan cuisine, which combine well with couscous, beans, lentils and vegetables in a variety of tasty dishes. If buying lamb sausages, check the level of chemical preservatives and don't eat too many or too often.

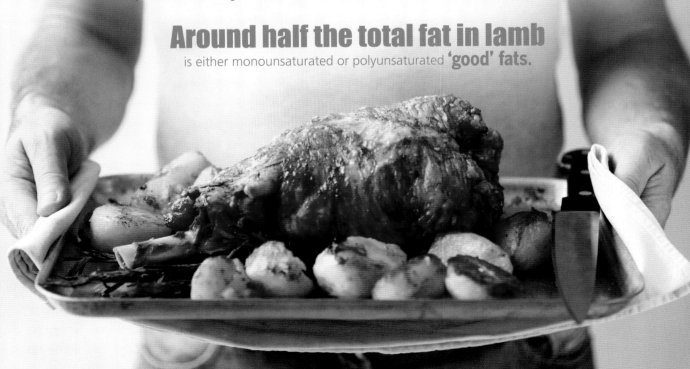

Around half the total fat in lamb is either monounsaturated or polyunsaturated **'good'** fats.

Pork

Pork is the cheapest of the red meats but equally delicious and a particularly good source of vitamin B$_1$. It is also the basis of a huge variety of cured meat products.

How does it get to us?

Like chickens, modern breeds of pigs can be reared intensively indoors, which is why their meat is cheaper than pork from free-range animals. Different production systems result in pork defined as follows:

➤➤ **Free-range pork** Less than five per cent of pork in Australia and New Zealand is free-range. The breeding sows live outdoors in fields – usually in metal arcs with straw bedding. The piglets are born outdoors and remain with their mothers until weaned at about a month old, when they are moved to separate fields until ready for slaughter. The meat is excellent but this is a relatively slow and costly way to produce pork.

➤➤ **Outdoor-reared/outdoor-bred pork** The breeding sows live outdoors and the piglets remain with their mothers until weaned. Outdoor-bred pigs are then taken indoors in sheds where they are fattened up for slaughter in the same way as indoor-reared pigs. Outdoor-reared pigs spend more time outdoors but are similarly fattened up indoors.

➤➤ **Indoor-reared pork** Most of our pork comes from indoor herds of up to 1,000 pigs, often living on concrete or slatted metal floors which are easier to clean than straw bedding. Breeding sows give birth and feed their litter in farrowing crates. When weaned at three to four weeks old, the young pigs are fattened up on feed made from grain and soybeans.

Buy the best

Good butchers will be able to tell you the source of their pork and how the animal was raised. Some butchers and farm shops sell pork from traditional breeds. However, it may be easier to source premium pork at farmers' markets or direct from a farmer by phone or online.

A better life means better meat

In many parts of the world pigs are bred in overcrowded conditions and fed large quantities of antibiotics to keep disease levels down. Poor welfare can affect the quality of meat, while overuse of antibiotics contributes to antibiotic resistance in humans – both sound health reasons to buy pork from humanely reared animals. From 2015, New Zealand will ban the use of metal cages known as 'stalls' to confine large numbers of pigs, and in Australia the plan is to phase them out voluntarily over the next few years.

● **The tastiest pork** comes from organic or free-range pigs, which are often traditional breeds such as Wessex Saddleback, Tamworth, Large Black and Hampshire. They grow more slowly than the typical modern pork pig and the meat has enough fat to ensure that it is tender and succulent when cooked.

● **The most nutritious pork** is probably from organic or free-range animals, as research suggests that pork from pigs with the opportunity to eat pasture-based fodder is richer in vitamins than the meat from indoor-reared pigs fed on grain and soybean.

● **The leanest pork** comes from modern breeds of pigs that are bred to be extremely lean. But it can be bland and disappointing with a rather ropey, dry texture, so it is important not to overcook it.

How can I use it?

Fresh pork freezes well for four to six months; if stored in the fridge, use it within two days.

➤➤ **Roast it** Leg is the traditional cut for roasting, but rolled shoulder, roasted slowly on a rack to allow the fat to drain, is succulent and more economical.

➤➤ **Simmer it** For an unusual main course, cook lean fresh pork (loin, leg or chump) in the Italian style, by simmering it in milk flavoured with the zest of an unwaxed lemon, a teaspoon of lightly crushed coriander seed and three plump cloves of garlic.

➼ **Stew it** Pork is particularly delicious cooked in cider, with onions and apple.

➼ **Grill it** Pork chops or kebabs can be grilled with tomatoes, zucchinis, capsicums and mushrooms.

➼ **Stir-fry it** Thin slices of lean pork make an excellent stir-fry with ginger and garlic, snowpeas, broccoli and sliced waterchestnut.

Bacon & ham

Traditionally, pork has been cured – probably more than any other meat – to produce a supply that keeps for much longer and still provides a valuable source of protein, minerals and vitamins. This has brought us a vast and delicious variety of cooked hams, bacon and pancetta, and cured raw hams.

How do they get to us?

There are two ways of curing pork:

➼ **Dry-cured**
● **The best-tasting** bacon, ham, salami and other products are dry-cured. The fresh pork is rubbed with salt and, almost always, a nitrate preservative to inhibit growth of bacteria – usually potassium or sodium nitrate or nitrite – plus seasonings and often something sweet such as honey or marmalade.
● **Air-dried** In the southern European tradition, dry-cured ham is then air-dried for several months. The whole process takes up to three years for the best hams.
● **Smoked** Bacon and ham may go on to be smoked for varying lengths of time: for bacon the smoking process lasts from hours to days, sometimes weeks.

➼ **Brine-cured**
● **The more common way** to cure fresh pork is to soak it in a liquid brine solution of the same ingredients used in dry-curing mixed with water.
● **In cheaper types of bacon and ham** polyphosphate chemicals are often added to the brine to make the meat absorb and retain more water.
● **Smoked** Brine-cured bacon and ham may also then be smoked.

Mass-market cooked hams may contain 25% or more added water plus other extras including sugar and preservatives.

What to look for

● **A good-quality cooked ham** will be a delicate pink in colour with a soft, slightly dull surface. Avoid bright pink, glossy or moist-looking ham – it will almost certainly have been brine-cured with polyphosphates and contain a lot of added water.
● **More natural cooked ham** may be irregular in shape, a sign that it has been sliced from one whole cut of cured pork. If ham is even in size and shape it has most likely been made by re-forming pork from different cuts with water, gelatine and additives; the even shape makes it easier to slice. This mass-market re-formed ham won't taste as good as natural ham.
● **Choose good-quality dry-cured bacon** rather than brine-cured. Although it is usually more expensive, it has a firmer consistency. Brine-cured bacon gives off white liquid as it cooks, which makes it difficult to get rashers to crisp up. It also shrinks visibly in the pan, so it's debatable whether it is ultimately better value than dry-cured.
● **Some pre-packed bacon or pork** products have vitamin C (ascorbic acid) added, which may help to counteract any potentially cancer-causing effect of the preservatives.

How much can I eat?

● **Bacon, ham and other cured pork** products come within the dietary recommendation for red meat (see page 225), but because the chemical preservatives have a cancer-causing potential, they should be no more than a small proportion of the total red meat in the diet. Bacon, ham and other cured products also typically contain high levels of salt, another reason why it is unwise to eat them in large amounts.
● **The latest health advice** is to limit consumption of cured pork products or cut them out altogether. If you can't face giving up the culinary pleasures of bacon and ham, the answer is to eat them sparingly and treat yourself to the best you can afford.

How can I use them?

These meats are so full of flavour a little goes a long way. Enjoy them in small amounts and accompany them with fruit and vegetables rich in vitamin C. Bacon keeps for three to five days in the fridge, or a month in the freezer; vacuum-packed should be fine for at least a week in the fridge, three months in the freezer, but once opened treat as loose bacon. Fridge storage for ham varies with type, from three to five days for sliced cooked ham to up to three months for air-dried. Check 'use by' dates on packaging and avoid any product that smells 'off'.

At breakfast Keep the classic bacon and eggs as a once-a-week treat at most and serve it with fresh orange juice. For a change, fry a little diced bacon and add chopped fresh tomatoes, rich in vitamin C; heat through and serve on wholemeal toast.

In soups Smoked ribs and hock are inexpensive cuts of ham on the bone, ideal for flavouring hearty soups, such as lentil or minestrone. A few ribs or a small piece of smoked hock, boiled with pumpkin and squash, cabbage, kale or leek, with perhaps a little potato, will make a large quantity of soup.

To add flavour A little diced pancetta, the firm streaky bacon from Italy, will add delicious flavour to soups, stews and quick pasta sauces, such as carbonara with lots of chopped parsley adding vitamin C.

To add texture Crispy-cooked bacon crumbled over a leafy salad, with slices of avocado, adds texture as well as flavour and protein.

As a treat Prosciutto di Parma and jamón ibérico are the best air-dried hams from Italy and Spain, and are served sliced very thinly.

In 2011 Australians ate 111kg of meat per person,
divided into 43kg of chicken, 33kg of beef, 25kg of pork and 9kg of lamb.

Sausages

Three-quarters of all sausages sold in Australia are made of beef, followed by pork, chicken and lamb, in that order. Many sausages are quite high in fat and salt, and most contain preservatives so it is best not to eat them too often.

What types are there?

Sausages may be fresh or cured: when buying fresh, seek out a quality butcher who makes his own without added colourings and preservatives. Read labels carefully for details of additives, and go for sausages with a high meat content. Each country has it's sausage specialities. These are just a few:

- **Bratwurst**, a German smoked sausage of pork or veal, sold raw and cooked. Can be simmered in hot water for 10 minutes, then finished off by grilling.
- **Chorizo**, a spicy Spanish pork sausage, flavoured and coloured with paprika, which can be smoked or unsmoked; some are raw and require cooking. A small amount packs a lot of flavour in a stew, soup or sauce.
- **Sucuk**, a spicy garlicky beef sausage used in Turkey and elsewhere in Central Europe. Usually fried in thin slices or used in small pieces to season other dishes.
- **Frankfurter**, a highly seasoned German sausage of mixed pork and beef that has been much abused as the hot dog.
- **Salami**, varieties of salami are made all over Europe, mostly from pork. They are hung to 'mature' for at least a few weeks and are highly flavoured.
- **Lap cheong**, a Chinese dried pork and liver sausage often used in small pieces to season rice or noodle dishes.

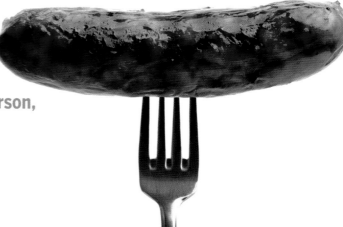

Veal

The meat of veal calves is low in fat and high in protein, with similar vitamins to other red meats, but less zinc and iron, particularly if the calves are fed a milky diet.

How does it get to us?

Veal is inextricably linked with the dairy farming industry, which depends on cows having calves in order to produce milk. Most female calves live to be the next generation of milkers, but male dairy calves are of no further use to the dairy farmer and are quickly sold on to be reared for veal.

➤➤ White veal calves in Europe are reared in **intensive indoor systems**, on a milky diet to keep the meat **pale in colour**. Kept at first in separate cubicles, from eight weeks calves are housed in groups, ranging from five to ten to indoor herds of up to 80. They live on concrete slatted floors without straw, as this would colour the meat if they ate it. However, this is not a good environment for the calves and regulations in Australia and New Zealand do not permit the production of this kind of veal.

➤➤ Rosé veal or pink veal calves Calves are fed **green, plant-based foods**, in addition to the milk-based diet. This more natural diet turns the meat **rosy-pink in colour**. Most calves **graze outside** for at least part of the time, but some are 'loose-housed' in barns so that they can move around and bedded on straw. Most are slaughtered between eight and 12 months. The younger the animal, the **milder and more tender** the meat; older veal is sometimes called 'young beef'.

➤➤ In the best, often organic systems calves stay with their mothers or are placed with a 'retired' cow who acts as a 'wet nurse', and they graze on pasture with the cows.

What to look for
● **Choose veal with a rosy colour** – it has a better nutritional profile than white veal and the calves are more likely to have had a better life.
● **The healthiest veal** comes from calves that have grazed outside, which results in more omega-3 fatty acids and conjugated linoleic acid in the meat, plus more iron and zinc.

How can I use it?

Veal keeps for two to three days in the fridge, nine to 12 months in the freezer (three to four months for minced). As it contains very little fat, it needs a liquid, sauce or stuffing to keep it moist and juicy.

➤➤ Roast it Leg is a prime roasting cut; if boned and stuffed, this helps to keep the meat moist. Loin is another good roasting cut.

➤➤ Grill or braise it Veal chops and cutlets cook well this way.

➤➤ Stew it Cubes of shoulder or shin, cooked gently and slowly, make good stews and pies.

Is veal cruel? Veal got its cruel reputation from the veal crate system devised to produce white veal, in which calves were kept, often chained, in tiny darkened cubicles for their three month lives. The veal crate is banned in Europe, the UK and in Australia and New Zealand, but it is still used in some countries, including some parts of the USA and in Switzerland. White veal, and some rosé, still comes from intensive rearing farms, and calves are taken from their mothers at an extremely young age – within hours, at most days, of being born – and sometimes transported huge distances, causing stress and injury.

Liver & kidneys

All offal is highly nutritious, but only liver and kidneys are still widely eaten today. Some specialist butchers still stock a range of offal; you may need to search online.

Good to know

Most types of offal – brains, heart, sweetbreads, tongue, tripe, trotters – are good sources of protein, vitamins and minerals. Liver is particularly high in vitamin A, but should be avoided in pregnancy as too much vitamin A has been linked to birth defects.

How can I use it?

Liver is an excellent source of vitamins A and B (especially B_2, B_3 and B_{12}), plus several minerals including copper, zinc, phosphorus, iron and selenium.
- **Calf's liver** is a super-nutritious pick-me-up food, which is usually quickly sautéed. Try this: season sliced liver, sear it briefly, then deglaze the pan with balsamic or sherry vinegar, and serve with a folate-rich vegetable such as spinach, broccoli or kale.
- **Lamb's liver** has a stronger flavour than calf's and is cheaper. Try thin slices quickly pan-fried for 3 to 4 minutes at most, combined with slow-cooked onions, then served with mashed potato and a green vegetable. Or try it in a casserole or stew.
- **Pig's liver** has a soft texture and strong flavour, and is a good choice for pâtés and terrines.

Kidneys are particularly rich in vitamin B_{12}, but are high in energy compared to liver.
- **Lamb's kidneys** are tender enough to grill or fry. Slice in half and cut out the white core of the kidney before cooking.
- **Ox, calf's or pig's kidneys** have a stronger taste and are better in casseroles and stews. Their flavour combines well with herbs, mushrooms, mustard, olives, capsicums and tomatoes.
- **For a classic steak and kidney pie** mix ox's, pig's or lamb's kidney with braising steak, fried onions and gravy, then add a pastry topping.

Venison

With more protein and less fat, venison is one of the healthiest red meats you can eat.

How does it get to us?

Venison comes from four breeds of deer: red (the most common), sika, fallow and roe. All taste quite similar, although chefs and game dealers often rate the smaller roe deer highly for the tenderness and fine-grained texture of its meat. If the carcass is hung, the meat develops a distinctively gamey flavour; otherwise it is very similar to that of grass-fed beef.

Wild venison is from deer shot in the wild, on a traditional game 'shoot', or as part of an organised cull. An annual cull keeps numbers at manageable levels and prevent deer from doing too much damage to forests and cultivated crops.

Farmed venison is from deer fenced in on large expanses of land where they roam and graze freely. In a hard winter, they might need extra food – preserved grass, root vegetables, grain – or even be brought indoors to keep them in good condition.

A 70g serving of venison supplies 50 per cent of daily protein needs.

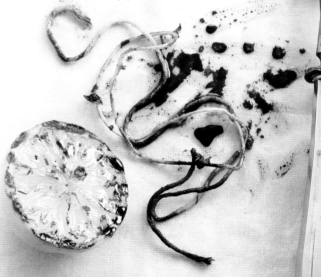

Where and when to buy it

- **Butchers with a game licence** sell wild and farmed venison. You can often find farmed venison in farm shops or farmers' markets, or buy direct through mail order or online. Venison is still considered a minority taste, so it's rare to find it in supermarkets.
- **Farmed venison** is more consistent in quality throughout the year, although traditionalists swear that it never comes up to the best wild venison.
- **Most venison is sold fresh** although you may see venison sausages, burgers and pâtés. A few products are cured, and so contain tiny amounts of potentially dangerous chemical preservatives.

How can I use it?

Venison often works well in dishes more usually made with beef or lamb, or try out specific venison recipes. It is a very lean meat, so you may need to add a little extra oil.

Braise it in a slow-braise casserole cooked with sweet fruits, vegetables and nuts: try it with quince, blackberries, root vegetables or chestnuts.

Roast it Prime roasting cuts such as loin or haunch (leg) can be cooked pink, just like beef. Roast it quickly and allow it ample time to rest before carving.

Mince it Use it as a change from beef in burgers cottage pie, spaghetti Bolognese or chilli con carne.

Spice it Venison has the depth of character to match the strongly aromatic spices of Indian, Malaysian and Thai curries, as well as fiery Mexican dishes.

In a warm salad Season a small piece of loin with black pepper, sear on all sides, then leave to rest for 5 minutes; slice thinly and serve over salad leaves.

Try it raw For an excellent carpaccio, chill a small piece of loin, slice thinly, then beat the slices between two sheets of greaseproof paper until paper-thin. Arrange the slices on a plate, drizzle with olive oil and lemon juice, and top with parmesan shavings.

Rabbit

Classed as a white meat, rabbit supplies lean protein. It is one of the best sources of vitamin B_{12}, a good source of vitamins B_3 (niacin) and B_6 (pyridoxine) and has high levels of iron and zinc, plus phosphorus.

How does it get to us?

Wild rabbits live a natural life, centred on underground warrens, and are trapped or shot. You can buy wild rabbit from a game dealer, a butcher or farm shop with a licence to sell game, by mail order or online, and often at farmers' markets.
- **The meat should be pale pink**, without any darkened or bruised flesh which could indicate that the animal had not been cleanly shot. If lead shot remains in the meat, it will smell 'high' and taste bitter.

Farmed rabbit is more common than wild in Australia and New Zealand, due to diseases prevalent in the wild. Farmed rabbits are caged and fed on a grain diet. The meat is softer and has more fat than that of wild rabbit and its flavour is milder.

How can I use it?

Because freshness is crucial, wild rabbit should be cooked on the day you buy it. Freezing wild rabbit is not recommended; farmed rabbit can be frozen. Wild rabbit is so lean that it can be dry, so cook it quickly or add a little fat to keep the meat succulent. The best meat is the saddle and the back legs.

Casserole it Brown joints of rabbit and cook in the oven with bacon, garlic, vegetables and herbs.

Roast it Marinate rabbit legs overnight in olive oil, lemon juice, rosemary, thyme and pepper, then roast at a high temperature for 25–30 minutes. The saddle is delicious wrapped in thin slices of dry-cured ham, then roasted.

Use in paella Rabbit is one of the meats used to make an authentic paella Valenciana.

Poultry & game birds

All types of poultry supply excellent protein.
With the exception of duck and goose, poultry is lower in fat than red meat.

How do they get to us?

The term 'poultry', strictly speaking, refers to domesticated birds reared for the table. By far the most popular is chicken, which in less than half a century has gone from being a rare treat to one of the cheapest, most ubiquitous meats in the world – largely as a result of factory-farming on an industrial scale.

➡ **Indoor-reared** About 85 per cent of the half a billion chickens reared annually for meat in Australia and New Zealand are kept in large sheds in flocks of up to 50,000 birds, with artificial light and ventilation. They are fed soy- and cereal-based feeds until they reach the desired weight at about five to six weeks old. A small proportion of indoor poultry is reared in smaller-scale operations, with fresh air, natural light, more room per bird and some sort of 'environmental enrichment' such as straw bales to perch on and peck at. Both types of indoor operation are sometimes referred to as 'barn-reared'.

➡ **Free-range** The birds have constant daytime access to a green, outdoor area so they can exercise and peck around for natural food in addition to the grain-based diet. Flocks can be large, but indoor space per bird is more generous than for indoor-reared birds. The birds take longer to reach target weight.

➡ **Organic** These birds are always free-range, and are kept in small flocks.

They must be fed only organically grown feed and their outdoor range must be on organically farmed land.

➡ **'Game' birds**, by tradition, are hunted and shot in the wild, but in Australia and New Zealand, native birds are generally protected by law. Introduced species such as pheasant and partridge are farmed for sale as meat, and a few are farmed specifically for use in recreational shooting events.

Different types

Most birds have lean meat that contains some healthy monounsaturated fat, but their skin contains saturated fat and is often best removed either before cooking or eating. Wild game and free-range birds are generally leaner than farmed birds. Here's an A to Z of types.

➡ **Chicken** is one of the most versatile and widely used foods in the modern diet. All grades of chicken supply protein, vitamins and minerals (*see* page 224), but the nutritional quality declines with lower welfare standards and price. **Poussin** is the term use for a small, immature chicken. It has less flavour than chicken and serves only one person.

Why is free range better? Just as with other meats, the more natural food in the bird's diet, the higher the levels of desirable omega-3 fatty acids and conjugated linoleic acid. Physical activity also helps produce a healthier fat profile, and free-range birds get more exercise. So the healthiest meat comes from birds that have been able to roam outside and have some pasture-based, foraged diet. Meat from indoor birds fattened up as quickly as possible on cereal- and soy-based feed, with little opportunity or motivation to exercise, will not have such a good nutritional profile.

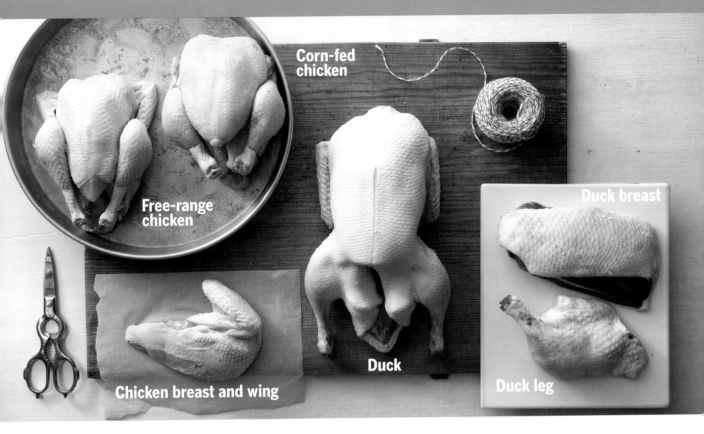

Corn-fed chicken

Free-range chicken

Duck breast

Chicken breast and wing

Duck

Duck leg

Duck is a mid-sized bird with delicious, rich, dark meat. As a water bird, it has a lot of fat in and just under the skin: the meat is 10 per cent fat, but with the skin it's a whopping 29 per cent fat, which makes it even more important to remove the skin from duck before eating (comparative figures for chicken are four and 18 per cent). Most of the 10 million ducks farmed each year in Australia and New Zealand are reared indoors in shed conditions similar to chickens.

Goose is a large bird with dark, rich, almost gamey meat, usually only available at Christmas. A water bird, it has even more fat than duck. Traditionally the fat was rendered out during roasting and saved for use in cooking and also for home remedies.

Guinea fowl is smaller breasted than chicken, with slightly firmer, darker meat that is low in saturated fat. The meat has a flavour somewhere between chicken and pheasant.

Partridge is available from specialty butchers in Australia and New Zealand. It is a small, mild-tasting game bird that is low in fat and high in protein – almost 37g per 100g of meat.

Pheasant is farmed in Australia and New Zealand and is relatively high in fat for a game bird at 10 to 12 per cent, but most of it is monounsaturated. The breast meat is drier than chicken and the legs chewier, so care is needed in cooking, but the result can be delicious as well as nutritious. A 100g serving of roast pheasant supplies 32g of protein and virtually all of your daily iron requirement.

Quail is a very small game bird now bred for the table. It has delicately flavoured meat that tastes a little like chicken.

Squab is the farmed version of pigeon. A small bird with dark red meat, it has a flavour more

Surprise ingredients in processed 'chicken' When you pick up a fast-food chicken meal, you will almost certainly get more than the chicken you bargained for. In one popular supermarket chain, a dozen ingredients are listed for the 'chicken' in their 'crispy chicken strips'.

The same is true for the chicken (and turkey) in many other supermarket products. Whether in chicken ready meals, or pizza with a chicken topping, even sandwiches and salads, the chicken itself often contains water, salt and sometimes added cornflour or another starch.

Processed products, such as turkey 'ham', chicken kievs or some chicken nuggets, also carry the same potential risks from chemical preservatives and salt as other processed meat products (see page 58). It is therefore wise not to eat them too often.

● **Some free-range and organic producers specialise** in more mature birds and breeds with more flavour. Duck breeds known for flavour include Aylesbury, Pekin and Muscovy, while Standard Bronze is a favoured breed of turkey. Turkeys, ducks and geese have superior flavour if they are hung for a few days after slaughter, and usually this is only done by small independent producers. To seek out this wider choice try farmers' markets or research them online.

● **When buying game birds**, check with the butcher or game dealer that the bird has been cleanly shot. If lead shot is in the meat the bird will taste bitter and you risk breaking a tooth.

How can I use it?

like beef or venison than chicken. It is very rich in iron – just 50g cooked squab supplies the full daily requirement. Usually only the breast is eaten.

➤ Turkey is a favourite Christmas bird; organic and free-range turkeys are often only available at this time. The white breast meat is similar in taste to chicken. The dark leg meat is fattier, but contains more than double the iron and zinc. Most turkey joints and mince, which are widely sold, are from intensively reared birds.

What to look for

● **Whole birds** should have fresh, unblemished skin and meat; avoid birds with bruises, or dry, torn or discoloured skin. Make sure the wrapping on a pre-packaged bird is not torn or leaking.

● **Free-range birds taste better** than indoor-reared because they are a few weeks more mature by the time they are killed, which makes for a better flavour in the meat – as a general rule, the older the bird, the better the flavour. They also have a better nutritional profile, so buy free range if possible.

● **Increasing amounts of chicken** are sold pre-butchered in packs of breasts, thighs or drumsticks. This may be more convenient, but whole birds offer better value if you use every bit of the bird. With a sharp knife and kitchen scissors, jointing a chicken is not difficult; the breasts and legs can be made into separate dishes, or frozen until needed, and the carcass used to make stock.

Refrigerate poultry as soon as possible after buying it. If you are cooking it that day, you can leave it in its shop wrapping. If not, unwrap it, remove any giblets from inside a whole bird, then put it in a loosely covered container, or on a large plate covered with foil or greaseproof paper. Put the bird on the bottom shelf and don't overcrowd the fridge around it. Cook poultry within two days of purchase, or by its 'use by' date, whichever comes soonest. (*See* Safe eating, right) Better still, use it or freeze it the day you buy it.

➤ Roast it Roasting is one of the healthiest ways to cook poultry and game birds, because it allows fat to drain off during cooking. Most types of bird roast well, with cooking times and techniques varying with the size and type of bird.

● **The classic roast chicken** is still a special meal made with a good-quality free-range or organic bird.

● **Leftover roast meat** can be used in risotto, curry, a salad or sandwiches, and the carcass boiled up with onion, carrot, celery, peppercorns, bay leaf and herbs to make stock.

➤ Braise it A popular example is coq au vin – jointed chicken slow-cooked in red wine with garlic, onions, mushrooms and herbs, then enriched towards the end of cooking with a scattering of crispy bacon lardons and soft-cooked shallots.

It is perfectly legal to inject chicken breasts with water and protein from cows or pigs if the products are labelled accordingly.

Poach it Cook a whole chicken or chicken pieces in water with added spices and seasonings; the poaching liquid can be kept to use as a stock. Use the meat in a salad or, to make a pie, cut it up and use in a creamy sauce with mushrooms, peas or leeks, topped with puff pastry. Or try making Moroccan pastilla, a nutty filo pastry pie traditionally made with squab but also good with chicken.

Casserole it For a quicker cooking method than slow-braising, brown pieces of chicken in olive oil with onions, celery and garlic, then add vegetables of your choice – sun-dried capsicums and chopped tomatoes, for example, or carrots and leeks – plus extra liquid if needed, and simmer till cooked.

Curry it The leg meat from chicken or turkey works well in homemade curries. For the best flavour, cook chicken legs with the bones left in, then remove them just before serving. As in casseroles, the amount of meat can be stretched with vegetables to suit.

Sear it For a warm autumnal salad, sear breast of duck, slice thinly and serve over a green salad dressed with vinaigrette and crunchy croutons.

Safe eating

Chicken and turkey are one of the most common causes of food poisoning as a result of contamination with bacteria such as campylobacter and salmonella. Both of these bugs are killed by cooking, so the most important rule is to make sure poultry is fully cooked through. However, because most poultry is lean, you should not overcook it or it will become dry.
● **To test for doneness by eye**, plunge a sharp knife or skewer into the thickest part of the meat. For chicken, turkey and goose, the juices that run out must be completely clear; if they are at all pink the meat needs more cooking. (Duck and some game birds may be served rare, in which case the juices will be pink.)

● **To test for doneness by temperature**, a more precise way of checking, use an instant-read thermometer. At the end of the recommended cooking time, push the probe into the thickest part of the meat. For chicken and turkey, the white breast meat should have reached a temperature of 71°C; the leg meat should be at least 75°C.

Kangaroo

A high-protein, almost fat-free meat, kangaroo is increasing in popularity in Australia and overseas.

How does it get to us?

Kangaroo is a wild meat, harvested from Australia's national parks on a quota system based on yearly population audits.

How can I use it?

As kangaroo is very low in fat, it can dry out quickly, so the best cooking methods either add moisture or keep the meat rare with brief cooking. It can be used as a substitute for other red meat in most recipes.

Mince it for rissoles, shepherd's pie and spaghetti Bolognese. It can be used as a leaner substitute in any minced beef recipe.

Roast it Kangaroo fillet should be cooked rare or no more than medium-rare for maximum tenderness, and rested well before carving.

Braise it Long, slow cooking creates a tender, flavoursome dish. Sweet, tangy and earthy flavours go particularly well with kangaroo – try beetroot, plum, red currant, orange or dried fruits.

2 Fish & seafood

Fish and shellfish are the last major resource of wild, protein-rich food left on the planet but over-fishing and pollution have taken their toll. Fish farming has expanded to fill the gap. China is the worlds largest producer; two thirds of its fish come from aquaculture.

What does it do for me?

Fish is one of the very best foods you can eat for health, a real nutritional treasure trove that supplies:

➡ High-quality protein All fish and shellfish are excellent protein sources, with less fat and saturated fat than meat, and especially in the case of oily fish, high levels of beneficial oils.

➡ Vitamins All fish and seafood supply significant amounts of B vitamins (B_3, B_6, B_{12}), which help the nervous system and brain to function properly.
- **Oily fish** is the best food source of vitamin D, and a good source of vitamin A – important for vision.
- **Fish liver oils** are rich in vitamins A and D, as well as vitamin E which works as an antioxidant.
- **Fish roes** are extremely nutritious. Mullet, lumpfish, salmon and flying fish roe are amongst those available for cooking.

➡ Minerals Fish and seafood are rich in trace elements and minerals, including: potassium (regulates blood pressure); **iron** (gives energy, prevents anaemia), **zinc** (supports the immune system); **selenium** (may protect against some cancers); **iodine** (regulates metabolism and thyroid gland); phosphorus (for healthy teeth and bones). Whitebait, canned salmon and other fish eaten with the bones are good sources of calcium.

➡ Omega-3 oils Oily fish and shellfish, crab in particular, are the best dietary sources we have of two omega-3 fatty acids: EPA (eicosapentaenoic acid) and DHA (docosahexaenoic acid). Cod liver oil is another very rich source.
- **EPA and DHA** are thought to have a number of beneficial health effects; these include protecting against heart disease and stroke, helping to build brain and eye tissue, supporting the immune system and brain function, and ensuring the healthy development of the unborn child.
- **Most canned fish** – including tuna – retains its EPA and DHA omega-3 fats, according to a recent UK analysis. Canned fish such as salmon or sardines also deliver more calcium because their softened bones are included and usually eaten as well.

Canned tuna isn't nutritionally inferior
New UK food analysis suggests it is as rich in omega-3 fats as fresh tuna.

Fish farming is now a $100 billion worldwide industry but the impact of intensive farms on rivers and coastal areas and the **high levels of drugs and pesticides** often used concern health and environmental experts.

Is eating fish good for the brain? Eating fish may not make you cleverer but it may well help maintain brainpower throughout life. The human brain is almost 60 per cent fat, much of this the beneficial omega-3 DHA, and people who eat fish rich in DHA tend to experience less dementia and fewer problems with memory as they get older. Research backs up these claims. Two Dutch studies involving several thousand people reported that regular consumption of fish protects against age-related brain impairment and dementia. Another found that adding DHA to the diet of children with attention-deficit hyperactivity disorder (ADHD) improves behaviour, reading skills and concentration.

What types are there?

▶▶ **White fish** Includes barramundi, bream, catfish, cod, flake, flathead, flounder, John Dory, ling, monkfish, mullet, skate, snapper and whiting. Flake is actually a small shark.
● **Flavours vary** and textures range from soft (flounder, whiting), through flaky (bream, snapper, flathead) to relatively firm (barramundi, cod, monkfish).

▶▶ **Oily fish** Includes all the fish with steely, silver or blue-grey skin: herring, mackerel, salmon, sardines, swordfish, tuna and trout. It also includes the tiny, silvery-blue anchovy, which is usually canned or salted rather than fresh, and whitebait, actually young herring, eaten bones and all.
● **Oily freshwater species** include brown trout, rainbow trout, salmon and carp.
● **They contain more healthy omega-3 fats** than white fish, with the fat spread throughout the body and muscle tissue; in white fish it is concentrated in the liver. With the exception of rainbow trout, oily fish has a stronger flavour than white.

▶▶ **Crustaceans** include:
● **All shellfish species** with a crust-like shell and legs, such as crab, yabbie, lobster and prawns.
● **The flesh is sweetly flavoured**, while textures go from slightly firm flesh (lobster, prawn) to soft and flaky (crab).

▶▶ **Molluscs** include:
● **Bivalve shellfish**, such as clams, mussels, oysters and scallops; they have complex marine flavours and textures that vary from fleshy (mussels, oysters) to more muscular (clams, scallops).
● **Cephalopod molluscs**, such as squid, octopus and cuttlefish, which have large heads and tentacles. The cephalopods have a flavour somewhere between a white fish and a scallop, but with a more muscular, slightly chewier texture.
● **Gastropod molluscs**, better known as snails: edible sea snails include whelks (often called 'mud whelks'), which are caught in whelk pots, and winkles, which can be harvested from rocks and mud flats at low tide.

How does it get to us?

The ocean harvest Wild fish is mostly caught by sea-going fishing vessels, ranging from small boats that go out for hours or days at a time, returning to port with a fresh catch, to huge factory ships that spend weeks at sea, processing and freezing the fish as it is caught. Various methods are used to catch different species, some more controversial than others:

- **Trawler nets and seine nets** dragged behind vessels scoop up large numbers of shoaling fish. Mid-water trawler and seine nets catch fish that shoal not far below the surface, such as anchovy, herring, sardine and mackerel. Bottom trawlers target bottom-dwelling flat fish such as flounder, and prawns, and deep-water fish such as cod and squid. Bottom trawling has been criticised for damaging the seabed and indiscriminately hoovering up everything that lies in its path.
- **Line fishing** ranges from individual rod-and-line, used commercially for bass, for example, to long-line fishing with hundreds of hooks per line targeting large fish such as tuna, as well as smaller species such as mackerel. Long-line fishing has been much criticised for the large numbers of unwanted fish and seabirds such as albatross, that are also caught.
- **Dredging** involves dragging a chain net over the seabed, which can cause damage. Oysters, scallops, crabs and some types of clam are caught this way.
- **Baited traps or pots** are used to catch crabs, crayfish and lobsters.
- **Harvesting by hand** Cockles are often hand-picked from the sands at low tide and scallops are hand-picked from the seabed by divers.

Fish farms and aquaculture Fish farming has been with us since ancient times, but its rapid growth in recent decades is unprecedented; some see it as the marine equivalent of intensive farming on land. Asia and the Pacific region accounts for almost 90 per cent of the worlds aquaculture.

Sustainable freshwater carp farming
Not all species of farmed fish depend on wild fish for food. The carp, a fast-growing omnivore that can thrive on a mostly vegetarian diet, provides excellent nutrition and is widely farmed across the world. The World Wildlife Fund has highlighted China's success in developing aquaculture to provide its people with a protein-rich, low-cost diet in an eco-friendly way, minimising the need for artificial feed. In Europe, particularly Eastern Europe, where carp is traditional Christmas Eve fare, sustainable management of pond aquaculture is also being strongly encouraged. Being environmentally responsible makes good business sense, say Food and Agricultural Organization consultants in a 2011 report.

- **Commonly farmed species include** salmon, tilapia, carp, catfish, trout, prawns, mussels and oysters, and the number of species is growing. Some of these – rope-grown mussels, for example, and oysters – are farmed very successfully, resulting in high-quality products without damaging their environment. Some methods, however, have been strongly criticised:
- **Tiger prawn farming** has destroyed large areas of mangrove forest, a unique habitat, and polluted the coastal waters around the farms, with high levels of pollutants found in some of the prawns. The Marine Conservation Society recommends buying tiger prawns only from suppliers that can ensure their product is sourced from farms that comply with environmental standards for habitat protection and impacts of production. The easiest way to do this is to buy organic tiger prawns.
- **Commercial salmon farming** depends on large quantities of wild fish being caught and processed for feed, depleting the ocean food chain. It is also accused of polluting local waters and spreading disease among wild fish. Ask your supplier whether what you are buying is wild or farmed, and if the source is sustainable. Organic salmon is fed on waste offal and trimmings from the commercial fish catch.

Aquaculture has been the fastest-growing sector of food production for six decades,
averaging growth of **almost 7% a year.**

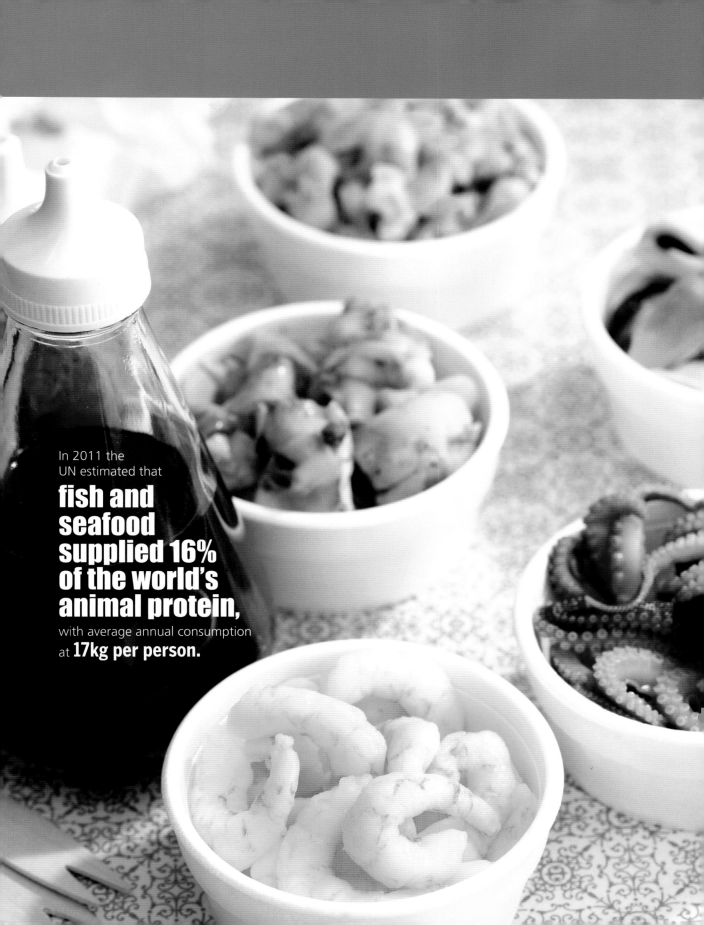

In 2011 the
UN estimated that

**fish and
seafood
supplied 16%
of the world's
animal protein,**

with average annual consumption
at **17kg per person.**

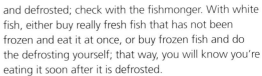

Buying and handling

Whether you buy from a traditional wet fish shop, a market fish stall, a fish counter in a supermarket, or are visited by a travelling fish van, there are two general points to keep in mind when choosing fish:

● **Seasonality** Many fish are seasonal foods, which taste better – and are better for you – at certain times of year. Some seafood is simply not available fresh at certain times. Check with your fishmonger, who will be able to recommend what is particularly good for the time of year.

● **Freshness** For fish and shellfish to be at its best – and for shellfish to be safe – it must be really fresh, so its important that your fishmonger has a good, quick turnover of stock. Fish should have a pleasant marine smell, but never smell pungently fishy, which is a sign that the fish is old.

What to look for

■▶ **White and oily fish** A whole fish tells you a lot about freshness.

● **A fresh fish will have clear eyes and bright red gills** (the bit below the head). It should look athletic and svelte, with a skin that is moist and sparkly, not dry or matt.

● **Fillets are harder to judge for freshness** Look for those with a nice gloss; dull-looking fillets, may have been lying around for too long. Any that are sitting in water may have been previously frozen

and defrosted; check with the fishmonger. With white fish, either buy really fresh fish that has not been frozen and eat it at once, or buy frozen fish and do the defrosting yourself; that way, you will know you're eating it soon after it is defrosted.

● **Oily fish must be fresh when you buy it**, because freezing is rarely successful (salmon and sea trout are exceptions to this rule). Ideally, you will first see the fish whole so you know it is fresh, then watch the fishmonger gut and prepare it for you. Oily fish, such as mackerel and herring, deteriorate faster than white fish and develop a strong fish oil smell that many people find off-putting. It is best to cook oily fish and eat it the day you buy it.

■▶ **Seafood**

● **Fresh wild prawns** are delicious but hard to track down and expensive; check that apparently fresh prawns have not been previously frozen and defrosted. Frozen prawns usually have added salt and will also contain a lot of water, known as an ice glaze. When deciding which to buy, go for frozen prawns that state their weight after defrosting (deglazed weight), otherwise you can end up with almost as much water as prawns.

● **Scallops are best bought fresh**, too, because frozen scallops often contain a lot of water. If they look softly plump and watery, they may have been soaked in water to plump them up. Opt for smaller scallops that haven't been soaked: they may be more expensive, but will be better value for money.

● **Mussels and clams**, and other bivalve shellfish, should have shells that are clammed shut – this is a sign of freshness. Never buy or use bivalves with smashed or broken shells: they haven't been transported properly. On average, from a kilo of mussels you might expect to throw two or three away; any more and the mussels aren't fresh enough.

Storage and safety tips

● **All fresh fish and shellfish** should, ideally, be eaten on the day of purchase. If this is not possible, store fish in the bottom of the fridge for no more than 24 hours. Place live molluscs in a large container and

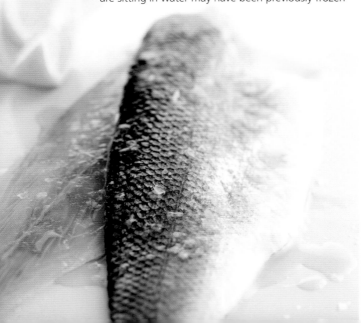

clear eyes and bright red gills.

Ideally, cook and eat fresh fish and shellfish the same day that you buy them.

cover with a damp cloth before placing in the fridge. Never leave live molluscs in fresh water as they will die.

● **Freeze only fresh white fish** To preserve its delicate texture, wrap it tightly in foil and freeze at the lowest possible temperature, preferably on fast-freeze. Once frozen it can be stored for up to three months at −18°C. Other than salmon and trout, do not freeze oily fish as its oils cause it to spoil rapidly.

● **Use a separate clean chopping board** when preparing fish and shellfish, to avoid transferring potentially harmful bacteria to other foods. Always wash your hands before and after handling fish.

● **While preparing fish fillets** run your fingertips over the cut side to feel for any bones and use clean tweezers to pluck out any that you find.

● **Before you cook mussels**, scrub them well under running water and remove the beards. If any of the shells are slightly open, give them a tap: if they close immediately, they're fine to eat; but if not, throw them away. Discard any broken shells as well.

How much can I eat?

Fish and seafood are highly nutritious, with a wealth of attributes that promote good health and protect against illness, so in principle it is a good food to eat as often as you like. But both are under constant threat from pollution and over-fishing, so some caution is required. Make sure your fish and shellfish come from a sustainable source and unpolluted waters, and be aware of the following:

● **Oily fish** are the richest source of beneficial omega-3 fats, so its consumption is generally recommended. But, because pollutants from industry and dumping of waste can build up in the fat of oily fish, pregnant and breastfeeding women, as well as children under 12 and women trying to conceive, are advised to eat no more than one 150g serve per fortnight, with no other fish consumed that fortnight. All other adults should stick to one serve per week, with no other fish consumed that week.

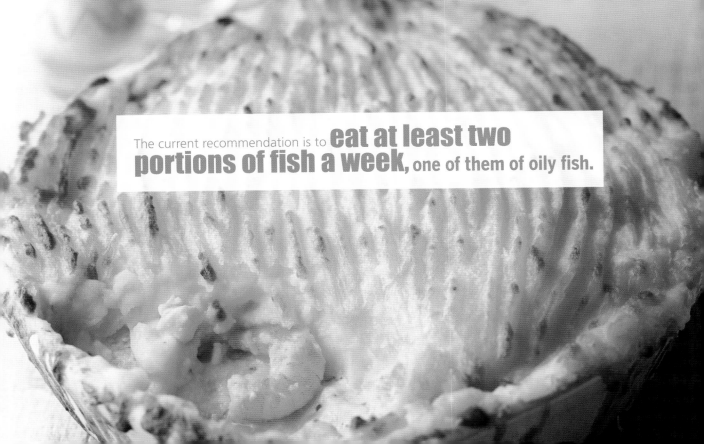

The current recommendation is to **eat at least two portions of fish a week,** one of them of oily fish.

- **Farmed prawns and fish** Buy fresh and organic if possible. The World Wildlife Fund has criticised high levels of pollution from waste, chemicals and antibiotics and widespread disease in intensive prawn farming. Similarly, intensive fish farms often make heavy use of antibiotics and pesticides. As in animal farming, overuse of antibiotics can contribute to antibiotic resistance in humans.

- **Bivalve shellfish** Mussels and clams feed themselves by filtering microscopic organisms from seawater, which brings a small risk that harmful bacteria and viruses, such as gastroenteritis, as well as natural toxins from the marine environment may build up in their tissues. Rope-farmed mussels generally have high standards of purity and consistent quality, but to minimise any potential risk follow the advice in Storage and safety tips, page 244.

- **Salt** Many seafood products, such as smoked salmon and smoked mackerel, are heavily salted, which is not good for anyone with high blood pressure. Most prawns and shellfish are naturally high in sodium, so should be eaten in moderation.

- **Allergies** Although not as common as allergies to milk, eggs or peanuts, shellfish allergy affects about one in 100 people, and fish allergy about 1 in 200. It occurs more often in adults than children, and once triggered tends to last for life.

- **Fish bones** An obvious risk if swallowed – *see* Storage and safety tips, page 244. Fish is often served on the bone, but even if it is filleted don't assume that any cooked fish set in front of you is bone-free: keep your eyes peeled for the bone that got away.

- **Cholesterol** Although low in fat, shellfish is high in dietary cholesterol, which was once considered harmful. Research now suggests that cholesterol in food does not clog arteries as previously thought.

How can I use it?

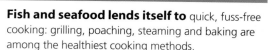

Fish and seafood lends itself to quick, fuss-free cooking: grilling, poaching, steaming and baking are among the healthiest cooking methods.

▶ Steam it Whole fish steams well – so well that a special piece of equipment, the fish kettle, was designed for the purpose (and for poaching). Rolled fillets or fish portions can be cooked in a steamer, perhaps set on a bed of vegetables such as samphire. In the classic French dish moules marinières, mussels are steamed in a little white wine or stock.

▶ Poach it Smoked haddock poaches beautifully, either in milk or water; try it for a special breakfast with a poached egg on top. Salmon is delicious poached in a little white wine, with a bay leaf and strip or lemon zest added.

▶ Grill it For a special treat, grill whole John Dory on the bone, sprinkled with a little olive oil and lemon juice, turning the fish once.

▶ Bake it Both whole fish and individual portions cook beautifully in oven-baked parcels – in essence, another way of steaming. Place the fish with finely cut vegetables (carrot strips, red or green capsicums, spring onions) and herbs to taste on a piece of foil, drizzle with lemon juice and olive oil (or Chinese flavourings, perhaps), then fold the ends of the foil together to seal, leaving plenty of air round the fish. Salmon, cod, sea bass and many other fish cook well this way. For a quick, delicious dish, spread a little basil pesto over fish fillets and bake in foil.

▶ Blitz it Smoked trout or mackerel makes a delicious pâté, mixed with cooked beetroot, low-fat cream cheese and lemon; or try smoked salmon with low-fat cream cheese, horseradish and dill; or brown and white crab meat mixed with a little mayonnaise, lemon and chives.

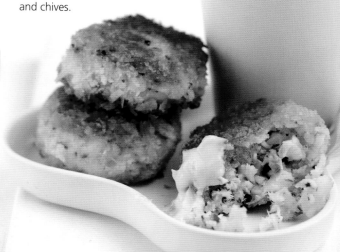

Sea vegetables

Some call them superfoods – these marine plants are full of good nutrients and virtually fat-free.

What do they do for me?

➨ Sea vegetables include samphire, sea aster and seaweeds – kelp, kombu, arame, wakame, dulse, nori, hijiki. They contain many vitamins, notably C, B group, including some B_{12}, and E, but because we eat them only in small quantities, they are not a significant source. Some seaweeds (kombu, wakame, bladderwrack, nori) also contain vitamin K.

● **Sea vegetables have useful amounts of minerals**, including iron (essential for healthy blood), calcium (which builds strong bones), iodine (which the body uses to make thyroid hormones), vanadium (which may help to regulate blood glucose levels) and zinc (which boosts the immune system). The dried seaweeds are a particularly good mineral source.

● **They contain fucoidans**, sulphurous starchy substances that some research suggests have anti-viral, anti-inflammatory and anti-thrombotic actions.

➨ Sea vegetables are good for you, but be aware that, like fish, they can be contaminated by heavy metals, such as arsenic, lead and mercury, which sometimes pollute the marine environment. Some suppliers regularly test their dried seaweeds to ensure they are free of contaminants and will indicate this on the packaging, so look out for assurances of quality and purity.

Where do I get them from?

● **Sea vegetables are harvested by hand** They are available fresh during the summer months, when they are sold in fishmonger shops and at the wet fish counter of supermarkets. Ask the vendor about their source to ensure they come from clean waters.

● **Dried sea vegetables and seaweeds** are available from wholefood shops. Choose brands that offer assurances about purity and check that dried seaweed products don't contain any unwelcome additives, such as artificial colourings.

How can I use them?

Samphire can be steamed; **sea aster** can be wilted in a small amount of butter. Dried **seaweeds** need to be soaked and rehydrated before using.

➨ With fish Buttery samphire or sea aster goes well with any white fish.

➨ In a vegetable mix Add a little samphire or sea aster to other green vegetables (peas, asparagus, spinach, green beans) to make a more unusual vegetable selection.

➨ In sushi You can buy ready-made nori-wrapped sushi, or try your hand at making your own.

➨ As tasty flakes Sprinkle flaked dried seaweeds over soups and salads.

➨ In salads Soak and rehydrate dried seaweeds and use them in small amounts with other vegetables in salads. Samphire and sea aster work well in a salad with asparagus and green beans.

Foods from the sea are the best sources of iodine,
with seaweed being the most reliable natural source.

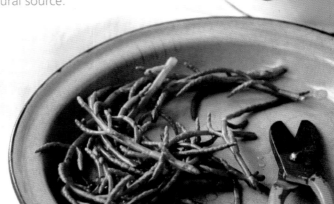

3 Fruit & vegetables

Low in fat, delicious and packed with goodness, fruit and vegetables should play a key role in your diet. Each has its own combination of vitamins, minerals and phytochemicals; eat a variety to benefit from them all.

Why seven-a-day?

⏩ **A slogan centred on five-a-day** was adopted by the US government in 1991 to increase public awareness of the health benefits of eating fresh produce; later it was picked up by the World Health Organization. Other countries such as Australia and New Zealand have chosen a higher daily target based on more recent research.

⏩ **How much is ideal?** A Spanish study published in 2013 found a six per cent decrease in risk of death for every extra serve of vegetables consumed. Eating a varied seven-a-day could reduce risk for diseases such as cancer, heart disease and stroke.

Is the sugar in fruit bad for me?
Recent studies have suggested that eating too much fructose – the predominant sugar in fruit – contributes to weight gain, obesity and 'metabolic syndrome', increasing the risk of cardiovascular disease and diabetes. In fact, the research focused on high consumption of fruit juice and drinks with added high-fructose corn syrup (HFCS), rather than on whole fruit. You would have to eat mountains of sweet, sugary fruits to approach the amounts of fructose involved. But a chilled soft drink or two, or a large carton of fruit juice soon adds up to a lot of concentrated fructose.

Many think we should aim even higher: Canada recommends up to ten and Japan a huge 17 serves.

⏩ **Fewer than half** of the population in Australia and New Zealand achieve the daily seven-a-day target according to consumption surveys. Intake is particularly poor amongst low-income families and people living in rural and remote areas.

Eat whole fruit
Whole fruit contains fibre, vitamins and micronutrients These are thought to neutralise, or compensate for, the effects of the fructose – the type of sugar in fruit.
- **Fruits with edible skins and seeds** have more fibre which slows the absorption of the fructose. High-fibre fruits include apples, pears, passionfruit, raspberries, pomegranates, blackberries and peaches.
- **Fruit juice** delivers fructose without the fibre of whole fruit, so don't count more than one occasional small glass towards your seven-a-day. For a longer drink, dilute it with water.

Does cooking destroy vitamins?

⏩ **It's common knowledge** that the heat of cooking reduces the vitamins and nutrients in vegetables. But is it correct? In fact, it is only partly true.
- **Cooking makes vegetables more digestible**, which means we absorb their nutrients more easily.
- **Many nutrients survive cooking**, vitamins E and K, for example; some actually become more available – such as vitamin A in the form of beta-carotene and lycopene.

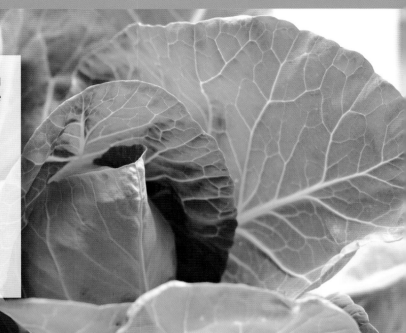

The now familiar 'seven-a-day' health slogan was coined in the late 1980s by **Californian fruit growers to help market their produce.**

Beware of pesticides Always wash fruit and vegetables thoroughly before use. Pesticide residue will be removed with the skin on vegetables that require peeling; others need to be washed for as long as you would wash your hands. Adding a small amount of salt or vinegar to the water can help remove residues, then rinse thoroughly. Commercial produce washes are also available. **Six fruits and vegetables** often found to have **high levels** of pesticides are strawberries, peaches, capsicums, cherries, apples and greens. Organic produce – not always a practical or affordable option – is pesticide-free but should also be washed to get rid of any bacteria.

Both fruit and vegetables contain soluble fibre, which aids digestion and helps

slow the release of glucose into the blood, producing a steady release of energy.

● **Some nutrients are water-soluble** so they leach into the liquid when cooked in water – this happens with some of the B vitamins, for example.
● **Some nutrients are destroyed by heat** – vitamin C is vulnerable because it is also water-soluble.

▶ Best ways to cook vegetables Much scientific effort has gone into finding the best ways to cook vegetables to conserve their valuable nutrients. Here are a few of the findings:
● A study of 12 different vegetable types found that **vitamins B_1 and B_2** were better retained when vegetables were roasted and steamed, rather than blanched or fried.
● A study of broccoli concluded that of all domestic cooking methods only steaming did not cause

significant losses of chlorophyll, **vitamin C** and beneficial **plant compounds**.
● Another broccoli study noted that more **antioxidant vitamins** were retained after microwaving than boiling. Cooking in water caused a leaching effect, which increased with cooking time.
● A study of the impact of cooking methods on folate found that boiling destroyed over half the **folate** in spinach and broccoli, but no significant decrease occurred as a result of steaming.

To get the most benefit from vegetables
● **Use them as fresh as possible**, because really fresh vegetables have more nutrients to start with.
● **Don't overcook them** – overcooking is the surest way of destroying vitamins and other nutrients such as fibre.
● **Steaming** and, to a lesser extent, roasting are better methods for retaining nutrients than boiling or frying.
● **Steam vitamin C-rich vegetables**, such as cabbages and spinach, for the shortest time possible.
● **Use the cooking liquid** from vegetables cooked in water to make sauce or gravy, or in a soup, so the water-soluble nutrients are not lost.
● **Eat vegetables raw** whenever you can – in salads, with dips or as snacks.

See also pages 84–91 and pages 142–143.

Apples & pears

What do they do for me?

Apples and pears are a good source of vitamin C and several beneficial micronutrients – quercetin, epicatechin and chlorogenic acid. Research suggests that these may reduce the risk of cancers, heart disease, asthma and diabetes, adding more truth to the adage 'an apple a day keeps the doctor away'.

How do they get to us?

These are orchard-grown outdoor fruits that are ready for harvesting in autumn. Fruits are picked by hand to prevent bruising. Apples are picked ready to eat, pears while still hard, before they ripen.

● **Most apples and pears are stored** soon after picking in cool, dark rooms in air that is modified by removing oxygen, the gas that causes fruit to rot. Because of improved preservation techniques, stored fruits can have a good flavour and retain most of their nutrients. Wash them thoroughly before use.

Freshly picked, newly harvested apples are fragrant and delicious. Eat them as soon as possible – don't refrigerate them as this reduces the aroma and taste. To find more traditional varieties, look in farm shops and farmers' markets.

● **Apples from cold storage** are best kept in the fridge to preserve their crunch. Take them out to warm up to room temperature before you eat them, as they will smell and taste better.

To enjoy pears at their best choose large, hard fruits and let them ripen at home, which can take up to a week in a cool room. As they ripen, they become more fragrant. When the flesh feels ever so slightly soft under the skin, they are ready – eat them straightaway as they soon spoil.

How can I use them?

Apart from the simple pleasures of eating them fresh and whole, both apples and pears can be enjoyed in a variety of dishes at any meal:

Breakfast Grate apples to make a Swiss-style Bircher muesli with soaked oats and yogurt. Sweeten breakfast cereal with a spoonful of apple purée, rather than sugar. Slice up a pear to add natural sweetness to cereal.

Poached For a delicious dessert, poach pears in red or white wine, port or marsala.

Baked Core apples and stuff the holes with chopped dried fruits, nuts and spices, then pop them in the oven until fluffy. Bake pears sprinkled with sugar and dusted with nutmeg or cardamom. Or make a tarte tatin, the upside-down French dessert of sliced apples (or pears), caramelised in butter and a little sugar, then topped with pastry and baked until golden.

As a crumble Stewed apples don't need much added sugar; adding oats and finely chopped nuts to the topping makes it more nutritious.

Savoury The sharpness of pear or apple compote complements roast pork, duck or goose.

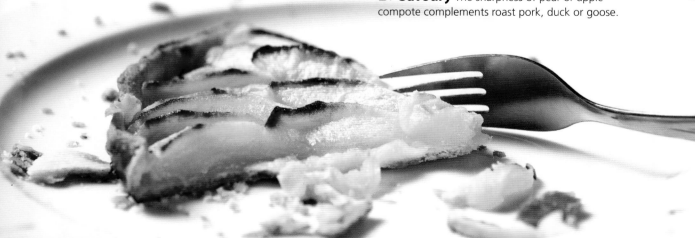

Berries

{ Raspberries, strawberries, blueberries, blackberries, blackcurrants, redcurrants, gooseberries }

What do they do for me?

➡ **All are an excellent source** of vitamin C and rich in micronutrients.

● **Anthocyanin compounds** in berries may have health-boosting effects, including strengthening the immune system, lowering blood pressure and reducing the risk of type 2 diabetes. The **tannins** are thought to be good for the heart and to promote longevity.

How do they get to us?

➡ **All berries are hand-picked**, which largely explains why they are often expensive. They require careful handling and packaging to avoid spoilage in transport.

● **Blueberries**, blackberries, blackcurrants, red-currants and gooseberries all grow on bushes in open fields.

● **Raspberries** grow on tall canes, and are increasingly cultivated under plastic canopies to protect the berries' appearance and to extend the growing season.

● **Strawberries** are ground plants. Some are still grown in open fields, but – to extend the season – now more usually in polytunnels, either in the ground or in grow bags on raised shelves which makes picking easier. Many are grown in hydroponic systems, in which the nutrients the plants need are dissolved in water.

➡ **For maximum fragrance and sweetness**, buy local berries fresh in the growing season (spring and summer). Store in the fridge, but give them time to warm to room temperature before serving to maximise the fragrance and bouquet.

● **As berries are** often pricey it can be worthwhile buying large quantities when the crop is plentiful and at its best as well as cheapest. Spend an hour or two at a pick-your-own fruit farm, or check out local markets and farm shops. Treat family and friends to a fresh berry 'splurge', then freeze the rest for future use.

● **Some berries freeze well whole;** spread raspberries, gooseberries, currants, blueberries and blackberries out on a tray to freeze quickly, then transfer to plastic freezer boxes or bags. Strawberries are better frozen as a fruit coulis (puréed, with the pips sieved out) – this is also good for raspberries, blueberries and blackberries. Redcurrants, blackcurrants and gooseberries freeze well as a compote (whole fruits softened in a little sugar).

How can I use them?

At the height of the berry season, enjoy them fresh from the punnet at any time of day. When cooking tarter berries, add as little sugar as possible.

➡ **Breakfast** Have them with low-fat natural yogurt, chopped nuts and seeds, or on top of cereal with milk. Stir frozen raspberries, summer berries, or a spoonful of blackcurrant compote into hot porridge.

➡ **Berry salad** A bowl of mixed berry fruits, with a dusting of sugar and a squeeze of lemon juice, makes a low-effort dessert that everyone loves.

➡ **Summer pudding** When berries are plentiful, this traditional pudding – mixed berries macerated in a bowl lined with white bread – is the flavour of summer.

➡ **Crumbles** Fresh or frozen berries add colour and flavour to an apple or pear crumble. Try apple-raspberry, pear-blackcurrant, pear-blueberry or apple-blackberry.

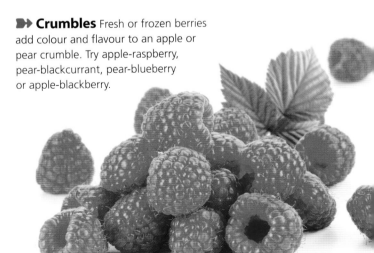

Citrus fruits { Oranges, lemons, limes, grapefruit, mandarins, kumquats, pomelos, tangelos }

What do they do for me?

➡ Citrus fruits – are one of the best sources of vitamin C, an antioxidant which helps to protect against disease and infection.

● **The pith of citrus fruits is rich in beneficial plant compounds**, such as hesperidin, which is thought to be anti-inflammatory, and limonene and quercetin, which research suggests may help to combat cancer.

How do they get to us?

➡ Citrus are tropical or sub-tropical fruits grown in orchards in sunny climates where there is little or no risk of frost.

● **Most oranges are a winter fruit**, and in season are fragrant, deliciously ripe and heavy with juice. Small fruits, such as mandarins, with leaves still attached will have been freshly picked. Don't be too concerned with appearance: the least attractive fruit can taste the best.

● **After they have been picked** citrus fruits are routinely treated with waxes containing chemical fungicides to help them keep for months in cold storage. The waxes are not suitable for human consumption. If you intend to use the zest of citrus fruits, make sure to buy organic fruits, which are never waxed, or fruit that is labelled 'unwaxed'. Alternatively, scrub the fruit with a vegetable brush before using.

How can I use them?

➡ It's healthier to eat the whole fruit rather than drinking citrus fruit juices because many of the beneficial plant compounds are in the yellow-white pith just beneath the skin, which is lost in the juicing. Juicing also destroys the fruit's beneficial dietary fibre and depletes other nutrients.

➡ After drinking citrus juice, rinse your mouth with water if possible. Do not brush your teeth with toothpaste for at least 30 minutes after eating or drinking citrus, to allow saliva time to neutralise the acid. If you're having fruit juice or citrus fruit at breakfast time, brush your teeth before the meal rather than just after it.

➡ Slice them When oranges and grapefruit are at their best, serve them simply peeled and sliced. Or serve segments of grapefruit with a raspberry coulis.

➡ Squeeze them The juice of lemons, limes, Seville oranges or grapefruit give slightly different flavours to a marinade – on fish for a ceviche, for example.

➡ Zest them Mix grated lemon zest with finely chopped garlic and parsley and sprinkle over meat dishes before serving. Use orange/lemon zest and juice to flavour cakes, or to make a syrup to drizzle over a warm cake, when it has cooked.

➡ Warm lemon Pour hot water onto a slice of lemon and sip as an alternative to tea and coffee. With more slices of lemon and a little honey, this is a classic soothing remedy for colds and sore throats.

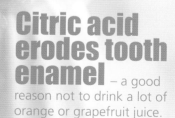

Citric acid erodes tooth enamel – a good reason not to drink a lot of orange or grapefruit juice.

Rhubarb

What does it do for me?

▶▶ **Rhubarb is a good source** of vitamin K, which is important for blood clotting and strong bones. It also has useful amounts of vitamin C and calcium.

● **What makes rhubarb particularly attractive** is that it is available early in spring or even in late winter, when other fruit options are becoming limited.

How does it get to us?

▶▶ **Outdoor rhubarb** grows in many back gardens, and is also grown commercially. It is at its best in late spring, when at least half the stalk is red and the stalks have not yet become too coarse.

▶▶ **Buy whole stalks** rather than cut rhubarb because they keep better. Take the stalks out of any plastic bag (which encourages them to rot) and put in the fridge.

How can I use it?

▶▶ **Use only the stalks** – do not eat the leaves, which are poisonous.

▶▶ **Add sweetness** Rhubarb needs added sugar to make it palatable, so should not be eaten too often. A mixture of rhubarb with apple or berries requires less sweetening. Add only the smallest amount of water, if any, as rhubarb contains a lot of moisture, which comes out in cooking

▶▶ **Bake it** One of the simplest ways to cook rhubarb is to peel the stalks, cut them to the desired length, then sprinkle them with sugar and bake in the oven.

▶▶ **Simmer it** Put peeled, chopped rhubarb into a pot, sprinkle with sugar, cover with a lid and leave to

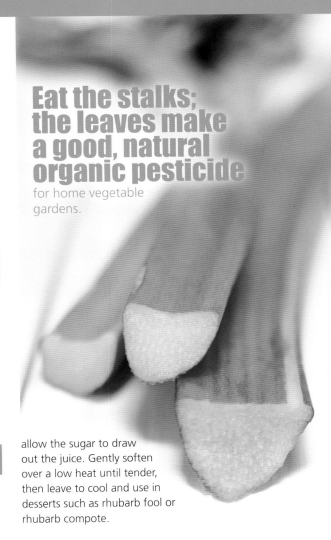

Eat the stalks; the leaves make a good, natural organic pesticide for home vegetable gardens.

allow the sugar to draw out the juice. Gently soften over a low heat until tender, then leave to cool and use in desserts such as rhubarb fool or rhubarb compote.

▶▶ **Roast it** A little roasted rhubarb is a good sharp accompaniment to mackerel or roast pork.

▶▶ **Preserve it** Use the coarser, greener stems of outdoor rhubarb to make chutneys and relish. Or add a little stem ginger and make jam.

▶▶ **Add some sparkle** Turn cooked, sweetened pink rhubarb into syrup, put a little in the bottom of a glass and top up with sparkling wine.

Stone fruits & grapes

{ Peaches, nectarines, apricots, cherries, plums, grapes, avocados }

What do they do for me?

▶▶ Stone fruits contain modest levels of vitamins and minerals, but are excellent sources of protective phenolic compounds. The cyaninin and chlorogenic acid in plums and peaches, for example, may help combat cell damage that can lead to diseases such as cancer, and the resveratrol and quercetin in grapes may inhibit the growth of certain cancers. Levels of phenols are highest in the skins of dark plums, cherries and black grapes.

▶▶ Avocados, a different type of stone fruit, are a good source of vitamins A and E, which support the immune system and fight infection, and vitamin K, which helps build bone mass.

How do they get to us?

▶▶ All stone fruits are tree-grown and hand-picked. Avocados grow only in hot regions. Peaches, nectarines and apricots need warmth and sun to ripen.

● **Grapes** grow on vines and need sunny warm summers to ripen. Grapes available during winter are imported.

▶▶ All of these fruits are best eaten in summer and autumn, when they are in season locally.

● **Nectarines and peaches** will ripen considerably if you buy them hard and keep them at room temperature. Larger, more mature fruits usually ripen better than small ones, and generally taste sweeter. Fruits sold as 'ripe and ready to eat' are more expensive because they require more elaborate packaging and may have been air-freighted. Never store nectarines and peaches in the fridge as it spoils their texture.

● **Apricots** for eating raw must be ripe when picked – they don't ripen much after picking. Use harder fruits for cooking. Apricots keep quite well in the fridge.

● **Plums** usually ripen and become sweeter at room temperature. Once ripe, they can be kept in the fridge.

● **Cherries** are best stored in the fridge and brought out an hour or so before you want to eat them.

● **Grapes** are freshest in summer when they are harvested; after that, they are put into cold storage and fumigated with sulphur, which can give them a dank, damp smell which washing should remove. Keep them at room temperature and they will sweeten slightly.

How can I use them?

▶▶ Bake them Halve and stone larger fruits, then sprinkle with sugar, dot with butter and bake until the juice starts to run. Serve as dessert with yogurt.

▶▶ Stew them Underripe fruits can be made into compote by gently stewing them with a splash of water, a little sugar and a flavouring such as vanilla, orange-flower water, orange liqueur or port.

▶▶ Preserve them Make jam from apricots, peaches or plums to enjoy in winter.

▶▶ With cheese Grapes and apricots go well with rich salty cheeses.

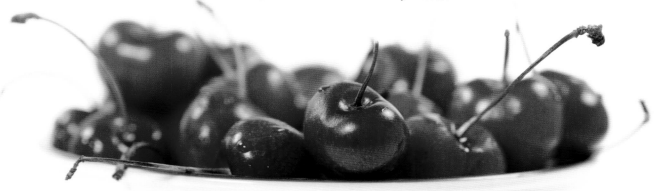

Tropical fruits

{ Bananas, pineapples, mangoes, papayas, passionfruit, pomegranates }

What do they do for me?

➤➤ Tropical fruits usually have a high GI so not the first fruit choice for anyone with diabetes or watching their weight. But they do supply excellent nutrients, for example:

● **Bananas** are a good source of vitamin B_6, which helps the nervous system function properly and aids energy production.

● **Pineapples** are a rich source of vitamin C, which supports the immune system, and manganese, important for blood clotting and thyroid function. They also contain bromelain, an enzyme thought to be anti-inflammatory and helpful for digestion.

● **Mangoes** are a good source of beta-carotene – important for vision – as well as vitamin C and fibre.

● **Papayas and passionfruit** are good sources of vitamin C and beta-carotene; papayas also supply vitamin E and their enzymes papain and chymopapain are thought to have an anti-inflammatory action.

● **Pomegranates** contain punicalagin compounds which have disease-fighting antioxidant properties.

How do they get to us?

➤➤ Some fruits can be picked underripe while others must be harvested as ripe as possible.

● **Bananas** for shipping they are harvested underripe, then ripened in storage with ethylene, a gas given off naturally by ripe fruit. Leaving underripe bananas in a bowl among riper fruits will encourage them to ripen.

● **Mangoes** are air-freighted ripe as they don't ripen well once picked. Choose fruit with fragrance and a slight 'give' under the skin. Store at room temperature.

● **Papayas** are tree-grown, picked unripe and often air-freighted. They ripen slightly at room temperature.

● **Passionfruit** grow on vine-like plants and are harvested when about three-quarters ripe. They will ripen at room temperature, then are best stored in the fridge as they have a tendency to dry out.

● **Pineapples** grow in soil and are harvested when about two-thirds ripe. They are shipped in cold storage. To test for ripeness before buying, pull on one

of the green spiky leaves at the top – it should come away fairly easily. The fruit should have a nice, light pineapple fragrance and no browning on the skin.

● **Pomegranates** are tree-grown in the Middle East and Spain and picked and shipped ripe. They should have a deep red skin. Store at room temperature and allow the skins to harden slightly and 'sink' before you eat the fruit – they will be sweeter and juicier.

How can I use them?

➤➤ Snack on them Make sure they are as ripe as possible and enjoy them as they are.

➤➤ Salads Try thinly sliced pineapple with celery or fennel; mango with avocado and coriander; or to use underripe mango or papaya, try it thinly sliced in a piquant Thai-style salad with chilli and fish sauce.

➤➤ Cakes Banana bread, pineapple upside-down cake, passionfruit icing. Overripe bananas can be frozen in their skins for future use in baking.

➤➤ Homemade smoothies Blend banana/ pineapple/mango with natural yogurt.

➤➤ Unusual desserts Bake bananas in orange and passionfruit juice, with a little sugar.

Cabbage family

{ Cabbages, cauliflowers, broccoli, brussels sprouts, spring greens, bok choy, kale }

What do they do for me?

➡ **Cruciferous vegetables** contain a group of natural compounds such as sulforophane and diindolylmethane, which appear to protect against various cancers.

➡ **All vegetables in the cabbage family are an excellent source of vitamin C** (important for the immune system); vitamin K (for strong bones and blood clotting); vitamin A (good for skin and eyesight); and folate (helps prevent anaemia).

How do they get to us?

➡ **All are field-grown**, with different varieties suitable to different seasons throughout the year.
● **Buy seasonal**, local cruciferous vegetables if possible: these are likely to be the freshest and most nutritious.

How can I use them?

➡ **Grate them** Raw red or white cabbage, radishes or brussels sprouts, finely sliced or grated, will all make a healthy and tasty coleslaw.

➡ **Steam them** to retain most of their nutrients. Try cooling steamed cauliflower florets then adding a garlicky yogurt dressing and a sprinkling of parsley or mint. Dress warm broccoli florets with lemon juice, olive oil and toasted pine nuts or pumpkin seeds.

➡ **Roast them** Kale is delicious steamed till just wilted, then briefly roasted in a little oil in a hot oven; remove the tough ribs when preparing kale.

➡ **Blend them** Cauliflower and broccoli make velvety, liquidised soups. Kale is good in chunky broths made with beans, a little ham and chopped tomatoes. Bok choy and Chinese greens can be added raw, or wilted, to fragrant Asian soups and broths.

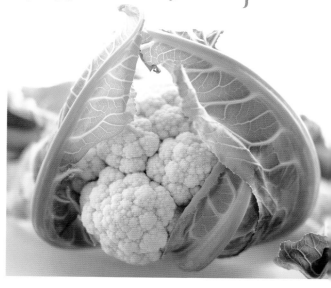

Other green vegetables

{ Celery, asparagus, fennel, globe artichokes, spinach, silverbeet }

What do they do for me?

➡ **This catch-all group** is delicious and nutritious in lots of different ways.
● **Celery and asparagus** are both rich in vitamins C, K and folate. Celery also contains significant levels of minerals and plant compounds, such as ferulic acid, that are thought to help lower blood pressure.
● **Fennel** contains the aromatic compound anethole, thought to have an antibacterial, antifungal action, hence its reputation for freshening the breath.
● **Globe artichokes** have nutrients similar to those of celery and asparagus, but also contain silymarin (milk thistle), thought to be beneficial for the liver.
● **Spinach and silverbeet** are excellent sources of the antioxidant vitamins A, C and E, with a useful

Was Popeye right about spinach?

Recent Swedish research has shown that eating spinach can improve the performance of muscles by reducing their demand for oxygen, making active muscles more energy efficient. A 300g serving of spinach reduced oxygen requirement by up to five per cent – an effect noticed in as little as three days. But it's not, as was once thought, the iron in spinach that improves performance. It's the abundance of nitrates in spinach acting 'like a fuel additive for your muscles – it makes them run much more smoothly and efficiently', says Dr Eddie Weitzberg, who led the study.

amount of K. Spinach is a good source of folate and of iron and its vitamin C helps us to absorb the iron.

How do they get to us?

▶▶ **Celery, asparagus and globe artichokes** are mostly field-grown, although some asparagus is now grown in polytunnels to extend its growing season. Spinach and silverbeet can be field-grown, but are also grown under cover in polytunnels.

Buying and storing

● **Asparagus needs to be eaten** as soon as possible after it is cut. Look for spears with juicy, firm stems. The asparagus season is spring.

● **Globe artichokes, celery and fennel** all keep quite well in the fridge for a few days. Spinach and silverbeet are at their nutritional peak when very fresh but keep quite well in a plastic bag in the fridge.

How can I use them?

▶▶ **Asparagus alone** Steam, roast or grill it and enjoy with a little melted butter.

▶▶ **In salads** Sliced raw fennel, asparagus, small artichoke hearts and celery bring juicy crunch to salads.

▶▶ **In gratins or soups** Bake celery and silverbeet in cheesy sauces. Celery or spinach make delicious soups.

Pea & bean family

Peas, snowpeas, sugarsnap peas, broad beans, green beans, runner beans

What do they do for me?

▶▶ **All are good sources of vitamin C,** which builds resistance to infection; B vitamins, which support the nervous system; vitamin K, which helps build bone mass; and folate, which helps prevent anaemia and neural tube defects in newborn babies.

▶▶ **They are also useful sources** of carotenoid compounds, zeaxanthin and lutein, which aid vision and eye health.

How do they get to us?

▶▶ **Traditionally, leguminous veg are field-grown,** ready for eating at slightly different times throughout summer and into autumn. Many are now grown in polytunnels to give them protection and extend the growing season. Most of the crop of freshly harvested peas is blanched and frozen.

How can I use them?

▶▶ **Eat them in season as fresh as possible,** lightly cooked, when sweet and new. Refrigerate if not to be eaten immediately. Many leguminous vegetables, especially peas and broad beans, freeze extremely well.

▶▶ **In salads** When young and small, all these vegetables can be eaten raw (or lightly steamed), finely chopped or thinly sliced into salads.

▶▶ **In meat-free mains** Use mashed cooked broad beans to make veggie burgers. Or try a

Peas and broad beans are higher in protein
than other vegetables.

vegetable stew with braised peas and thinly sliced runner beans, tomatoes, garlic, olive oil and onions.

➡ In pâté Lightly cooked broad beans or peas can be mashed, then mixed with herbs (mint, basil, parsley, chives) and low-fat thick yogurt or light cream cheese to make a verdant green pâté.

Corn

What does it do for me?

➡ It contains useful plant compounds such as lutein and cryptoxanthin, which are good for vision and eye health, and ferulic acid, an anti-inflammatory. But it contains more carbohydrate and is higher in energy than most other vegetables. Of its many varieties, yellow corn – fresh, frozen or in tins – and baby corn are the most familiar.

How does it get to us?

➡ Corn is a field-grown crop. Baby corn in Australia is a mix of home-grown and imported.

Buying and storing
● **Look for** corn-on-the-cob that has slightly moist outer leaves, enclosing glossy plump, firm niblets; dull, puckered corn is old. Store whole in the refrigerator.

How can I use it?

➡ Steam it Keep corncobs in their husk and microwave whole for four minutes per cob. Serve fresh cobs with a little butter and freshly ground black pepper – the niblets should be tender but still have a little bite.

➡ Stir fry it Baby corn spears are a great addition to mixed stir-fried vegetables.

➡ Scatter it Canned corn kernels scattered in or over salads add colour and nutrition. Corn is also a tasty addition to omelettes and soups.

Onion family
{ Onions, shallots, leeks, spring onions, garlic }

What do they do for me?

➡ All members of the onion family are excellent sources of health-promoting sulphur compounds which appear to have antibacterial, antiviral and antifungal actions, and may help protect against heart disease and cancer. The stronger-smelling the allium, the more of the compounds it is likely to contain.

How do they get to us?

➡ These are all field-grown crops With the exception of spring onions, after harvesting they are stored in a cool place to dry out slowly. Most alliums are locally grown but garlic is sometimes imported.

Buying and storing
● **Garlic** stays fresh for one to four months depending on how well it is stored. A fresh bulb will feel firm. Avoid bright white bulbs, which have usually been treated with bleach.
● **Store onions, shallots and garlic** in a cool dark place, but not in the fridge as the low temperature affects the flavour and the smell may taint other foods.
● **Use spring onions and leeks promptly**, but store in the fridge for a few days if necessary. Leeks must be washed thoroughly to remove any grit.

How can I use them?

➡ Fry them Softened in a little oil, onions, shallots or garlic add flavour to casseroles, stews and soups.

➡ Bake/roast them Use soft-cooked sliced onions in savoury quiches or tarts. Bake blanched leeks in a cheese sauce. Roast onions with root vegetables such as parsnips and carrots. Roast fresh garlic, then spread on toast.

Mushrooms

What do they do for me?

▶▶ **Mushrooms are fungi**, so strictly speaking they're not vegetables at all. Their beneficial nutrients include:

● **Plant sterols which convert to vitamin D in sunlight,** making mushrooms the only natural non-animal source of vitamin D – albeit in small amounts.

● **B vitamins,** which support brain function and energy levels; mushrooms are also a good source of potassium, which helps combat high blood pressure.

● **Beta-glucans** which appear to boost the immune system and may help combat cancer.

● Some research suggests that the conjugated linoleic acids in mushrooms may inhibit the development of breast cancer.

How do they get to us?

▶▶ **Cultivated mushrooms are grown in dark** sheds and tunnels. An artificial growing medium is inoculated with mushroom spores. Varieties include white, button, chestnut, flat, field, enoki, shiitake and oyster, ranging in taste from mild to a meaty, savoury flavour.

▶▶ **Wild mushrooms grow naturally, usually in woods** Pine mushrooms, chanterelles, ceps/porcini, and slippery jacks are all types of wild mushrooms. They have a meaty savoury taste and are more pungent than cultivated varieties.

▶▶ **Mushrooms are cheap, tasty and healthy**, so eat them in abundance, but be sure that wild mushrooms are from a reliable source.

● **Choose mushrooms that are firm and dry** Cultivated mushrooms are best stored in the fridge in a paper bag. Take them out of plastic packaging because this tends to make them go soft and slimy.

● **Use cultivated mushrooms soon after you buy them** and always wash cultivated mushrooms before eating.

● **Wild mushrooms should be brushed gently** to remove moss, grass or leaves. If damp from rain, lay them in a single layer on newspaper or kitchen paper to absorb the moisture, then store in a paper bag in the fridge. Wild mushrooms can be left in a warm place to dry out, which intensifies the flavour.

How can I use them?

▶▶ **Grill them** and serve as part of a cooked breakfast or as a side dish.

▶▶ **Add them to omelettes, casseroles, pies** – almost any savoury dish.

▶▶ **Cream them** Soften chopped mushrooms in a little oil, add stock, cook through and blend into soup. Serve them with a swirl of yogurt and chopped parsley. A dash of truffle oil adds a touch of luxury.

▶▶ **Vegetarian stock** Sauté fresh mushrooms and onions, with a few slices of dried porcini, then add water and simmer to make a stock for soup, risotto, stew or gravy.

Do not pick wild mushrooms
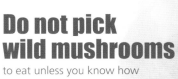
to eat unless you know how to identify them: to amateurs, edible and deadly, poisonous types can look alike.

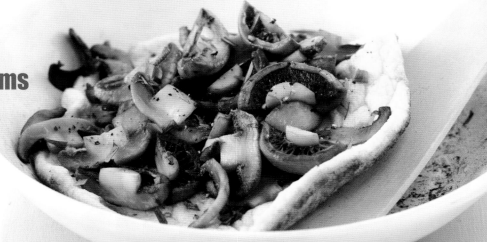

Root vegetables

{ Carrots, celeriac, swedes, parsnips, beetroot, Jerusalem artichokes, sweet potatoes }

What do they do for me?

This group is rich in vitamin C, beta-carotene (vitamin A) and vitamin E, which are protective against damage from free radicals that are the precursors of illness and disease.

● **Carrots** are rich in carotenoid compounds, zeaxanthin and lutein, which are good for vision and eye health. In older carrots, more of the nutrients are available when they are cooked than eaten raw.

● **Beetroot** contains betacyanin, a purple-coloured plant compound that has been found to have an anti-cancer effect. Beetroot is also a good source of folate.

● **Orange-coloured sweet potatoes** and Jerusalem artichokes are both good sources of fibre and potassium, too.

If you are watching your weight, let root vegetables play second fiddle to other vegetables in your diet as they are high in carbohydrates. Otherwise, eat as many as you like.

How do they get to us?

All are field-grown, with the edible part developing underground. After harvesting, they are usually stored; if they no longer have green leaves, you can tell they have been stored. Stored root vegetables are larger and sweeter than freshly harvested 'new' root crops.

How can I use them?

When you buy root vegetables they should be firm to the touch, with a smooth taut skin. Store them in a cool, dark place, away from light and eat them while their texture is still firm and crunchy.

Grate them As well as the familiar grated carrot, raw beetroot is good grated in salads. Or try celeriac dressed with mayonnaise and natural low-fat yogurt, flavoured with wholegrain mustard.

Dip them Cut carrot, beetroot or celeriac into batons and use as vegetable crudités with dips; they are a good inclusion in your children's lunch boxes.

Roast them Cut into chunks, root vegetables roast beautifully with olive oil and herbs. Oven-bake or microwave sweet potatoes as you would potatoes.

Bake with them Carrots and sweet potatoes work well in cakes: try parsnip and beetroot, too.

Blend them Make delicious and warming root vegetable soups. Use beetroot in traditional borscht.

Try sweet potatoes in place of regular potatoes as chips, baked, roasted, mashed or in soups. They add more beneficial nutrients to the dish.

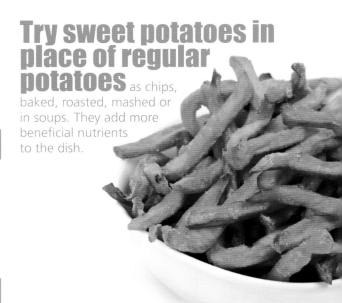

Potatoes

What do they do for me?

Potatoes supply vitamins B_6 and B_1, important for brain function and energy; vitamin C, which protects against disease; and folate, which helps prevent anaemia. But they are starchy with more kilojoules and fewer nutrients than other vegetables.

How do they get to us?

▶▶ **Potatoes**, strictly tubers rather than root vegetables, are a field-grown crop.

● **New potatoes are newly grown**, freshly harvested potatoes with thin, flaky skins which scrape off easily. Mainly available in spring, they tend to have a firm, slightly waxy consistency.

● **Main-crop potatoes are older potatoes**, with thicker skins, that are stored after harvesting. The consistency of the potato varies with the variety. These are available all year round.

Buying and storing

● **Potatoes, whether old or new**, should be firm, unwrinkled and have no greenness on the skin.

● **Even stored under the best conditions**, potatoes lose some quality the older they get. They should be stored in an opaque bag in a cool, dark place with good air circulation and used within ten days.

● **Do not put potatoes in the fridge:** cold temperatures convert starch to sugar, giving potatoes a strange sweet taste.

● **Choose the right potato for your recipe**. If you want creamy mash, you need a floury potato. For rosti, choose a waxy potato that holds together well. Most supermarket potatoes indicate their suitable uses.

How can I use them?

▶▶ **As an accompaniment** Perfectly boiled new potatoes or light and fluffy mash provide delicious carbohydrate in many meals. If roasting, par-boil first for quicker, crispier results.

▶▶ **Blended into soups** Potatoes add body to other vegetables in soups (celery, leek, Jerusalem artichoke, onion, spinach), whether left chunky in a broth, or liquidised to a smooth soup.

▶▶ **In potato salad** Serve chunks of boiled new potatoes, chopped spring onions and gherkins with a thick yogurt, mayonnaise and mustard dressing.

Pumpkin family

{ Butternut, jap and blue pumpkins, zucchini, marrows, squashes }

What do they do for me?

▶▶ **Orange-fleshed pumpkins and squash** are excellent sources of the antioxidant vitamin A, and are also good sources of B vitamins.

▶▶ **Plant compounds**, such as cryptoxanthin, lutein and zeaxanthin, found in some orange-fleshed pumpkins, are also good for vision.

▶▶ **Pumpkins and squashes** provide useful levels of minerals such as calcium and phosphorus, which build bone strength, and potassium which helps regulate blood pressure.

▶▶ **Zucchini, marrows and bitter melon** have a high water content and contain more modest amounts of vitamins (mainly A and C) and minerals.

▶▶ **Spaghetti squash** can be used with sauce as a low-joule alternative to spaghetti.

How do they get to us?

▶▶ **Squashes and pumpkins are field-grown;** zucchini are grown either outside or in polytunnels or glasshouses. All are warm-weather crops.

Storing

● **Hard-skinned pumpkins**, such as butternut, are stored whole after harvesting and keep well for several months in cool, dark conditions.

● **Orange-skinned pumpkins may look solid**, but they should be used no more than a few days after purchase, or they will start to soften and eventually rot.

● **Use zucchini as soon as possible** after picking; they develop a slightly bitter flavour the longer you keep them. Smaller zucchini are usually sweeter.

How can I use them?

Roast them Chunks of pumpkin roast well in olive oil with sage leaves; or try chunks of zucchini with oregano, garlic and cherry tomatoes.

Marinate them For a simple raw salad, thinly slice small zucchini and marinate in lemon juice and olive oil for 30 minutes, then top with a spoonful of smooth goat's cheese and a sprinkle of chopped mint.

Blend them Squashes and pumpkins make satiny-smooth liquidised soups; adding grated melting cheese and croutons makes them more substantial.

Char them Slice zucchini lengthways and char them on a cast-iron grill. Season with pepper and olive oil and serve with olives, anchovies, cured ham or salami as antipasti.

Bake them Use pumpkin purée to make pumpkin pie. Grated zucchini are good in muffins.

Fruit vegetables

{ Tomatoes, capsicums, chillies, eggplant, cucumbers }

What do they do for me?

Tomatoes and red capsicums are excellent sources of vitamin C and beta-carotene. as well as lycopene, which may protect against prostate cancer.

Chillies are rich in vitamins and minerals, but are so hot that we only eat them in small amounts. They also contain a substance called capsaicin, which is used in topical ointments to relieve muscular pain.

Eggplant contain the antioxidant compound nasunin, which some research suggests may inhibit the growth of cancer.

Cucumbers are not especially rich in nutrients but their high water content makes them both refreshing and low in kilojoules.

How do they get to us?

All can be grown outdoors, especially in warm climates, but many are cultivated in greenhouses or in polytunnels, to protect them, encourage faster growth and ripening, and to extend the season.
- **Tomatoes** ripened naturally on the plant in the sun taste sweetest. Leave them in a bowl at room temperature and they will continue to ripen and sweeten a little, as will capsicums.
- **Capsicums, chillies, eggplant and cucumbers** are grown in polytunnels and greenhouses, and vary little throughout the year. Unlike tomatoes, they keep well in the fridge and make a handy stand-by for vegetable dishes.
- **Chillies** vary enormously in strength, from green jalapeños which are fairly mild, to scotch bonnet which are extremely fiery. They can be dried or preserved in oil. Take out the seeds and ribs from fresh chillies if you want to remove some of the piquant heat. Wash your hands after handling chillies and do not rub your eyes.

How can I use them?

Eat them raw Tomatoes, cucumbers and capsicums are classic salad vegetables, while a finely sliced de-seeded chilli adds piquancy to salsa.

Roast or grill For a tasty dip, blend roasted and peeled tomatoes and capsicums with Greek-style yogurt or ground toasted nuts. Char-grill eggplant and mash the flesh with olive oil and tahini (sesame paste).

Stuff them Fill capsicums with leftover pilaf, or cooked grain mixed with chopped dried fruit and nuts, a little olive oil, tomato juice and water.

Curry them Eggplant and tomatoes are used in many Indian dishes. Chillies add fire while grated cucumber with yogurt makes cooling raitas.

Salad leaves & herbs

What do they do for me?

➡➡ **Most of these leafy vegetables** contain useful amounts of a range of minerals and vitamins, but are an especially rich source of vitamin A and beta-carotene, which converts to vitamin A in the body, important for healthy skin and vision.

➡➡ **They are an excellent source of vitamin K**, essential for strong bones.

➡➡ **They contain significant amounts of zeaxanthin**, thought to offer protection against age-related macular degeneration in the eyes.

➡➡ **Parsley, watercress and salad leaves** of the mustard family stand out as having particularly high levels of nutrients.

How do they get to us?

➡➡ **Salad leaves are cultivated in** open fields and also hydroponically. More than half of Australia's hydroponic lettuce is grown outdoors. (Australia is currently the largest hydroponic producer of lettuce in the world.)
● **Watercress** is grown outdoors in shallow gravel beds of clean, preferably running water.
● **In packing factories** different lettuce varieties are broken up and washed, then packed in bags of mixed leaves. The sealed bags have a 'modified atmosphere' (air with the oxygen removed) to keep the leaves fresh and extend their shelf life.
● **Leafy salad greens** are best eaten as fresh as possible after they are picked. Whole lettuces of the crunchier type (cos, iceberg) may look fine after several days in the fridge, but become more bitter the longer they are kept.

Modified Atmosphere Packaging (MAP) is now widely used to extend the life of food, especially salad, and does not need to be declared on the product. MAP removes most of the oxygen in a bag or container, and replaces it with nitrogen or carbon dioxide. There is no evidence that the use of MAP decreases the nutritional value of food, but leaves wilt and droop very quickly after the bag is opened, so they are best used straightaway. MAP is also used with packaged cheeses; many small speciality cheeses are preserved in this way.

● **This is one group of vegetables** where practically everyone can grow their own. Try sowing mixed salad leaves, rocket and herbs in pots on the patio or even in a sunny window box and use them to spice up bought lettuce.

How can I use them?

➡➡ **Dress them** Serve a well-dressed green salad with or after hot savoury dishes.

➡➡ **Cook them** Quartered hearts of cos lettuce or iceberg can be gently braised in stock with herbs and spices. Lettuce and watercress make unusual soups

➡➡ **In sandwiches** All add freshness and zing to staple sandwich ingredients.

➡➡ **Blitz them** Blend handfuls of parsley, mint and basil with olive oil and lemon juice to make salsa verde to serve with fish, or over grilled haloumi cheese or meats.

➡➡ **Chop them** A handful of chopped fresh herbs (parsley, coriander, mint, dill, chervil, chives) brings life to all sorts of meat, fish and tomato dishes. Add them at the last minute to enliven soups.

4 Eggs & dairy foods

Eggs are one of the healthiest, most affordable foods available. Dairy foods, too, offer excellent nutrition and value. But mass production of both has become a source of concern and can affect their nutritional quality.

Eggs

Designed by nature to be a complete nutritional package for the growing chick, eggs are a first-class food – enjoyed by humans for thousands of years.

What do they do for me?

▶▶ **Eggs** offer us a wide range of important nutrients, including:
● **High-quality protein** with all the amino acids necessary for body metabolism: one large egg contains about 6g of protein. Eggs are not high in fat and almost two-thirds of it is unsaturated.
● **Almost all vitamins except for vitamin C** Eggs give us vitamin A (good for skin and eyesight); vitamin D (which helps the body absorb and regulate calcium); vitamin E (helps combat heart disease, cancer, stroke); many B vitamins, especially B_2 (niacin, needed to metabolise food), B_{12} (essential for making blood cells, releasing energy and maintaining the nervous system), and choline (essential for cell function growth, so particularly important during pregnancy).

Eggs contain high levels of the eye-protective pigments

lutein and zeaxanthin which many studies suggest can help prevent macular degeneration.

● **Minerals in eggs include** iodine (important for thyroid function); calcium and phosphorus (for strong teeth and bones); selenium (essential for healthy immune system function); iron (vital for making haemoglobin which transports oxygen in the blood); and magnesium (protects against heart disease, high blood pressure, stroke and type 2 diabetes).

How many can I eat?

▶▶ **For years, health experts recommended** the restriction of eggs in the diet to three or four a week because the cholesterol they contain was thought to raise blood cholesterol levels. Research now shows that for most people dietary cholesterol has little, if any, effect on blood cholesterol; in fact, the vitamin D in eggs may boost heart health.
● **The current recommendation** from the Heart Foundation is that eggs are nutritious and safe to eat.
● **Young children, pregnant women and the elderly**, however, are advised not to eat raw or undercooked eggs.

What types are there?

● **The vast majority are hens' eggs;** specialist shops and farm outlets may sell larger duck eggs, and smaller bantam and quail eggs.
● **All eggs taste pretty much the same**, irrespective of their type and size: quails' eggs, for instance, taste just like small hens' eggs.

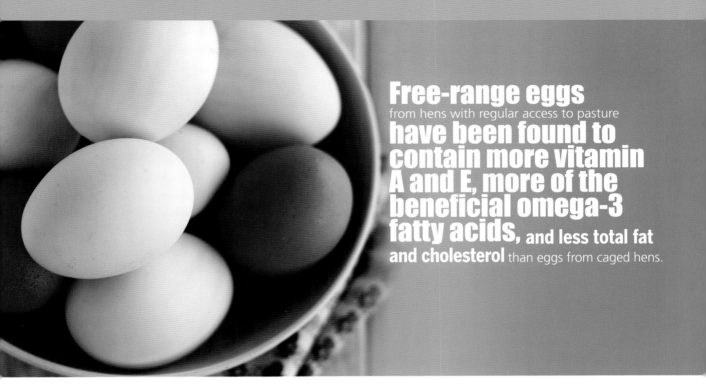

Free-range eggs from hens with regular access to pasture **have been found to contain more vitamin A and E, more of the beneficial omega-3 fatty acids,** and less total fat and cholesterol than eggs from caged hens.

● **Duck eggs have firmer whites** which take a little longer to whisk and cook; but they make particularly good meringues and fluffy sponges.

Does shell colour matter?

No. Shell colour depends on breed but makes no difference to the egg inside. In the past, most eggs were white-shelled, but brown are now preferred. Across the world, the preferences are about 50:50. Duck eggs vary from near-white to pastel greeny-blue. Quail lay pretty speckled eggs.

How do they get to us?

➡ **The egg carton indicates** the method of farming and which farm or production site the eggs came from.

● **Organic eggs** The hens are kept in small flocks, in free-range systems where they can exercise and forage. They have easy access to outdoors, onto pasture that is free of pesticides and artificial fertilisers, and therefore certified as organic.

● **Free-range eggs** The hens are housed in barns with constant daytime access to grassy land outdoors, where they can forage and exercise. However, the term 'free-range' is a broad one. In the best systems the hens live outside during the day, and only come back inside for protection at night. In contrast, some systems with very large flocks offer little more than theoretical access to outdoors via a small hatch through which relatively few birds can actually get out.

● **Barn eggs** These come from hens that are loose-housed in barns where they lay their eggs in nests. They have enough space to move around and flap their wings, and there are places to perch, but conditions are usually crowded and the hens are never allowed outside.

● **Eggs from caged hens** The bare battery cage system, where hens are tightly packed in wire cages, is now banned in some countries. Such cages are not large enough for the hens to be able to flap their wings and the hens are at increased risk of disease. Such eggs must be labelled 'eggs from caged hens'.

What to look for in eggs

▶▶ **Eggs should be truly fresh when you buy them**. Make sure they're well within their 'use by' date: by law, that's 28 days from being laid.

● **Free-range and organic hens** are not kept in close confinement or in large flocks, so their eggs are far less prone to salmonella and other diseases common in factory farming conditions.

● **Eggs eaten uncooked** – in fresh mayonnaise, for example, or a chocolate mousse or frozen dessert – should be within the first week of their 'use by' period to avoid food poisoning from bugs such as salmonella.

● **Eggs are safe when cooked** because cooking kills any food-poisoning bacteria. But the end result won't be quite as good with old eggs as with really fresh eggs.

● **When you crack a really fresh egg the yolk will stand up slightly**, supported by a thick, jelly-like white. In an older egg the yolk is more likely to break into the white, which will be runny.

● **Older eggs float in cold water** Another test of freshness is to place eggs in cold water: fresh eggs sink, while older eggs float.

▶▶ **Good eggs have strong thick shells** that don't shatter easily. Goose and duck eggs have particularly thick shells.

● **A deep ochre or orange-coloured yolk** usually indicates that the bird had a healthy diet foraging on grassy land as the chlorophyll colours

Should I go for eggs with 'extra omega-3'? Some brands of eggs make a selling point of having more health-promoting omega-3 fatty acids than standard eggs. These are produced by including fish oil or oil-rich seeds in the hens' diet. If you already buy eggs from organic or free-range birds with access to pasture forage, the eggs will already be naturally high in omega-3 fats, so there's no need to buy the more expensive omega-3-enriched eggs.

the yolks. The eggs also taste richer. However, some producers of indoor eggs use feed with synthetic colourings, so check the source of your eggs, too.

● **Pale yellow yolks and thin, fragile shells** are often a sign of eggs from cereal and soy-fed birds that are never outside on grass, although free-range eggs may also be more fragile and have paler yolks in winter.

How can I use them?

▶▶ **Eggs need to be kept cool** in the fridge. Leave them in their box, pointed end down to keep the yolk in the centre and prevent it from settling into the air pocket within the shell.

▶▶ **Breakfast** Eggs offer a highly nutritious breakfast option. Boiled, poached, scrambled, or occasionally fried – preferably in a little olive oil.

▶▶ **Lunch** Eggs make inexpensive, easy lunches whether at home or at work. Egg with mayonnaise and cress or lettuce is the cheapest healthy option in sandwich shops, or prepare your own. Or make a nutritious omelette, with a little cheese, tomato, or mushrooms.

▶▶ **Meat-free mains** An omelette, frittata or Spanish tortilla; pancakes; a soufflé, perhaps with cheese; hard-boiled eggs with a vegetarian curry are just a few of many options.

▶▶ **Dessert** Egg desserts bring added protein to a light dinner – baked custard flavoured with nutmeg, crème caramel or bread-and-butter pudding with dried fruit. Or use eggs to make custard to serve with fruit purées and compotes.

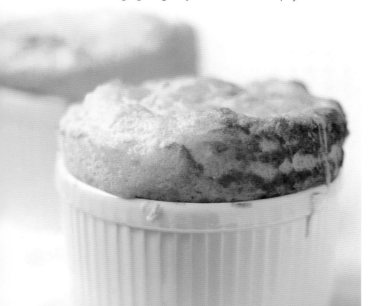

Milk & yogurt

What do they do for me?

Dairy foods are deliciously varied, highly nutritious and usually good value as well. They supply:

▶▶ **Protein** A 200ml serving of milk – skim, low-fat or full cream – provides more than 6g of protein. A small (150g) tub of natural yogurt supplies 7.5g protein.

▶▶ **Vitamins** – especially vitamin A (supports immune system and vision; skim and low-fat milk have less than full-fat). The levels of other vitamins and minerals are higher in the lower-fat milks: thiamin (for the heart and nervous system); B_2 (for good skin and energy); B_3 (niacin, regulates energy and metabolism); and B_{12} (brain function, energy, red blood cell production).

▶▶ **Minerals** – milk and yogurt are known as good sources of calcium; in addition they supply phosphorus (important for healthy teeth and bones); iodine (regulates metabolism and the thyroid gland); magnesium (essential for skeletal development); zinc (fights infections and promotes wound healing); and potassium (helps regulate blood pressure).

▶▶ **Friendly bacteria** – unsweetened natural yogurt contains 'good' bacteria and has been credited with a variety of health benefits, including protection from the harmful bacteria that cause food poisoning. Yogurt is also thought to boost the immune and digestive systems, reducing constipation, stomach acidity and diarrhoea; research suggests that eating probiotic yogurt can reduce inflammation in people with inflammatory bowel disease.

How does it get to us?

▶▶ **Cow's milk comes in** whole (full-fat), low-fat and skim varieties, and makes up the vast majority of milk sold.

Organic or otherwise, **milk from cows eating fresh grass** has a superior **omega-3 fatty acid profile,** with more conjugated linoleic acid, than milk from animals fed conserved grass such as silage.

● **The image of the herd of dairy cows** grazing on pasture is still with us, but increasingly dairy cows are being taken indoors into factory-farm conditions, just as animals raised for meat and eggs were before them. The import of US-style mega-dairies is highly controversial, largely driven by the supermarket demand for cheap milk.

● **Most of the milk in Australia and New Zealand** is now produced by a handful of breeds that have come to dominate the dairy industry because of their high milk yield.

● **Indoor dairy farming** uses large barns, and the cows rarely, sometimes never, go outside. They are given grain-based feed, with no access to grass. Milking is automated and in some systems goes on round the clock. This system is used in some parts of Asia and Europe.

● **Grass-fed cows live outside most of the time when the weather is mild enough**, grazing on fresh pasture, and are milked twice a day. In winter they are housed in large barns and fed on silage, hay and some form of supplementary cereal and protein feed, to ensure they get a balance of vitamins and minerals.

● **Organic cows live outside for at least six months** when the weather is mild enough, grazing on organic fields that cannot be sprayed with either pesticides or chemical fertilisers. Organic herds tend to be smaller and the milk is a little more expensive but has been shown to contain more beneficial nutrients.

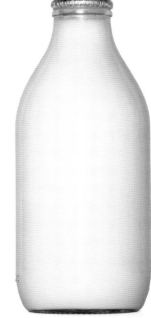

Full-fat milk and yogurt are not really very fatty –

cow's milk is usually around 3.7% fat, with full-fat natural yogurt containing around 4.5% fat.

How is it processed?

▶▶ Pasteurisation is a rapid heat treatment that kills bacteria in milk, making it safe to drink. By law, all milk in Australia (and virtually all milk in New Zealand) is pasteurised as a precaution against food poisoning and tuberculosis. Some vitamin and mineral content is lost in the process but pasteurisation greatly increases the shelf-life of milk.

▶▶ Unpasteurised milk, also known as 'raw' milk, can be sold in New Zealand only in small amounts from a very few farms. It is illegal in Australia. Proponents argue that it retains a higher level of nutrients than treated milks and that with its full complement of good bacteria and health-promoting enzymes, it is easier to digest, better for the immune system and healthier than pasteurised milk. One Swiss study suggests that raw milk may have protective effects against childhood asthma. However, pregnant women are warned against consuming unpasteurised milk or milk products, such as unpasteurised cheeses. Raw milk must be kept refrigerated

▶▶ Homogenised milk This milk is processed so that the cream is evenly distributed throughout the milk and doesn't settle on the top.

▶▶ Long life (UHT) and sterilised milk This describes milk that has been heated to a temperature that kills off all bacteria. This has the longest shelf-life of all and does not need to be refrigerated until the carton has been opened. This process is also used for some types of cream and yogurt as well as juices and other products.

What other types are there?

▶▶ Sheep's milk Richer in protein and calcium than cow's milk, but also higher in fat. Some people who cannot digest cow's milk find they can tolerate sheep's milk (*see also* page 269).

▶▶ Goat's milk Like sheep's milk, this is often popular with people who find it difficult to digest cow's milk.

▶▶ Buffalo's milk This is another alternative to cow's milk, but hard to find – it is mainly used to make cheese (mozzarella, ricotta).

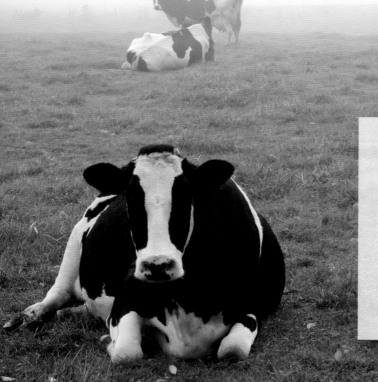

Is organic milk better? Several scientific studies suggest that it is more nutritious. One study found, on average, 68 per cent more omega-3 fatty acids in organic than non-organic milk. Research in the UK, Norway and Sweden also shows that free-range and organic farms achieve the same level of disease prevention and better animal health than intensive production systems where antibiotic use is considerably higher. However, it is reportedly as much as 40 per cent lower in iodine than milk from cows whose feed contains it.

How is yogurt made?

- **Natural yogurt is made by stirring live beneficial bacteria** – such as *Lactobacillus acidophilus, casei, bulgaricus* or *bifidus* – into milk, then incubating the milk for several hours at about 42°C. The bacteria thicken and ferment the milk, producing a pleasantly sharp flavour. After cooling, the finished yogurt can be poured in tubs.
- **The type of yogurt depends on the type of milk used** – whole milk makes full-fat yogurt, low-fat milk makes low-fat, skim milk makes fat-free.
- **Fruit and flavours are added** when the yogurt is ready to pot up; or for set yogurt, the inoculated yogurt is poured into the tub then left to ferment. Strained yogurt is thicker because most of the whey (milk protein) is taken off.

How much can I have?

➡️ **The Healthy-Eating Plate** shows dairy foods – including milk, yogurt and cheese – occupying a little under a sixth of total daily food intake (*see* page 120). For those who can enjoy and tolerate milk and dairy products, a daily portion of milk and live yogurt is a convenient and inexpensive way of getting excellent nutrition. Babies under a year old should not be given cow's milk as a drink but from six months may be given foods made with full-fat milk.

- **To maximise the potential benefits** of milk and yogurt, choose milk (and yogurt) from grass-fed cows. It is likely to have a richer, more complex flavour, thanks to the animals' more varied diet. To cut down on fat, go for lower-fat varieties, which still deliver the important nutritional benefits.
- **Watch out for unwanted added ingredients in yogurts and yogurt drinks** These often contain high levels of sugar or other sweeteners, starch, plus additives such as colourings and flavourings. Some yogurt-type drinks, such as kefir and ayran, are very natural but many are highly processed foods with extra ingredients that have no nutritional benefit.

- **Probiotic bacteria are present in all live, natural yogurt**, so it is not necessary to buy more expensive yogurt drinks to benefit from the health-promoting bacteria.
- **Look for single-origin brands** that come from a named farm, where particular pride is taken in the quality of milk. Most milk and yogurt is made from pooled milk, that is, milk from a number of different farms mixed together by the processor.

What if I cannot drink milk?

Many people are lactose-intolerant (cannot absorb the sugar in milk) because they lack the digestive enzyme, lactase, required to digest it. The incidence of lactose intolerance is highest in those parts of the world that do not have a long tradition of

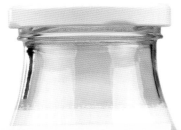

A1 or A2 – what type is your milk?

Scientists have been examining the two different proteins in milk – so-called beta-caseins and referred to as A1 and A2 proteins – for potential links to milk intolerance. It is thought that some people find cow's milk with A1 protein less digestible than milk with A2 protein. Milk from today's Holstein-Friesian herds has predominantly A1 protein. Milk from traditional breeds has predominantly A2 protein. If you think you may suffer from milk intolerance, try Guernsey milk, or milk marketed as A2, and see if you feel any better on it. Other scientists disagree with the A1/A2 theory, saying there is no evidence for it. The jury is out, so be your own judge.

It is estimated that **65 per cent of people around the world are lactose intolerant** to some degree.

dairy production: in China, for example, up to 90 per cent of the population may be lactose-intolerant to some degree.

● **Cow's milk can cause food intolerance** in some people even where dairy foods are a traditional part of the diet. Not liking milk is often the first sign. A food intolerance can manifest itself in conditions such as asthma and skin problems.

● **Anyone having problems digesting milk** could first try organic cow's milk or milk from grass-fed cows (see page 269). If things do not improve, try sheep's or goat's milk or lactose-free milk. If symptoms still persist, it may be best to avoid milk – there are alternative dietary sources for the nutrients in milk. Some people find they can still digest yogurt.

How can I use them?

Milk and dairy foods can be enjoyed in many forms and work in numerous dishes. Taste different types of milk and yogurts to see which you prefer.

➤➤ **Breakfast** Hot porridge made with milk on a cold winter morning or a summer bowl of muesli soaked in milk and topped with yogurt and fruit are both delicious and filling breakfasts.

➤➤ **Snacks** A tub of low-fat natural yogurt with fruit, chopped nuts and seeds makes an excellent snack.

➤➤ **Sauces** Milk can be used to make roux-based sauces: white/bechamel, parsley or cheese sauce. Spoon a little low-fat natural yogurt onto spicy dishes, either as an instant sauce or to calm down excess heat.

➤➤ **Desserts** Many inexpensive, traditional desserts – rice pudding, semolina, bread-and-butter pudding, crème caramel – are made with milk.

➤➤ **Shakes** Children (and adults) love milk shakes made with banana, chocolate (a little cocoa), strawberry and mango.

➤➤ **Low-fat substitute** Serve thick, low-fat yogurt instead of cream with desserts. Use yogurt, or part yogurt, instead of mayonnaise in potato salad.

Cream, butter & cheese

These are nutrient-rich foods but relatively high in fat. Enjoy them for their taste but not to excess.

What do they do for me?

All supply some important nutrients and, in moderation, can be part of a healthy diet.

➤➤ **Protein** Cheese is an excellent protein source. Hard cheeses are higher in protein than softer cheeses.

➤➤ **Vitamins** Cream, butter and cheese are all rich in vitamin A (good for skin and eyesight) and the fat they contain helps us absorb it. They contain useful amounts of vitamin E (helps reduce the incidence of heart disease, cancer and stroke); vitamin K (needed for blood clotting and to prevent bone loss); and vitamin D, which helps the body absorb calcium.

➤➤ **Minerals** They are all good sources of calcium and phosphorous (for healthy teeth and bones); potassium (helps regulate blood pressure); and magnesium (essential for skeletal development).

➤➤ **Cream, butter and cheese contain conjugated linoleic acid (CLA)**, which is thought to have cancer-fighting properties. Products from grass-fed cows have higher levels of CLA than those from cows housed indoors and fed on cereals.

What types are there?

➤➤ **Cream**
● **Pure cream** – contains no less than 35 per cent fat. Use for pouring or whipping.
● **Double cream** – a thicker cream that can be whipped very stiff; it contains no less than 48 per cent fat. Double cream can be cooked without curdling.
● **Whipping or thickened cream** – lighter than double; it contains no less than 35 per cent fat and gelatine for thickening. It does not curdle when cooked.

- **Clotted** – a rich cream, no less than 55 per cent fat, with a thick crust on top. It is a speciality of England's West Country, traditionally served in a Devonshire tea with scones and jam; it can also be used in cooking.
- **Light cream** – a thin cream, it contains 18 per cent fat. Use for pouring. Will not whip.
- **Sour cream** – soured with bacterial cultures to give it a slightly sharp taste. The cream can curdle if allowed to boil.
- **Sterilised** – cream that has been heated to a high temperature, which destroys nearly all bacteria so once canned it keeps, unopened, for several months. The high temperature gives the cream a caramelised flavour; it has no less than 23 per cent fat.

▶ Butter
- **Unsalted** As the name implies, it contains no salt.
- **Salted** This contains 3 per cent salt; lightly salted butter contains 1.5 per cent salt.
- **Easy spreading/spreadable** Vegetable oil, olive oil, air and/or more liquid parts of the fat are incorporated in the butter so that it remains soft when cold.

- **Clarified butter (ghee)** is butter with the milk solids removed so it can be heated to high temperatures without burning; it is useful in cooking and traditional in Indian and Middle Eastern cooking.
- **Continental or lactic** is the French style of butter in which the cream is ripened with lactic cultures to give a pleasantly fresh, almost slightly sour taste.

▶ Cheese
- **Soft, mild, fresh cheeses**, such as mozzarella, ricotta, cottage cheese, fromage frais and goat's curd are useful for cooking, quite neutral and milky in flavour. They need to be eaten by their 'use by' date as they don't keep.
- **Semi-hard cheeses** such as cheddar, gruyère, comté, pecorino and manchego are cheeses that have been salted and matured so they will have a more distinctive flavour and keep for some time. They can be eaten after their 'use by' date if any mould that has formed is pared off.
- **Heavily salted, strong-tasting white cheeses** such as fetta and haloumi are best used in small amounts to add a salty, savoury note.

Full-fat or reduced fat? Most official healthy-eating guidelines continue to advise us to eat fewer animal fats to protect against heart problems. But there is some conflicting scientific evidence. Certain studies have shown the potential of medium chain fatty acids found in dairy products to reduce body fat. Other research has linked a high saturated fat diet with reduced coronary artery disease in women; another study suggests that high intakes of full-fat dairy foods rich in conjugated linoleic acid (CLA) may reduce the risk of colorectal cancer. In addition, the trans-palmitoleic acid in full-fat dairy products may protect against diabetes: one study found that people with higher levels of this compound were 60 per cent less likely to develop type 2 diabetes. Eating too many fatty foods, however, can lead to excessive weight gain, which is never advisable.

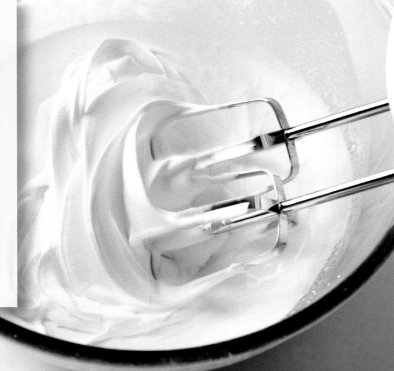

- **Blue cheeses** such as Stilton, gorgonzola and Roquefort are usually quite salty and have special moulds that give a characteristic strong 'blue' flavour.
- **White cheeses with a velvety rind** such as brie and camembert are firm when young, but best eaten when they are riper and have developed a pleasantly pungent smell.
- **Washed-rind cheeses** such as taleggio and reblochon have an orange rind and a pungent aroma but often don't taste as strong as they smell.
- **Matured hard cheeses** – such as parmesan, aged pecorino and vintage cheddar are dry textured, intensely savoury, salty cheeses to be used in small amounts.

How do they get to us?

Cream is simply fat separated from milk, usually produced by rotating the milk at high speed. Whipping cream is made by mixing cream with air to roughly double the volume. Crème fraîche and sour cream are treated with lactic bacteria to give them a slightly sharper taste. Clotted cream is heated in shallow pans, then allowed to cool and form a crust.
- **The taste of cream varies according to how the cows were farmed**. Cream from grass-fed and/or organic cows will look more golden in colour, with a more nuanced flavour than cream from cows kept mainly indoors, which will have a simpler, creamy taste and look white by comparison. If you always buy the same brand of cream, it could be interesting to swap around, compare and contrast. You may be surprised by how different they are.

Butter is produced by churning cream, then the fat globules are pressed and kneaded together. Adding salt, a preservative, will ensure that the butter keeps for two or three months longer but may also mean that it is less fresh than unsalted.
- **If you buy salted butter, most brands will taste quite similar** because the salt masks the subtler dairy flavours. If, on the other hand, you like unsalted butter, the biggest taste differences are between continental-style butters, which tend to be slightly sharper and more lactic, and the uncultured sort, which are more neutral in taste. For more traditional styles

of farm butter made with whey, or from cream ripened to develop its flavours, check out farmers' markets where small producers sell their specialty dairy foods.

Cheese is made in slightly different ways depending on the type, but there are common stages: (1) Milk is warmed; (2) Lactic bacteria is added; (3) Either animal rennet or a vegetarian coagulant is added causing the milk to curdle, separating into white curds and liquid whey; (4) The curds are cut (or pulled and twisted in the case of mozzarella), then drained, salted and put into moulds; (5) Blue cheeses are pierced with needles to introduce air and bacteria that cause the blue mould to develop; (6) The cheeses are matured to develop their flavour and firm up; the longer the maturing process, the stronger (and more expensive) the cheese.
- **For cheap, standard cheese** for sandwiches, supermarkets offer many rindless cheeses cut from a block. These tend to be sold by fat content – everything from full to reduced fat – and by maturity/strength which is indicated by a number from 1 (mild) to 5 (strong).
- **For more unusual, specialty cheeses**, a more adventurous selection can be found in specialist cheese shops or delicatessens as these tend to stock more small-scale, hand-made cheeses. They are usually run by enthusiasts with expertise in storing, maturing and handling cheese.

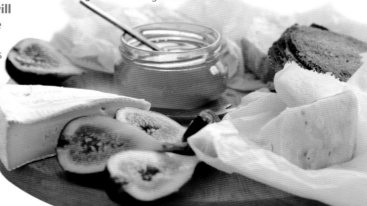

> ### Butter or alternative spreads?
> Many wholefoods practitioners say that butter is far more natural than the artificial alternative, which is made from oil that may have been hydrogenated, bleached, deodorised, emulsified, fortified and coloured to resemble butter. This may be true, but excess saturated fat may be harmful even if its source is a 'natural' one, so it might be worth reconsidering your need to put any kind of yellow fatty spread on your food!'

How should I use them?

These are rich foods so enjoy them in moderation While cheese falls into the dairy food group, for most people full-fat dairy foods and fats such as butter and cream should be occasional foods only.

▶▶ **Sauces** Cream makes an almost instant sauce. Use it to bake fish; to thicken the pan juices from a meat sauté; to enrich thin, runny cooking juices/gravy; to mellow a dish that's too spicy. Butter and eggs are the basis of creamy emulsified sauces, such as Hollandaise and Béarnaise, for special occasions.

▶▶ **Soups** Gently sweating/softening vegetables (carrot, celery, leek, onion, Jerusalem artichoke, potato, cauliflower, broccoli, watercress) in a little butter for 10 minutes will produce a deeper, sweeter taste in soups that you intend to liquidise.

▶▶ **Baking** From shortbread to sponges, butter adds an unbeatable melt-in-the-mouth taste to home-made cakes and biscuits.

▶▶ **Meat-free meals** Use cheese to make vegetable-based dishes tastier and more substantial: grilled haloumi on roasted vegetables; grated hard cheese in home-made veggie burgers; grated parmesan on chunky soups and pasta; salty mature cheeses (blue, goat's cheese) in salads.

▶▶ **When serving cheese at home**, remember to take it out of the fridge some time before you eat it, anything from 1 to 3 hours depending on the temperature of your home. Refrigeration dulls the taste of cheese and by allowing it to come back up to room temperature, you will get much more from it: richer aromas and deeper flavours.

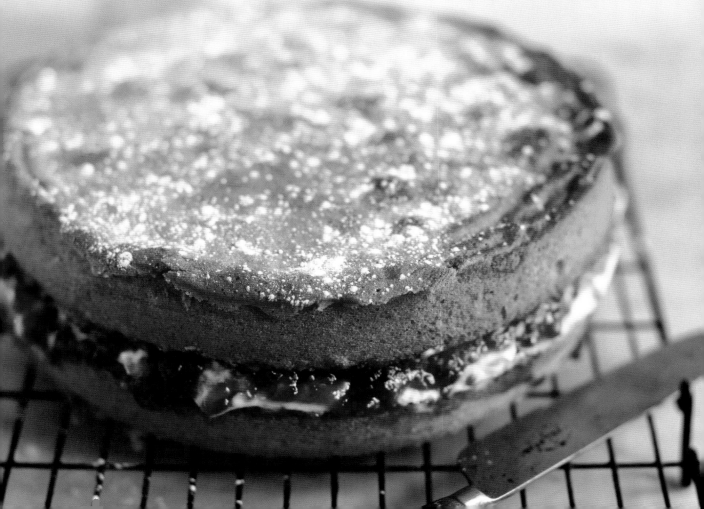

5 Pasta, legumes, grains & seeds

Starchy carbohydrate foods such as pasta and grains are staple fare throughout the world and highly nutritious; they play a key role in our daily diet. Tasty legumes usefully combine protein, carbohydrate and vegetable, while seeds are rich in protein and healthy oils.

Pasta

For thousands of years humans have eaten dough-based foods such as pasta and noodles. Today, varieties once associated with specific parts of the world have travelled across all frontiers.

What types are there?

Pasta divides broadly into Asian and Italian types. Both are easy and quick to prepare, inexpensive and versatile. Wholemeal varieties contain more fibre and other nutrients.

▶▶ Italian pasta is based on starchy dough, traditionally made in southern Italy from durum wheat semolina, and in northern Italy from flour mixed with eggs. Today, by law, all Italian pasta is made with durum wheat; some types contain egg,

The story that Marco Polo brought pasta back to Italy from China is a myth. The first known reference to pasta in Italy dates to 1154 in Sicily, a century before the great traveller was born. It is now thought that pasta came into Italy with the Arab conquest of Sicily in the 7th century.

some don't; some pastas are coloured with various natural colourings (spinach makes green pasta, squid ink makes black). Dried pasta has a long shelf life; fresh pasta must be eaten within days.

● **There are more than 600 pasta shapes**. They retain their Italian names: conchiglie (conch shells), ditali (thimbles), farfalle (butterflies), fusilli (twists), penne (quills), spaghetti (strings) – to name but a few. 'Culinary' Italian is rich in suffixes indicating size: *-ini* means thin (as in spaghettini), the opposite of *-oni* (spaghettoni are thick strands of spaghetti); *-cino*, *-ello*, *-etto* all refer to small pasta types.

● **Gnocchi are made with potato**, as well as flour and egg, or sometimes with ricotta.

▶▶ Asian pasta is at least 4,000 years old; in 2002 archaeologists in China uncovered a bowl of the world's oldest known noodles, carbon-dated to around 2,000BC. Asian noodles come in many varieties.

● **Noodles can be made from various ingredients** including wheat flour (with or without egg); rice flour (used in Asian cuisines, including Thai); and other vegetable starches such as mung beans or soy which make thread noodles and cellophane noodles. Dried noodles usually contain salt.

● **Other examples of Asian pasta include** foods such as spring rolls and wontons.

● **Japanese noodles include** udon, somen (fine white noodles of wheat flour and oil), soba (made from buckwheat) and harusame (made from potato or mung bean starch).

What does it do for me?

▶ **Pasta is not a high-energy food** –
100g cooked pasta contains around 400kJ. It supplies
B vitamins – B_1 (thiamin), B_2 (riboflavin), B_3 (niacin) and
B_6 (pyridoxine) – and traces of minerals. It is a good
source of insoluble fibre, which helps to move waste
matter through the gut.

▶ **It is low to medium GI**, so it releases energy
into the bloodstream fairly slowly; thicker pasta shapes
score lower than thin varieties.

▶ **Pasta is low in both fat and salt** – it's the
thick, creamy sauces that can add plenty of both. A
simple tomato-based sauce is much healthier.

▶ **The eggs in egg pasta add protein**,
as well as vitamins and minerals, raising the nutrition
score whether the pasta is dried or fresh.

▶ **Durum or 'hard' wheat has a high
gluten content**, so is not suitable for anyone who
cannot tolerate gluten. Non-gluten alternatives include
pasta made from buckwheat, rice or beans.

▶ **Wholemeal pasta has more** B vitamins,
zinc, iron and selenium and slightly more kiljoules than
white pasta, and the wheatgerm supplies vitamin E.
Wholemeal also has more than twice the fibre and a
lower GI. Wholemeal pasta made from spelt or hemp
is more nutritious than wheat pasta, but may be more
difficult to digest.

How does it get to us?

▶ **Almost all dried pasta is imported
from Italy**, while Asian varieties come from across
Asia. You'll find plenty of choice at large supermarkets,
in Italian or Asian groceries, or healthfood shops, as
well as online. Try out artisan brands, but judge for
yourself whether they are worth the extra cost.
● **A lot of 'fresh' pasta is imported** Buy from
shops with a good turnover to guarantee fresh stock.

Is fresh better than dried?

No – it simply has different uses in cooking.
To make stuffed pasta such as ravioli, for example, the
pasta has to be fresh and soft.
● **Be wary of what passes for fresh egg
pasta in supermarkets** – it could be made with
pasteurised liquid egg, rather than fresh eggs. Check
labels for ingredients such as potato starch, whey
powder, acidity regulators and synthetic flavourings, all
of which contradict the 'fresh' description.
● **To really appreciate fresh pasta, make it at
home** – it's not as hard as you might think. Generally
pasta has little taste on its own, it's the sauces that
bring it to life, but a good freshly made tagliatelle is

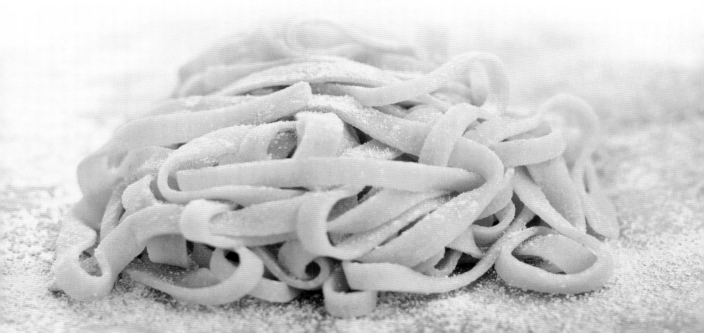

delicious with little more than a home-made tomato sauce, or at its most basic, a drizzle of good-quality olive oil and a sprinkling of torn fresh basil and finely grated parmesan.

Traditionally, in Italy pasta is served between the antipasti – a light first course with a good amount of vegetables and protein – and the protein-based secondi, the main course of fish or meat. It comes with a very small amount of sauce, just enough to coat the pasta, not to swamp it.

How can I use it?

▶▶ Pasta is compatible with almost any ingredient. It is most nutritious with sauces made using olive oil, tomatoes, fresh vegetables, garlic and herbs, with just small amounts of meat, fish or shellfish.

▶▶ Weigh out dry pasta before cooking: allow 75g–100g per person, which comes to around 1000kJ per serving when cooked. Portions vary according to quantities of other ingredients.

▶▶ The best way to cook pasta, whether dried or fresh, is in a pan of boiling water, large enough for the pasta to move freely. Allow at least 1 litre of water per 100g pasta. The water should be boiling when you add the pasta. Stir once to avoid sticking (oil is not necessary) and keep at a rolling boil. Drain in a large colander, then return to the pan and add sauce. Don't rinse pasta if serving hot – this washes off the starch that gives taste and texture; pasta may be rinsed for salads or for baked dishes.

▶▶ For al dente pasta – cooked until it's slightly firm and chewy, dried white pasta should be boiled for 8–12 minutes, 12–15 minutes for wholemeal. Fresh pasta cooks more quickly – anything from 1–5 minutes. Test it, if you are unsure. Al dente pasta has a lower GI than soft, well-cooked pasta.

▶▶ Experiment with different kinds as texture and colour make a difference. Generally, long thin strands go with simple sauces; thicker ribbon noodles take stronger sauces; tubes, twists or shells are good with chunky vegetables or in salads. Use different colours to visually complement other ingredients in the dish.

▶▶ Make sauces based on vegetables, small amounts of lean meat, fish, shellfish and herbs to boost flavour, colour and good nutrition. Or simply toss pasta with handfuls of chopped fresh herbs, such as basil, parsley, coriander, thyme, plus olive oil, lemon juice and black pepper.
● **Coat pasta lightly with sauce** so there's no pool left on the plate.

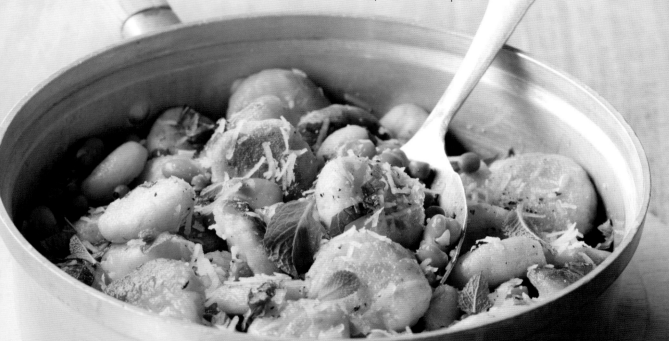

Most noodles can be boiled like Italian pasta, but take less time. Dried Asian noodles usually come in blocks or layers, which is helpful for portion control. They can be added to soups or stir-fries, served Italian-style with a sauce, or eaten as an accompaniment.

Cellophane noodles and rice sticks only need to be soaked in hot water. Crispy noodles are parboiled and dried before being deep-fried; they absorb fat during frying, so eat them only as a treat.

Use noodles in a stir-fry to create a well-balanced meal with lots of vegetables and a moderate amount of lean meat, poultry, fish, shellfish, tofu or legumes.

Bake spring rolls on non-stick baking trays, rather than deep-frying, to reduce the fat.

Pot noodles and three-minute noodles have a high sodium content, so don't eat them too often.

How should I store it?

● **Store dried pasta**, Italian or Asian, in an airtight container in a cool, dry place; keep the 'best before' date for reference.
● **Use home-made fresh pasta within 24 hours or freeze it** – it will keep frozen for up to eight months. Before putting fresh pasta in the fridge or freezer, leave it to dry to stop pieces sticking together.
● **Fresh Asian noodles can be kept in the fridge** unopened for up to three days. To freeze them, open the pack and spread them out on a tray, then pack into freezer bags when hard.

Legumes

Their high protein content makes legumes of all kinds an important food for humans and animals. They come from plants that yield edible seeds in a pod, which are then dried.

What types are there?

Beans, lentils, peas – there are many different varieties and names and definitions overlap. Most are excellent pantry standbys, easily transformed into nutritious meals. Here are some of the most widely used.

Beans include: adzuki beans; black-eyed beans (or peas); black kidney beans; borlotti beans; broad beans (aka fava beans); butter beans (aka lima beans); cannellini beans; flageolet beans; haricot beans (used to make baked beans); pinto beans; red kidney beans; soy beans.
● **Mung are the beans used to grow bean sprouts** – they're actually a dried pea and may be green, brown or black with yellow flesh.

Peas include: gunga peas (aka pigeon peas); marrowfat peas; split peas.
● **Chickpeas**, also known as garbanzo beans, are somewhere between a pea and a bean, actually another botanical species.

Lentils are distinguished by colour, shape and size. They range from black and dark brown, through different shades of green, to bright orange and yellow. They can be whole or split.

    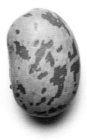 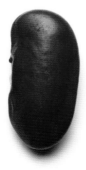 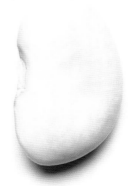

Australia is the world's leading exporter of chickpeas.

What do they do for me?

➥ Legumes are among the most nutritious of plant foods and a good replacement for animal and dairy foods. To get all the amino acids of animal protein foods, eat them with pasta or another grain.

➥ Most have a good balance of starchy complex carbohydrates and protein, and contain soluble and insoluble fibre. This combination makes legumes filling, keeping you satisfied for hours.
- **Legumes supply:** B vitamins (especially B_1 (thiamin) and B_9 (folate), vitamin E, minerals such as potassium, iron, zinc, magnesium and often calcium, plus a range of phytochemicals.
- **Most legumes are low in fat** (cooked soy beans have most at about seven per cent fat) and they have a low GI score, providing a steady source of glucose, so they can be a useful part of a diabetic diet.

➥ Key nutrients in specific legumes:
- **Chickpeas are a good source** of manganese, folate, iron and vitamin E, and, according to a report

---

Soy – superfood or health risk? Claims of soy's health benefits abound but its critics are equally vociferous. Some studies show that one to two daily servings (15–30g) of soy protein may protect against heart disease by lowering cholesterol and triglyceride levels; others suggest that it protects against several cancers. The anti-soy camp argue that eating soy could interfere with thyroid function and that the high content of isoflavones, a phyto-oestrogen plant compound, may increase the risk of tumours. Yet soy foods have been eaten in Asia for thousands of years, and the Okinawan Japanese, whose diet includes soy, are among the longest-lived people in the world. So, rather than treating it as a 'superfood' and eating excessive amounts, perhaps it makes sense to eat soy, as they do, in moderate quantities as part of a healthy diet.

Legumes supply about 10% of total protein

consumed around the world; they have twice the protein content of most grains.

in the *British Journal of Nutrition*, their protein quality is better than many other legumes.
- **Brown and green lentils** are more nutritious than split red and yellow lentils, with good amounts of B_6, folate and iron.
- **Protein in soy beans** contains all essential amino acids – the building blocks of protein – unlike other legumes, although these are less easily absorbed than those from animal sources. The beans also contain toxins, so they require special treatment to remove these (*see* box opposite).

How do they get to us?

➥ Most dried legumes are grown locally as open-field crops, with a few types imported. As they are not a perishable food, they are transported by road and boat. Most supermarkets stock dried and canned legumes, but for the best range – especially of organic varieties – go to wholefood shops. Asian grocers stock a wide range of lentils.

➥ What to look for when buying:
- **Dried legumes should have a bright colour and plump appearance**. If they look dusty and broken, these are signs of age (legumes get drier with age – the drier they are, the longer they take to cook and the more they fall apart). Pinprick holes could indicate insect infestation. Legumes should be evenly sized so they cook equally. Pricier legumes tend to keep their shape better when cooked.
- **Canned legumes are ready to use and convenient**, so no soaking or cooking are equired, and because they are pre-cooked you can be sure that they're toxin-free (*see* box opposite). Check the label for sodium content, which can be high: rinse them before using to reduce the salt. Also check the sugar content, which is often high in baked beans. Beans come through the tinning process better than lentils.

How can I use them?

▶ **Legumes are used in countless ways**, featuring strongly in Indian, Middle Eastern and Mediterranean food, and dishes such as dhal (made with lentils) and hummus (chickpeas) have travelled around the world. Here are some tips:

● **Soaking:** dried beans should usually be soaked in water for several hours or overnight before they can be cooked – soaking time depends on variety and size. Some, such as red lentils, don't require soaking at all. When the skins are smooth and unwrinkled the beans have soaked for long enough; discard any that float on the surface. Rinse well and cook in fresh water.

● **Don't add salt to the cooking water** – it toughens the skins as do sugar and acidic ingredients such as vinegar and tomatoes. Legumes should be fully cooked before these are added.

● **A 10-minute fast boil** is generally recommended at the start of cooking (except for lentils, peas and chickpeas). Then lower the heat and simmer until they are done.

● **Test for doneness:** for serving whole, the beans should be soft inside with the skin still slightly chewy; for purées, they should be soft right through.

● **Add beans to soups and stews** – they bulk them out into a sustaining, filling meal.

● **Replace meat with beans** – for example, lentils or black-eyed beans can replace half the meat in a shepherd's or cottage pie – making it cheaper but just as nutritious.

● **Eat with herbs** – serving legumes with plenty of herbs can help to prevent flatulence, a common side-effect of digesting legumes.

How to store

▶ **Dried legumes** store well in airtight jars in a dry cupboard. Take note of the 'best before' date.

● **Once cooked, legumes can be kept in the fridge for up to two days, or can be frozen**. As dried beans take time and effort to soak and cook, it is worth cooking more than you need for immediate use and freezing the rest in convenient portions for use later.

Kidney and soy beans are particularly high in toxins that can interfere with vitamin absorption, impair digestion and cause food intolerances. For safety, the dried beans must be thoroughly soaked and boiled.

● **Kidney beans** contain lectins, which can cause stomach pain and vomiting. To destroy the lectin content:

1 Soak the dried beans in water for at least 12 hours, changing the water at least once.

2 Rinse the beans and transfer them to a large pan, cover in fresh water and bring to the boil.

3 Boil the beans vigorously for 10–15 minutes, then simmer for 45–60 minutes until done.

● **Soy beans** contain a trypsin inhibitor, which prevents food being digested properly. This natural toxin is destroyed by the fermentation process used in making traditional soy foods, such as tempeh and miso, or it can be destroyed by soaking and boiling. To cook soy beans at home, follow steps 1 and 2 for kidney beans, but in step 3 boil the beans for 1 hour, followed by simmering for 2–3 hours.

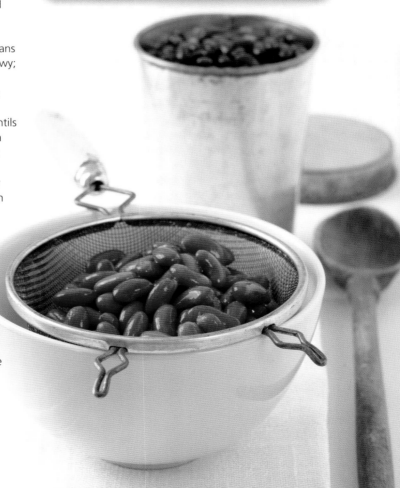

Grains

Cereal grains and rice are the basis of millions of foods around the world. Many of them are now highly processed which can quite drastically reduce their fibre content and nutrients.

New types of grain spring up all the time. Texmati® was developed in the USA as a cross between basmati and long-grain white rice. Wehani® is US long-grain brown rice. Doongara is an Australian version of basmati. Thousands of hybrid strains have been developed – some with better storage and cooking characteristics, or improved nutritional quality; some better able to withstand drought or other climatic extremes.

What types are there?

➤➤ **In their natural state** the many types of grain grown across the world offer a variety of tastes and textures and many nutritional benefits.
- **Cereal grains include:** amaranth, barley. buckwheat (aka kasha), corn, millet, oats, quinoa, rice, rye, sorghum, teff, triticale and wheat (including varieties such as khorasan and spelt).
- **Rice is one of the oldest cultivated crops** in the world. Varieties include: arborio, carnaroli and vialone nano (Italian risotto rice), basmati, Camargue red rice, Chinese black rice, jasmine (Thai rice), koshihikari (Japanese), pudding rice, sticky or glutinous rice.

What do they do for me?

➤➤ **All grains are a source of** complex carbohydrate, dietary fibre, protein, B vitamins, and minerals such as manganese, selenium and magnesium; levels of these nutrients vary between different varieties. Whole grains are more nutritious and make you feel fuller than refined grains.

➤➤ **Grains are low in fat and have virtually no sodium**. They also contain lignans and plant sterols, antioxidant phytochemicals, which may help lower cholesterol.

➤➤ **All grains are a useful source of protein**, especially for vegetarians. Higher protein levels are found in amaranth, buckwheat, khorasan, oats, quinoa, rye, spelt, teff and triticale.

➤➤ **When combined with** legumes such as beans and lentils, grains make up a complete protein, offering the full complement of amino acids we need.

➤➤ **Barley contains soluble fibre, zinc and magnesium**, but the grain loses much of its vitamins, minerals and fibre when it is pearled or polished.

➤➤ **The 'germ' of wheat**, the small reproductive part of the outer kernel – is a concentrated source of 23 nutrients, including vitamins A, B_1, B_3 and E, iron, zinc, magnesium, potassium and fibre.

➤➤ **The bran layer** on unrefined brown rice has a beneficial effect on digestion.

Grains in a gluten-free diet

➤➤ **Gluten in** barley, rye and wheat is a serious problem for anyone with gluten intolerance or coeliac disease. Those following a gluten-free diet must avoid these grains and their derivatives, including:
- **Burghul, a nutty and golden cracked wheat,** produced by cooking grains of wheat, minus the bran.
- **Couscous**, often thought of as a grain, but actually more of a small, grain-shaped pasta made from durum wheat, which is high in gluten.

➤➤ **Gluten-free grains include** rice, corn, millet, oats (high in soluble fibre), quinoa (higher in protein and lower in carbs than most grains), sorghum and wild rice.
- **Basmati, the 'king of rice'**, has the additional nutritional advantage of a lower GI than other kinds of rice. Wholegrain basmati is lighter and quicker to cook than other wholegrain rice.

Rice provides 20% of the world's dietary energy. It's the main staple food for 17 countries in Asia and the Pacific, nine in North and South America and eight in Africa.

- **Wild rice** – a type of aquatic grass with dark brown, long, pointed grains – has a higher protein content than actual rice and double the folate of brown rice. It contains the amino acid lysine.

- **Buying organic grains reduces exposure to pesticides**. Wholefood shops are a good source of organic grains, with the selection usually much wider than supermarkets.

How do they get to us?

▶▶ **Grains are field-grown crops** adapted to their local climate – some suitable for cool regions and others tolerant of hot and dry conditions. Certain crops, such as wheat, are rarely seen by consumers except in foods processed from them, such as flour, bread or pasta. Others, such as rice, are usually sold as grains, but will have had some form of processing.

- **Grains can be processed in various ways** – whole, cracked, rolled, milled, pearled, toasted, puffed, to name but a few.

- **Stone-ground grains** are nutritionally preferable to grains milled on a more industrial scale, as the friction and heat generated by steel rollers reduce the micronutrients.

- **Freshly harvested rice is known as 'paddy' rice or 'rough' rice.** It is dehusked by rubber roll sheller machines to produce brown rice (this doesn't affect the nutritional composition of the grain), and then can be further milled to produce white rice.

How do I use them?

▶▶ **At breakfast opt for porridge**, or a low-sugar, low-salt cereal such as Weetbix. Or try a bowlful of muesli made with soaked or dry rolled oats, nuts and seeds, topped with fruit and natural yogurt, which will keep your stomach satisfied for hours.

▶▶ **For lunch make up a healthy salad** – cold roast chicken, toasted pine nuts, chopped flat-leaf parsley served with quinoa or couscous.

▶▶ **For dinner try a Turkish dish** such as vine leaves stuffed with burghul and herbs, or an Indian lamb curry with lentil dahl and wholemeal basmati.

▶▶ **For dessert a good old-fashioned rice pudding** is easy on the digestion. Or try an Asian rice pudding made with sticky black rice, palm sugar and coconut milk.

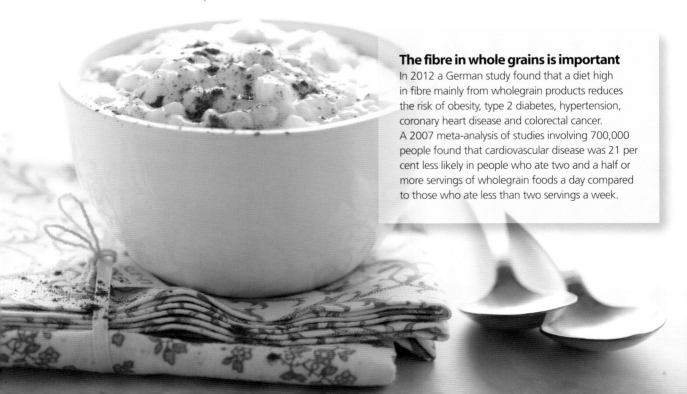

The fibre in whole grains is important

In 2012 a German study found that a diet high in fibre mainly from wholegrain products reduces the risk of obesity, type 2 diabetes, hypertension, coronary heart disease and colorectal cancer. A 2007 meta-analysis of studies involving 700,000 people found that cardiovascular disease was 21 per cent less likely in people who ate two and a half or more servings of wholegrain foods a day compared to those who ate less than two servings a week.

Cooking methods

➡ Before cooking many grains, particularly whole kernels, wash them to remove dirt and dust.

● **Boiling:** add grains slowly to generous amounts of boiling water – this washes off starch produced by cooking – then boil uncovered. When tender (10–15 minutes for white rice, 25–40 for wholegrain) drain in a sieve: be careful not to overcook.

● **Absorption:** this is suitable for most grains, whole or cracked; rye and whole wheat need soaking first. Grains are simmered in a precise amount of water, covered and without stirring, until they have absorbed all the liquid. Rice needs twice the volume of water to rice; most other grains (barley, oats, rye, quinoa, whole wheat) need three times as much water; millet needs four parts water to grain. Cooking times vary.

● **Steaming:** rice can be cooked in a steamer over boiling water; for best results soak it first.

● **Microwaving:** a variation of the absorption method, but in a bowl with a lid resting lightly on top. Long-grain rice needs 12 minutes, followed by 5 minutes standing.

● **Rice cookers:** if you eat a lot of rice, or have trouble cooking it, an electric rice cooker can effectively control the heat and the timing required.

Arsenic in rice – a health risk? A report of arsenic residues on rice led to some scary headlines in 2012, but the scientific consensus is that this does not pose any risk to most people. Arsenic occurs naturally in soil; rice will absorb it more than other grains because it spends part of its growing season in water. Levels of arsenic vary according to where the crop is grown, with rice from Egypt, India, Nepal and Pakistan having the lowest levels, and rice from the USA and France the highest. For those who rely heavily on rice, through culinary tradition or because of gluten intolerance, it may be advisable to source rice from low-arsenic areas. Yet even the higher levels are not thought to pose a health risk to someone who eats rice two or three times a week.

Different types for different dishes

➡ Use the rice type recommended in a recipe as each cooks in a slightly different way.

● **Long-grain rice, including basmati,** which becomes tender and fluffy when cooked, with separated grains, is used in many side dishes and often in pilafs where it is cooked in a seasoned broth.

● **Plumper, moister, medium-grain rice** is used in Italian risottos and also in sweet dessert dishes.

● **Short-grain rice** contains more starch and becomes stickiest of all. Varieties are used in risotto, paella, sushi and rice puddings. For sushi, rice is usually soaked for 30 minutes before steaming. Risotto is stirred constantly; paella is left undisturbed. Pudding rice needs long slow cooking, traditionally in milk.

How do I store grains?

➡ Check the 'use by' date and storage instructions.

● **Refined or polished grains** keep longer than whole grains – up to a year at room temperature.

● **For whole grains,** storage depends on whether the germ – the most perishable part of the grain – has been removed. Most intact grains keep for four to six months in a cool cupboard or fridge, but the shelf-life of buckwheat and millet is only around two months.

● **Wholegrain flours** have a shorter shelf-life than white. Most are at their best for two to three months, or up to six months in the freezer.

● **Take care with leftovers:** if cooked grains such as rice are left at room temperature, spores in the grains can germinate, causing bacteria to produce toxins that can cause vomiting and diarrhoea. Any leftovers should be cooled and refrigerated within an hour, then eaten within 24 hours.

Seeds

These tiny, highly nutritious foods are quite varied in taste. Many are used primarily as spices for flavour, while others make excellent snacks.

What types are there?

➤ A broad range of delicious seeds to explore and enjoy is now widely available in supermarkets and healthfood shops.
- **Seeds eaten whole include:** chia (a member of the mint family); linseeds; hemp seeds; pumpkin; sesame; sunflower – to name just a few.
- **Seeds used for flavour include:** aniseed, caraway, coriander, cumin, fennel, fenugreek and mustard.

What do they do for me?

➤ Seeds are rich in unsaturated oils, including omega-3 fatty acids in the form of alpha-linoleic acid (ALA). They are high in protein, B vitamins and vitamin E, and also minerals such as calcium, copper, iron, magnesium and phosphorus. They contain phytochemicals, have a low GI and are a source of soluble fibre. A few nutritional highlights of individual seeds include:
- **Chia seeds, whole and milled, are packed with** antioxidants, fibre, protein, calcium and ALA, which protects the liver and cardiovascular system.
- **Linseeds are an excellent source of** omega-3 and omega-6, vitamins E, B_6 and folate plus magnesium, phosphorus and copper. They are high in soluble fibre and a rich source of lignans.
- **Hemp seeds have a perfect balance** of three to one omega-6 to omega-3.
- **Pumpkin seeds contain cucurbitacins**, which have been shown to benefit prostate disorders.
- **Sunflower seeds are a good natural source of zinc,** which helps to boost the immune system.
- **Sesame seeds are rich in** calcium, magnesium, zinc, iron and fibre, vitamin B_1 and phosphorous, and also contain omega-6 and monounsaturated fats, plus lignans which may help to lower cholesterol.

How do they get to us?

➤ Most seeds are imported – China is the biggest source, but some come from the Americas, the Middle East and the Indian subcontinent.
- **The best selection is found in wholefood shops**, rather than supermarkets; to get the freshest, find a shop with a good turnover. Asian and Middle Eastern grocers stock a good range, too.

How can I use them?

➤ A little goes a long way: often all you need is a sprinkle. Keep small jars of seeds to hand. Their taste varies considerably, from neutral (linseeds), through mildly nutty (chia, sunflower, sesame), to stronger flavours (pumpkin, hemp).

➤ Sprinkle them raw over breakfast cereals and salads, or mix them into casseroles, soups or smoothies.

➤ Snack on them Seeds, such as pumpkin, sunflower or hemp, make an excellent portable snack.

➤ Bake or dry-roast seeds to enhance the flavour and make them crunchier. You can do this in a low-temperature oven, under the grill or in a dry frying pan. Shake them often so they turn evenly golden. Do not let them burn, as this degrades the oils and nutritional content, and creates a bitter taste.

➤ Enjoy them as spices Seeds used for spices in Indian and other cuisines – such as cumin, coriander, fennel or fenugreek – are dry-roasted, then ground. Mustard seeds are often used whole.

Storing
- **Some seeds**, such as chia, store well; others, such as linseeds, can go rancid. Always store in airtight containers and keep them out of the light. They should keep for two to four months in a cool cupboard, six months in the fridge and up to a year in the freezer.

6 Breads, snacks & treats

Billions of people around the world eat bread of some kind every day; there are now many delicious and nutritious varieties to enjoy beyond the mass-produced loaves of the West. Snacks can also contribute to good nutrition but too many can only be classed as treats. By definition treats are something to be enjoyed occasionally.

Breads

With a history dating back 30,000 years bread is our oldest, most familiar food – an essential, comforting staple of everyday life.

What does it do for me?

➡ All bread contains helpful nutrients – even the aerated, mass-produced white sliced loaf – although much commercial bread has an unhealthy level of salt. Both white and brown bread contain around 300kJ per medium slice.

➡ Commercial white bread is made from refined flour, which is usually chemically bleached. In many countries, certain vitamins and minerals must be added by law to wheat flour to replace those lost at the milling stage. In Australia and New Zealand, these include thiamin and folate.

➡ A brown loaf may be made with essentially the same ingredients, plus caramel added for colouring. So don't immediately assume it is more wholesome and healthier. Check the label for colouring agents such as 'caramel colour' to be sure.

➡ Wholemeal and whole-grain breads contain the outer husk and all the nutrients of the grain, providing fibre as well as vitamins B_1, B_2, niacin, B_6, folic acid and biotin, most of which are milled out of white flour with the bran and germ. The fibre and complex carbohydrates of wholemeal also make you feel fuller for longer.

➡ Bran-plus bread is usually white bread with added bran, which restores some of the fibre that is lost during the milling stage.

➡ Grainy bread is made from brown flour with malted wheat grains added. It is higher in folic acid (folate) than wholemeal, but lower in fibre.

➡ Multigrain is usually white bread with added whole grains, making it slightly more nutritious. (*See* pages 53–55 for further information about commercial bread processing.)

The smell of baking bread inspires feelings of warmth and wellbeing that **can help to sell a house,** according to estate agents.

Five secrets of shop loaves
(that a label does not reveal)

1 **They may contain natural L-cysteine**, a reducing agent produced from hydrolysed poultry feathers, hog's hair or (in China) human hair; a synthetic alternative is also used.
2 **Emulsifiers, used to create softness and an illusion of freshness**, include monoglycerides and diglycerides, which are sometimes synthesised from animal sources, including pork.
3 **Preservatives known as propionates (281, 282, 283)**, which inhibit the growth of moulds, have been linked to a wide range of allergic reactions, including migraine, eczema, gastro-intestinal symptoms and behavioural problems in children.
4 **'Processing aids' (not always listed)**, include amylase enzymes, used to promote crumb softness and to extend shelf life. Fungal alpha amylase is known to trigger asthma in bakery workers who inhale it. More rarely it can provoke symptoms in those who eat bread in which residues survive.
5 **Research into transglutaminase**, another enzyme, sometimes used to promote dough elasticity, has suggested that it may help to trigger coeliac disease (an immune reaction to gluten, *see* page 206).

Why you should bake your own

- **You decide what goes into it** and what does not – most shop-bought bread has too much salt.
- **You will never eat fresher bread**.
- **It will save you money**.
- **You can try making** a whole new range of breads, with different ingredients and types of flour.

Breads of the world

People make traditional breads all around the globe and there is a huge variety of them. A range of different flours and grains, oils and fats, plus other ingredients such as seeds, nuts, fruits and vegetables create distinctively different styles. The following are just a small sample:

- **Bagel, the 'roll with a hole'**, is boiled and then baked. Originally Polish and a Jewish staple, it's traditionally made with high-gluten wheat flour, although now in many varieties. Sizes vary; most have 1000kJ.
- **Baguette, the classic 'French stick'**. With a crispy crust and a fluffy texture inside, it is mostly carbohydrate and has around 800kJ per 70g.
- **Bara brith** is a crusty Welsh teabread, packed with dried fruit.
- **Boston brown bread** is a steamed loaf of rye, cornmeal and wheat flour, raised with bicarbonate of soda. It also contains milk, molasses and raisins.
- **Brioche** is a light yeasted roll or loaf, made with eggs, sugar and butter, and glazed with egg – half bread, half cake.
- **Challah** is an egg-glazed plaited loaf eaten on the Jewish Sabbath, containing sugar and traditionally a lot of egg. Dairy-free but may contain vegetable oil.
- **Ciabatta** is the slipper-shaped white Italian loaf, with a firm crust and open-texture. Made with olive oil; there is a wholemeal version (ciabatta integrale).
- **Cornbread** is made with cornmeal (aka polenta), salt, eggs, milk, oil and baking powder, but may also contain white flour. Yellow polenta is a good source of carotenoids such as lutein.
- **Crispbreads**, a Swedish favourite, are usually made from whole rye, providing fibre. A good pantry food, a typical crispbread has about half the energy of a medium slice of bread, but weight for weight bread has half the energy of crispbread.
- **Croissant**, the traditional French breakfast roll, is made from white flour, salt, sugar and butter, so is quite high in saturated fat.
- **Focaccia** is a rustic Italian yeast bread made from white flour, with olive oil.
- **Malt loaf** is a wheat-flour bread, sweetened with sultanas and honey and flavoured with malt.
- **Matzo** is a cracker-like flatbread, usually kosher, made from just flour and water, with scant nutritional value. It is eaten in place of bread during Passover.
- **Naan** is the soft flat Indian bread, made from flour moistened with yogurt.
- **Pain de campagne**, or 'country bread', comes in many regional variations in France. Different types contain unbleached white, wholemeal and rye flour.

- **Pita** is the Middle Eastern flatbread, made with white or wholemeal flour. It puffs out when warmed to form a 'pocket' for fillings. It has about 650kJ in 65g.
- **Pumpernickel** is German 'black bread', made from coarsely ground rye fermented with sourdough starter. True pumpernickel is dark from wholegrain rye and long baking; some versions use molasses. It has very little gluten, is high in fibre and has a low GI.
- **Rye bread** is made with sourdough starter because rye has insufficient gluten to make the dough rise. Studies suggest that it helps to maintain bowel regularity and reduce cholesterol. People with wheat sensitivity may be able to eat rye bread; check labels on wrapped 'rye' breads as some contain wheat flour.
- **Seeded breads** – seeds such as poppy, sunflower, sesame and caraway add nutrition to the basic bread.
- **Slimming bread** is white or brown bread which has been aerated to reduce the energy per slice to around 200kJ; it is also lower in nutrients and high GI. A better option is half a slice of wholegrain bread.
- **Soda bread** is a traditional Irish bread made with white or wholemeal flour, buttermilk and baking powder. It has no yeast, so is useful for those on a yeast-free diet.
- **Sourdough** requires a 'starter' made by soaking flour in water for several days to allow natural yeast and bacteria to ferment. The bacteria produce lactic and acetic acids, which make gluten proteins more digestible, so sourdough may reduce intolerance in people sensitive to gluten.
- **Tortillas** are the basic flatbread of Mexico, made with either wheat flour or cornmeal.

Snacks

Easily confused with treats, snacks should be a healthy way to fill a hunger gap. But so many commercial 'snacks' are strictly treats that it's remarkably easy to stray. Ask yourself, could I eat an apple? If the answer's no, you don't need a snack. If you do want to nibble, choose natural foods – fruit, nuts and seeds are ideal and will also keep you well.

Five tips for healthy snacking

1 **Plan ahead:** prepare nutritious snacks ahead of time, rather than reaching for a quick but often unwholesome filler when hunger strikes.
2 **Snacks by definition should be small** – place a limit of 500kJ.
3 **Avoid packaged snacks** if sugar is one of the first three ingredients on the label.
4 **Sit down to eat if possible;** eat slowly and chew properly. Have a glass of water or a cup of tea before you eat your snack.
5 **Snacks containing** wholegrain complex carbohydrates and protein will keep you satisfied for longer. (*See also* Healthy snacks, pages 168–179.)

Natural snacks

➡ Dried fruits are a healthy low-fat snack providing a higher concentration of some nutrients than fresh fruit, although others are lost in the drying process. Avoid fruits treated with sulphur dioxide as a preservative: sulphites can trigger asthma and allergic reactions.
- **Sultanas and raisins** make good snacks, supplying fibre, iron and potassium. They are high in fructose and around 500kJ per 25g.
- **Prunes** are dried plums, high in sugar and acidity, with around 150kJ per prune. They're a good source of iron, potassium and fibre, and a natural laxative.

➡ Olives are rich in monounsaturated oils, in vitamin E and other antioxidants, in iron, copper and fibre. Hydroxytyrosol, a phytonutrient in olives, may help to combat cancer and bone loss.

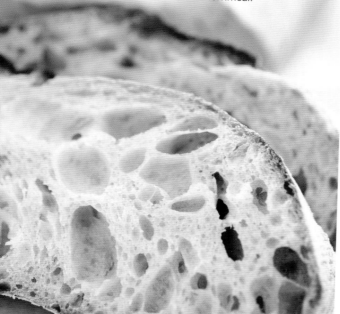

One drawback is that olives are high in salt from the preserving process, but are a useful occasional snack food at around 150kJ for ten.

➡ Seeds deliver protein, unsaturated fatty acids and a range of vitamins, minerals, fibre and antioxidants linked to health benefits. Some are particularly good to chew as protein-rich snacks, including pumpkin, sesame (with antioxidant compounds sesamol and sesaminol), and sunflower (antioxidant polyphenols such as chlorogenic, quinic and caffeic acids). *See also* page 283.

➡ Nuts are nutritional powerhouses.
Although high in energy, they may help to lower bad cholesterol, are an excellent source of protein and essential fats, and also minerals such as potassium, calcium, iron, magnesium, selenium and zinc.
● **They are best bought in their shells,** then cracked open as you want to eat them; this helps them keep longer and will mean you eat fewer. Small packs of ready-shelled nuts make good portable snacks.
● **Allergies to nuts, especially peanuts,** are quite common and potentially dangerous. If affected, you should avoid all nuts.

➡ Nut selection – kilojoules values are for a small handful 25g of shelled nuts:
● **Almonds** (500kJ) help to increase good (HDL) cholesterol. They are a rich source of vitamin E and B-complex, as well as phytonutrients.
● **Brazils** (650kJ) are a good source of vitamins E and B-complex and the highest natural source of selenium.
● **Cashews** (500kJ) are rich in vitamins B_5, B_6, riboflavin and thiamin. Sold ready shelled – look for creamy white, compact nuts, free from cracks.
● **Chestnuts** (200kJ) are high in carbohydrate, with some protein, and the only nut that contains vitamin C.
● **Coconut** (350kJ) is rich in copper, iron and manganese, but high in saturated fat.
● **Hazelnuts** (650kJ) and filberts/cobnuts are rich in folate and vitamin E.
● **Macadamia nuts** (750kJ) are rich in iron, copper, manganese and thiamin. High in fibre and monounsaturated fats.

● **Peanuts** (500kJ raw) have similar qualities to tree nuts. They're high in protein, fat, fibre, folate, niacin, thiamin, vitamin E, copper, iron and manganese. Roasting boosts antioxidants and helps eliminate aflatoxins (carcinogenic fungal contaminants).
● **Pecans** (700kJ) are rich in nutrients, notably vitamin E, thiamin, manganese, copper, iron and zinc.
● **Pistachios** (500kJ) are among the most nutritious nuts. They provide protein and fibre, and have twice the antioxidants of strawberries.
● **Walnuts** (650kJ) are a good source of protein and fibre, with vitamin E, copper, manganese and other antioxidants.

Packet snacks

➡ A healthy snack satisfies hunger, but
too many packet snacks are high in starch, sugars and salt that fuel cravings rather than supplying energy. We eat the whole bag; it's the manufacturer who decides the 'portion'.
● **A bag of crisps a day** adds up to consuming almost 5 litres of cooking oil a year purely in crisps.
● **Potato crisps top the list of foods that cause weight gain**, according to a study by Harvard researchers in the USA.
● **'Natural flavours' may not be what they appear:** some crisps and corn chips are labelled 'suitable for vegetarians' even though the flavour is roast chicken, smoky bacon or BBQ beef.
● **The buttery flavour in microwave popcorn** may come from diacetyl or 2,3-pentanedione (PD), chemicals that cause a respiratory disease called 'popcorn lung' in workers exposed to fumes in manufacturing plants.
● **High levels of monosodium glutamate (MSG)** have led the creation of 'clean-label' products using yeast extract instead. The only problem is that yeast extract contains natural glutamate, the active ingredient in MSG (*see* page 69).
● **One bag of crisps can contain** 500 times the maximum level of acrylamide designated safe in drinking water by the WHO. (*See also* page 157).

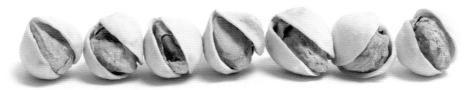

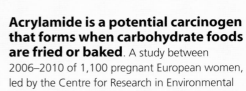

Acrylamide is a potential carcinogen that forms when carbohydrate foods are fried or baked. A study between 2006–2010 of 1,100 pregnant European women, led by the Centre for Research in Environmental Epidemiology in Spain, found a link between a high intake of acrylamide and low birth weight in babies. One of the researchers likened the effect of acrylamide to the well-known adverse effects of smoking on birth weight.

Around **6 billion bags of crisps are eaten** in the UK **each year** – that's almost 100 bags per person.

▶ Bags of variety – a small selection of packaged snack foods include:

● **Beef jerky** – strips of dried beef, often brined, processed and flavoured before drying. Good source of phosphorus and protein, but are high in salt and MSG.

● **Bread sticks** are typically made of refined flour with some fat; not very nutritious but not a disaster; around 80kJ a stick.

● **Popcorn** can be healthy, if prepared without a lot of butter and salt. The hulls are insoluble fibre and rich in polyphenols that protect against a range of degenerative diseases. But microwave popcorn is high in trans fats and the packaging may be lined with perfluorooctanoic acid which leaches onto the corn when heated. Popcorn has about 250kJ per 25g.

● **Potato crisps** get most of their energy from oil: a 25g bag of plain salted crisps contains 500kJ, compared to 80kJ in 25g of potato. Gourmet crisps usually have less fat relative to potato because they're sliced thicker, but even the finest hand-made crisps are basically fried starch. Tasty perhaps but it's best to wean yourself off them.

● **Pretzels** (hard, salted), have just a tenth of the fat in crisps and 400kJ per 25g, but are high in salt.

● **Root vegetable crisps** typically mix parsnip, sweet potato, carrot and beetroot. They have a few more nutrients than potato crisps, but are just as high in fat, salt and energy.

● **Salted peanuts are roasted**, which may enhance their health benefits, but they have high levels of fat and added salt; at around 1300kJ per 50g bag, their protein comes at a cost. Dry roasted peanuts are barely lower in fats and energy.

● **Salted pistachios** – the raw nuts are great snacks but salt is their downfall. Try them dry roasted, unsalted, at 550kJ per 25g shelled weight.

● **Stack crisps** are a highly processed, high-fat snack made from potato flour (less than 50 per cent) and other flours. They are best avoided.

● **Corn chips** are high carbohydrate and high fat, with about 900kJ per 25g before you start scooping up dips. But they're also a source of magnesium, as well as other minerals and vitamins including E and K, and a little fibre.

Sales of biscuits in Australia and New Zealand are over $1 billion a year and rising.

Biscuits

➠ It can be too easy to reach for biscuits to go with a cup of coffee or tea. Most mass-market biscuits contain refined flour and sugar, glucose syrup, palm oil, soy, trans fats, salt and chemical additives, so are not healthy snacks, but a few have redeeming features:
- **Fig rolls provide fibre and are fairly low in fat** with no hydrogenated fats; some of the sugar is from the figs. They have about 250kJ per biscuit.
- **Wheatmeal or digestive biscuits** are low in sugar and saturated fat, supply some iron and fibre.
- **Gingernuts are high in sugar**, but some of it comes from molasses, which also supplies iron.

➠ Biscuits made with wholegrain and/or organic ingredients can be a healthier, if more expensive, choice, but watch the sugar. And remember one biscuit, at a stretch two, is okay – more is not:
- **Macaroons** made with almonds or coconut are nutritional light bites.
- **Oats, oatmeal and raisins provide** fibre, vitamins and minerals, including iron.
- **Peanut butter** with wholemeal flour packs an energy punch.
- **Stem ginger** has the health benefits of ginger, but crystallisation adds sugar.
- **Wholemeal dark chocolate digestives** provide fibre and antioxidants.

➠ Cereal bars contain 'good' ingredients such as grains, nuts, seeds and dried fruits, but many are so high in sugars and fats, including high-fructose corn syrup and saturated fat, they don't deserve their healthy image. Analysis of one bar designed for children showed it to be 43.5 per cent sugars. Be choosy – carefully check ingredient labels to see what you're getting.

➠ Savoury biscuits are mostly refined white flour. Avoid varieties that are high in salt and flavourings such as dried, powdered cheese. Substituting a square of wholemeal bread provides more fibre and other nutrients.
- **Water crackers** are made of flour and water. They're fat-free with no salt, but scant nutritional value – a vehicle for cheese, but be careful how much.
- **Cream crackers** are refined flour with yeast and some fat with 130kJ each.
- **Wholegrain crackers** are a healthier choice, but recipes vary – check the labels carefully, some are rather salty.
- **Rice cakes** are made from puffed rice. They have about 200kJ a cake but are of little nutritional value. They are also high GI, so not suitable for diabetics.

Cakes & pastries

➠ Most cakes and pastries fall into treats but there are some snack options among them, especially if made with wholemeal flour.
- **Carrot cake** supplies a little vitamin A from the carrots. Extra ingredients such as oats, orange and walnut can raise the nutritional value.
- **Date and walnut** is a fairly sound choice – both are highly nutritious.
- **Muesli cookies and slices** can be high in sugar and fat, but the oats, nuts, dried fruit and seeds bring nutritional value.
- **Wholemeal scones**, whether cheese or fruit, are a satisfying and nutritious option – but limit the amount of butter you add.

Spreads

➠ A snack at home often involves some sort of spread on bread. This can be a healthy and nutritious option – or not – depending on bread and spread. Here's the low-down on some spreads:
- **Fruit butter** is a low-sugar substitute for jam. Apples, apricots, pears and other fruit are cooked to a pulp, sieved, sweetened and perhaps spiced; they are 80kJ a tablespoon. Offers few nutrients – mainly carbs.

- **Honey is high in sugars** (mostly fructose and glucose) but is probably healthier than refined sugar, with a lower GI and, weight for weight, fewer kilojoules. At its best, it's a powerful antibacterial with traces of B and C vitamins, magnesium, potassium, calcium, sodium chlorine, sulphur, iron and phosphate. However, in many commercial honeys modern heating and filtration destroy much of the goodness that gave honey a reputation as a wonder food. Locally produced raw honey (strained, not filtered) may help to build tolerance to local pollen, although this is not proven. Honey has 250kJ per tablespoon.
- **Jams are a traditional way of preserving fruit** with sugar, but the heat destroys much of the vitamin C. Marmalade is made with Seville oranges and other citrus fruits. Jams have 250kJ a tablespoon and offer sweetness but little more.
- **Peanut butter** and 'butters' made from cashews, almonds or hazelnuts retain most of the nutrients of the nuts, including vitamin E, B vitamins and fibre. They are more than 50 per cent fat, most of it the healthy monounsaturated and polyunsaturated type, but still high in energy. Look out for unwanted added ingredients such as cane juice, sugar and palm oil. Go for those made only with nuts, and no or very little salt. If you have a blender or food processor, you can make your own additive-free version by grinding roasted nuts until they form a butter that is smooth, wet and whipped looking. These butters contain 400kJ per tablespoon.

Ten terrific snacks

1 **Dips such as hummus and tzatziki** with raw vegetable sticks
2 **Yogurt with berries**
3 **Hard-boiled egg and tomato**
4 **Two wholegrain crackers** with nut butter
5 **Grapes** with a little cheese
6 **A handful of nuts, seeds and dried fruit**
7 **A slice of seedy wholemeal bread** with mashed avocado and sliced tomato
8 **Cottage cheese** with chopped raw vegetables
9 **A banana**
10 **Celery stick** spread with blue cheese

Treats

These are the many tasty foods that tempt us but we don't strictly need. The trick is to eat them occasionally and enjoy them to the full.

Beautiful baking

When we think of food treats, cakes are often the first things to come to mind. In fact, cakes can contain healthy ingredients – fruit cake is packed with dried fruit, eggs and nuts, for example – but also tend to be rich in sugar and fat, with a high kilojoule count. Traditionally, cakes mark special occasions, and this remains a good way to think of them – a celebration food to be shared with friends.

▶▶ **Popular treat cakes** that should not be everyday fodder include:
- **Brownies** made with dark chocolate contain antioxidants; up to 1500kJ in some servings.
- **Cheesecake** is based on cream cheese, sometimes with egg, supplying protein with extra carbohydrate in the base. Fruit often adds some vitamins and fibre, but this is a high-fat, high-energy food.
- **Cupcakes** are back in vogue – small sweet cakes topped with icing and glacé fruit. Not for everyday, and beware of inedible glitter.
- **Doughnuts** have few plus points – white flour, sugar inside and out, and deep-fried!
- **Muffins** are over-sized cupcakes that are high in sugar and fat; the blueberries can't possibly compensate. Typically they have 1500–2000kJ each.

Chocolate & confectionery

▶▶ **Chocolate is made from** the beans of the cacao/cocoa tree, fermented, dried and slow-roasted. Cacao contains proteins, fats, calcium, iron, carotene, thiamin and riboflavin, and is rich in antioxidant flavonols that help to lower blood pressure. Chocolate averages 600kJ per 25g. The quality of nutrients varies with type.

Chewing gum as an alternative to sweets brings potential health benefits. It can suppress appetite, relieve stress and boost memory performance. The act of chewing increases saliva, which combats the acids that cause cavities, while xylitol, a sweetener in some gums, has been shown to block tooth-rotting bacteria.

● **Dark chocolate contains little or no milk fat and the highest concentration of cocoa solids** – the higher the score, the better the chocolate as a source of flavonols. It also has useful amounts of iron, magnesium and potassium.

● **Milk chocolate is a solid form of drinking chocolate** first made by a Swiss confectioner in the 1870s. Mass-market bars generally have poorer nutritional quality, with refined sugar and fats. The addition of peanuts, hazelnuts and raisins slightly raises their nutritional profile.

● **White chocolate is made from cocoa butter,** milk solids and sugar; nutritionally, it scores the lowest.

➽ **Most sweets are almost entirely sugar**, which is bad for teeth. Many contain colouring, texturisers and sweeteners. Some luxury and hand-made confectioneries contain good natural ingredients:

● **Candied nuts** have nutrient-rich almonds or walnuts to compensate for the sugar coating.

● **Chocolate fudge** has some goodness from cocoa, butter and milk, and mineral traces.

● **Chocolate truffles** have nutrients from cream, butter and dark chocolate.

● **Florentines** have nuts and sometimes dried fruit.

● **Marzipan** contains almonds (in the paste) and whole egg.

● **Mint creams** contain eggwhites and the dark chocolate adds a few flavonoids.

Ice creams & sorbets

➽ **Real ice cream**, whether a luxury brand or home-made, contains only ingredients that our great-grandmothers would recognise – cream, milk, sugar, eggs, plus natural flavourings such as vanilla, fruit or chocolate. Although high in saturated fat and sugar, it has calcium and protein. Check labels to see what you're getting:

● **Fruit ice cream** may contain no real fruit at all, only flavours. If there is a picture of real fruit on the label, it should contain at least some fruit.

● **Sorbets and granitas** ideally contain just fruit juice and syrup; some sorbets also contain eggwhite and small amounts of milk fat and solids. Churning gives sorbets a 'snowy' texture. Granitas are stirred, creating crystals and a flaky texture.

● **Frozen yogurt** made with fruit can be a delicious alternative to ice cream, but watch the sugar content.

➽ **Cheap commercial ice cream** is not really a treat at all: it's made of oils, high-fructose corn syrup, monoglycerides and diglycerides, emulsifiers, flavourings and colours.

● **Soft serves** are partially reconstituted lactose, reduced whey protein concentrate, sugar, vegetable oil (some hydrogenated), dextrose, whey powders and additives. This is the confection sold from vans, squirted through a nozzle into cones. It may also contain lard (pig fat).

Ice cream trade secrets

● **The 'vanilla' flavour may come from piperonal (a chemical used in mosquito repellent)** or synthetic vanillin made from lignin, a by-product of wood pulp. In 2011 chef Jamie Oliver shocked American TV audiences with a claim that cheaper ice cream is flavoured with castoreum 'from rendered beaver anal gland'.

● **'Strawberry' flavouring may contain 12 or more synthetic organic chemicals** including benzyl acetate, also used as a solvent.

● **Manufacturers whip air** into it to make it lighter: regulations limit this to 50 per cent of the final volume of the ice cream.

According to one survey,

the average woman tells nine lies a week about her eating habits, with chocolate, crisps and cake the foods most lied about.

7 Hot & cold drinks

To keep our bodies healthy, we need to consume sufficient liquid each day to stay properly hydrated. Some of this essential fluid – the equivalent of six to eight glasses of water a day – comes from food, especially fruit and vegetables, but most comes from drinks of one form or another. What else is in those drinks can impact enormously on our health.

Water

What does it do for me?

▶▶ Readily available tap water is subject to rigorous checks ensuring that it is safe to drink. It can contain important minerals, such as calcium, magnesium, iron and potassium, but also traces of chemicals used to treat water:
- **Chlorine is added** to prevent the proliferation of bacteria and viruses.
- **Aluminium sulphate is used** to improve clarity – most, but not all, is filtered out.
- **Fluoride may be added** to combat dental decay. Critics say this 'mass medication' can be harmful but supporters note that the rate of dental caries in children in unfluoridated areas is double the rate in fluoridated areas.

▶▶ Filters can remove the 'baddies' but may also take away the 'goodies'. Activated carbon, distillation and reverse osmosis filters strip out many chemicals (although fluoride gets through activated carbon), but the minerals go with them, and the loss of dissolved oxygen can leave water tasting flat. A pinch of sea salt or mineral drops and a squeeze of lemon can replace minerals.

What goes into bottled waters

1 **They may contain more bacteria** than tap water, and are not subject to the same stringent standards.
2 **Almost half come from a municipal supply**, filtered or unfiltered, at up to 1,900 times the cost.
3 **Three litres of water** go into the making of one plastic litre bottle of water.
4 **Mineral waters from** subterranean sources contain dissolved mineral salts, elements or gases, but not necessarily any more than tap water.
5 **So-called vitamin waters** contain added vitamins; any potential benefits are outweighed by sugar, artificial colouring, preservatives and caffeine.

▶▶ In developed countries tap water is usually as good as, or better than, bottled. Instead of buying expensive water in plastic bottles, fill a glass or ceramic container or stainless-steel flask with tap water.
- **Elsewhere water safety can vary**, but even bacteria that are harmless to local populations may cause problems in a gut that has not built up resistance. When travelling, drink bottled water unless the tap water is boiled or purified. Avoid ice made from tap or well water.

Tea

All true teas derive from the *Camellia sinensis* plant, grown mostly in East and South Asia and Africa.

Five good reasons ...

... to drink tea

1 **It contains powerful antioxidants** known as 'flavonoids' and 'catechins', a flavonoid subclass thought to have many therapeutic effects.

2 **Despite a slight diuretic effect**, overall tea hydrates the body, and has additional health benefits.

3 **Tea may improve immunity** to disease through the amino acid L-theanine, which the liver breaks down to 'ethylamine', a molecule that primes immune blood cells.

4 **Tea-drinkers may be less prone to heart attack and stroke** due to antioxidants thought to help prevent cholesterol and free radical damage to arteries; flavonoids appear to restrict blood clotting.

5 **A catechin in tea** is credited with protecting DNA from cancer-causing changes and possibly inhibiting cancer cell replication.

What types are there?

▶▶ Tea choices – the various colours reflect differences in processing:

● **Black tea has the strongest flavour** and contains most caffeine. Some antioxidant catechin is lost in processing. It is best brewed for 5 minutes.

● **Decaffeinated tea** has all but a trace of caffeine removed and a lower antioxidant content.

● **Earl Grey is black tea** scented with oil from the peel of bergamot orange, reputed to have antiseptic, antidepressant and soothing properties.

● **Green tea is high in catechins** and contains vitamin K, important for blood-clotting. Its reputed benefits include combating cancer and heart disease.

● **Gunpowder is a type of green tea**. The leaves are rolled into pellets that unfurl in boiling water.

● **Jasmine, China's favourite scented tea**, is infused with petals – good if you don't like tea strong.

● **Kombucha is black tea** fermented with sugar, bacteria and yeast. Its fans claim it boosts immunity and liver function and combats cancer.

● **Lapsang souchong is Chinese black tea**, smoke-dried over pinewood.

● **Matcha tea is powdered green tea**, claimed to have the most health benefits as the whole leaf is ingested: one cup equates to ten of leaf tea.

● **Oolong is known in China as 'blue-green tea'**. It is thought to boost mental alertness and may also help to combat major diseases.

● **White tea** is made from buds and selected leaves that are steamed and dried. It is lower in caffeine than green tea, with higher levels of catechins.

Hot tea tips

▶▶ Take it 'black': according to one recent study, casein proteins in milk neutralise antioxidants in tea, countering its ability to improve vascular function.

▶▶ Make a pot: loose leaf tea has higher levels of beneficial chemicals than the leaf fragments, used in most teabags, and the space to expand allows the leaves to release more of their health-giving agents.

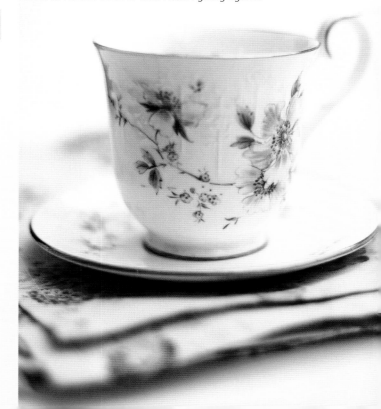

Herbal teas

Tisanes, **herbal teas** or 'infusions' are made from a range of herbs, fruit and spices.

What do they do for me?

➡ They are caffeine-free and may offer a variety of health benefits. Most herbal teas contain real herbs, but fruit teas may be made from synthetic ingredients. Check packet labels.

- **Chamomile contains** the amino acid tryptophan, which soothes the nerves and promotes good sleep.
- **Elderflower** is said to have anti-inflammatory properties and promote perspiration, which can relieve symptoms of colds, catarrh, chesty cough and sinus pain.
- **Fennel seed tea** calms an upset stomach.
- **Ginger** helps to reduce nausea and vomiting, including travel sickness. It may also relieve arthritic pain and may help reduce blood cholesterol levels.
- **Lemon balm** calms nerves and aids digestion.
- **Nettleleaf** is a pick-me-up that contains iron, calcium and magnesium.
- **Peppermint** aids digestion and relieves nausea.
- **Rooibos**, South African 'Red bush' tea, is made from a broom-like member of the legume family; it is rich in antioxidants and low in tannin.

Potential hazards of disposable cups

Using china or glass mugs or cups saves on waste, and may well be the healthiest choice, too.

- Paper cups may have a laminated plastic liner. This plastic has been linked to health problems due to traces of endocrine disruptors which may be released by hot liquid.
- Plastic cups may contain bisphenol-A (BPA), another endocrine disruptor that can leach into water at high temperature.
- Polystyrene cups are made from monostyrene, a liquid petrochemical. Styrene mimics oestrogen in the body and is considered a possible carcinogen.

Coffee

Coffee, like tea, has health pluses and potential minuses, too. It's important to take account of how it affects you, and adjust your consumption accordingly.

Five good reasons ...

... to drink coffee

1 **It's a good source of antioxidants** – one cup contains more than a serving of blueberries.
2 **It may help protect the heart and prevent stroke** – one to three cups a day has been shown to reduce the chances of serious abnormal heart rhythms and stroke by 20 per cent.
3 **It may reduce the risk of type 2 diabetes** and of colon and prostate cancers.
4 **It has been linked to** lower incidence of dementia and Parkinson's disease.
5 **Coffee drinkers** show lower incidence of cirrhosis and other liver diseases.

... but not too much because

1 **High coffee intake causes** calcium loss as the mineral is excreted in urine.
2 **Caffeine promotes alertness**, but too much can cause tremors, jitters, insomnia and stress.
3 **Cafestol and kahweol**, fatty compounds in coffee, can boost cholesterol synthesis in the liver which raises fat levels in the blood.

How is it made?

➡ Most coffee choices start with an espresso, made by forcing steam or hot water through the coffee grinds under pressure. This makes an excellent-tasting coffee and reduces the level of cholesterol-raising compounds. Any roast of bean may be used; darker roasts contain slightly less caffeine.

- **Americano** is an espresso diluted with hot water, with or without cold milk added.
- **Cappuccino** is milky espresso with a froth on top and sometimes a sprinkling of cocoa or chocolate.
- **Espresso** is a single shot of concentrated coffee, but has no more caffeine than a regular cup of coffee.

Decaffeinating coffee removes compounds that give coffee its distinctive flavour along with the caffeine. Because of this a stronger-flavoured bean, Robusta, is often used instead of the more usual Arabica. Compared to caffeinated coffee, decaf increases levels of fatty acids and cholesterol in the blood but, unless you drink a great deal, the effect is unlikely to be measurable.

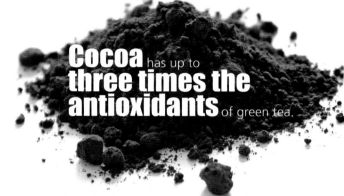

Cocoa has up to **three times the antioxidants** of green tea.

- **Filter coffee** is filtered through paper which eliminates the larger grounds and reduces the level of cholesterol-raising compounds.
- **Instant coffee** is lower in caffeine than fresh, and fatty substances are eliminated in processing, but it may contain higher levels of acrylamide (*see* page 288).
- **Latte** is espresso with hot milk – this adds nutrition but also kilojoules.
- **Machiatto** is espresso with a very small amount of hot milk added.
- **Mocha** is a latte with chocolate, often served topped with whipped cream.
- **Syrups** have become popular as a way of flavouring coffee, but these also add sugar and energy.
- **Turkish coffee** is made by boiling it in a pan and is served unfiltered. It has the highest concentration of cholesterol culprits cafestol and kahweol.

- **Commercial drinking chocolate** is made from cocoa powder, powdered milk and sugar.
- **Make your own:** try stirring a few cubes of rich, dark chocolate through hot milk. Delicious!

Hot chocolate drinks

What do they do for me?

➡➡ **Natural cocoa powder** contains flavonols shown to lower blood pressure and improve the function of cells lining blood vessels. In one Dutch study, men who drank cocoa were seen to halve their risk of dying prematurely from heart disease. Learn to love the bitter taste instead of heaping in sugar.

How are they made?

- **Some drinking chocolates** come as shavings or chunks of chocolate made with sugar and cocoa solids. The darker it is, the more antioxidants it contains.

Non-dairy milk substitutes

What do they do for me?

➡➡ **These can be useful for vegans** and for people who cannot tolerate lactose, as they are all plant-based and lactose-free. They are sometimes fortified with vitamins and calcium but usually lack most of the protein and nutrients found in milk. Many commercial brands contain added sugars, vegetable fats, salt, synthetic vitamins and minerals as well as lecithin, stabilisers and thickeners.

- **Almond milk** is principally water and almonds. It is lower in energy, protein and saturated fat than full-fat cow's milk.
- **Oat milk** tastes mildly sweet. It is made from water and oats, so is lower in energy, protein and saturated fat than full-fat cow's milk. It contains some soluble fibre that may help to lower blood cholesterol.
- **Rice milk** is made from water and brown rice, low in protein and fat, and relatively high in carbohydrates.
- **Soy milk** has good levels of protein. Commercial brands have similar energy, protein and fat content to full-fat cow's milk, but the type of fat and protein in soy is thought to be beneficial to heart health.

Sweeteners – what's in them?

➠ There are many low-energy alternatives to the empty kilojoules of sugar, but it's debatable whether any of them are a healthier option.

● **Acesulfame-K** is a derivative of acetoacetic acid, 200 times sweeter than sugar but not metabolised by the body so no energy is absorbed. There have been concerns about side effects, but it is approved as safe.

● **Agave nectar** is derived from the cactus-like agave plant. It's about 40 per cent sweeter than sucrose and higher in energy, but has a lower GI. Some adverse reactions have been reported in diabetics.

● **Aspartame**, produced from natural amino acids L-aspartic acid and L-phenylaline, is around 200 times sweeter than sugar and has no kilojoules. Sufferers of phenylketonuria, a rare genetic condition, must avoid it.

● **Coconut sugar** from coconut palm sap is mostly sucrose; high in minerals and B vitamins.

● **Fructose** is refined fruit sugar, sweeter than sucrose with lower GI; a range of health problems have been linked with HFCS (*see* page 46).

● **Saccharin** was discovered in the 1870s by a chemist working on coal tar derivatives. Fears that it is carcinogenic surfaced in the 1970s; it has been declared safe, but remains contentious.

● **Stevia** is a refined preparation of a herb long used as a sweetener in South America. May cause nausea and 'full' feelings, but generally recognised as safe.

● **Sucralose** is processed from sugar, but 600 times sweeter and said not to be absorbed by the body. Despite complaints of side effects, it is deemed safe.

● **Xylitol** resembles refined sugar but with fewer kilojoules and low GI. Mostly extracted from birch bark, but occurs naturally in certain fruits and vegetables. Some reports of side effects such as diarrhoea.

Yogurt drinks & milk shakes

What do they do for me?

➠ It depends what's in them; read the label. The ingredients that go into yogurt drinks can differ quite considerably.

● **Live, unpasteurised yogurt** has 'probiotic' bacteria that restore the balance of intestinal bacteria and boost immunity.

● **Brands 'enriched' with probiotics** confer some benefits, but scrutiny of health claims reveals a degree of hype. Some drinks are little more than watered-down yogurt with confected flavours and added sweeteners.

● **Drinks high in sugars**, including fructose and modified corn starch, are best avoided.

● **Those that contain both** bifidobacteria and lactobacilli provide a good balance of intestinal bacteria, but they must be consumed every day to reap the benefits.

➠ Exotic probiotics include:

● **Ayran**, a blend of yogurt and water, with added salt and sometimes fresh mint. Of Turkish origin, it is a refreshing drink in hot weather.

● **Kefir** is an enzyme-rich fermented drink made from kefir 'grains' – a mix of bacteria, yeasts, proteins, lipids and sugars – and usually milk. Contains good bacteria not usually in yogurt that can repopulate the digestive tract. Avoid brands high in sugars and additives.

● **Lassi** is yogurt thinned with water (or milk, in the Punjab). It is often salted, but may be flavoured with sugar, rosewater, honey, fruit and spices. Blend mango with water and live yogurt for a delicious mango lassi.

➠ A well-made milk shake can play a good role in a healthy diet, providing protein, calcium and vitamins from the milk, plus nutrients from added fruit.

● **Make your own** with different fruits, vanilla and spices. Whizz up equal parts of fruit and milk, with a few ice cubes and perhaps a little honey.

● **Commercial shakes** may contain no milk at all, and are often high in fats and sugars, with dozens of non-food additives. Best avoided.

contain 59 ingredients – but no strawberries.

More than 40 additives combined to synthesise the strawberry flavour.

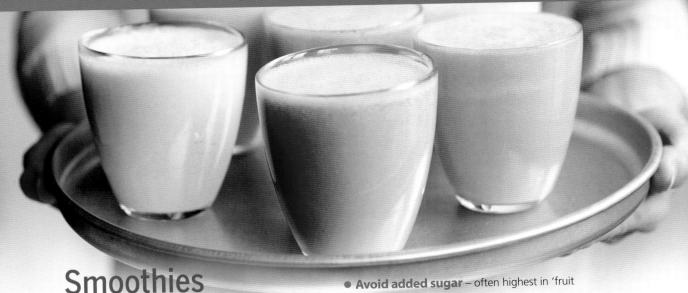

Smoothies

What do they do for me?

➡➡ **These blended drinks are made from a variety of ingredients** – fruit, vegetables, milk, yogurt, herbs, spices and supplements.
● **At their best** they contribute to a healthy diet; at their worst, they can be laden with fats, sugars, flavourings and other additives. Read the label.
● **Your own can be healthier and tastier** Try blending berries and low-fat yogurt with pomegranate juice, ice and a little banana. Experiment with your favourite fruits – but watch the quantities.

Juices

What do they do for me?

➡➡ **Drinking fruit and vegetable juices** is an easy way to get more vitamins and minerals into your diet, but there are downsides:
● **Juicing loses pulp and fibre** – juice never has as much goodness as the whole fresh fruit or vegetable.
● **Concentrates and pasteurised juices** are heavily processed. Opt for freshly squeezed juices.
● **Avoid added sugar** – often highest in 'fruit drinks' or 'fruit juice drinks'.
● **Juices increase the risk of kidney stones** due to their oxalate content.
● **Juices bathe your teeth in acid,** which damages the enamel.

What types are there?

➡➡ **Juice variety** – with a home juicer you can make your own. Here are a few healthy choices.
● **Beetroot juice** is rich in potassium, antioxidants and folic acid, and helps lower blood pressure. It may boost stamina and is quite low in energy. Wash or scrub the beetroot, then juice raw.
● **Carrot juice** supplies beta-carotene and juicing, like cooking, releases large amounts.
● **Cranberry** may be effective against urinary infections. **Caution:** cranberry can interact dangerously with blood-thinning medications.
● **Grapefruit** is high in vitamin C and potassium. It contains bioflavonoids and other phytochemicals that may protect against cancer and heart disease. **Caution:** can interact with some prescription medications.
● **Orange** is rich in vitamin C, although some of this is lost in juicing as it removes the white membrane under the orange skin.
● **Tomato juice** contains lycopene, a powerful antioxidant that may reduce the risk of prostate cancer.

Cordial

What do they do for me?

➡ **These fruity concentrates** are much cheaper than fresh juices but differ greatly in quality.
● **Go for high-fruit, low sugar-brands**. Dilute them well with water and add ice for a long, thirst-quenching drink.
● **Avoid cordials with artificial colours** and preservatives such as sodium benzoate, sodium metabisulphite and potassium sorbate, which have been linked to asthma, hay fever and dermatitis.
● **Be aware that 'sugar-free'** or 'no added sugar' often means they contain sweeteners such as saccharin or aspartame (*see* page 296). 'Contains a source of phenylalanine' suggests aspartame, which is dangerous for sufferers of phenylketonuria.
● **A better alternative to cordials is** to dilute fruit juice half-and-half with water.

Fizzy drinks

What do they do for me?

➡ **Sweet fizzy drinks don't belong in a healthy diet**. They are mostly carbonated water and sugar (including high-fructose corn syrup), with artificial sweeteners, flavourings and colourings.
● **They are 'empty kilojoules'** and a major contributor to obesity, type 2 diabetes and other ills. A 330ml can of regular cola contains around 500kJ.
● **Colas contain phosphates** that can impair calcium absorption, increasing the risk of osteoporosis.
● **Diet drinks contain no sugar and no energy** – yet there is mounting evidence that they encourage obesity.
● **Fruit-flavoured drinks** are often less than ten per cent fruit juice.
● **The ginger and lemon** in ginger beer may bring some benefits but the sugar content is high. Most commercial brands are flavoured carbonated water.

Five reasons to ...

... avoid low-joule diet drinks

1 **The low-joule label may tempt** you to reward yourself by drinking or eating more.
2 **Artificial sweeteners** can over-stimulate receptors in the brain, encouraging a 'sweet tooth' and cravings for sweetness.
3 **Daily consumption** of diet drinks increases the risk of developing type 2 diabetes.
4 **Two or more diet soft drinks a day** may accelerate decline in kidney function.
5 **A daily diet soft drink** increases the risk of stroke and heart attack by 43 per cent.

Energy drinks

What do they do for me?

➡ **Energy drinks are designed to boost energy, stamina and concentration**. Claims are made for ingredients such as B vitamins, taurine (an amino acid), and herbs such as ginseng and guarana, but their principal effect comes from high doses of caffeine, sugars and sweeteners. The drinks have been implicated in health problems and fatalities.
● **Some experts warn** that energy drinks shouldn't be used by anyone under 18, over 50, pregnant or breastfeeding, or with a family history of heart disease, high blood pressure, caffeine-sensitivity or glaucoma.

Why you might want to avoid them

● **Caffeine acts as a diuretic** It adds to dehydration during strenuous exercise and can cause palpitations.
● **There is no evidence that** B vitamins boost energy; health claims for taurine are not proven for the synthetic form in energy drinks.
● **Ephedrine** (a common ingredient) is a stimulant that can cause heart attacks, stroke and seizures.
● **People have reported** vomiting, tremors and chest pains after consuming these drinks.
● **Drinking them with alcohol** or during strenuous exercise has been linked to fainting and sudden death.

Alcoholic drinks

What do they do for me?

▶▶ **There is evidence that** a regular, small intake of alcohol may extend life, raising good (HDL) cholesterol while lowering bad, and reducing the risk of cardiovascular disease. However, exceeding safe limits quickly leads down the road to health problems (*see* page 72).

- **Drinking with food** is a better way to consume alcohol than drinking on its own.

Why no one should drink to excess

- **It increases the risks of** accidents, errors of judgement and violent behaviour.
- **It racks up empty kilojoules**, leading to weight gain and obesity.
- **Binge drinking** can raise blood pressure.
- **It is linked with** increased risk of cancers of the breast, mouth, pharynx, larynx, oesophagus, colon and, of course, the liver.
- **Chronic alcohol consumption** causes cirrhosis of the liver, lower fertility and malnutrition.

What types are there?

▶▶ **The risks of alcoholic drinks** tend to increase with the strength of the drink.

- **Beer** contains polyphenols, antioxidants that help to combat cancer. It supplies valuable iron – dark beers supply more than light – and silicon, which increases bone density: beers richest in barley and hops supply the most silicon.
- **Cider** is a rich source of catechins and proanthocyanidins – types of polyphenols, disease-fighting antioxidants dubbed 'lifespan essentials'. These are found in greater concentrates in cider apples than in dessert varieties. Rich in potassium and low in sodium, cider may also help to control blood pressure.
- **Cocktails contain a range of ingredients** which makes it tricky keeping track of the alcohol units – especially as these usually sweet drinks slip down as easily as the fruit juice they contain. When mixing your own, keep to just one shot of spirit.

Mixers served with spirits – bitter lemon, ginger ale, tonic water – are fizzy, with little if any nutritional value. Typically they contain sugar, sweeteners, flavouring and sometimes colour, and have around 150kJ per small can or bottle. Soda water is a kilojoule-free carbonated water that may help to settle an upset stomach.

- **Liqueurs are syrupy**, often strongly alcoholic drinks that are best avoided – or reserved for a rare after-dinner treat. A 50ml glass of creamy liqueur contains around 600kJ.
- **Spirits average 37–40 per cent alcohol** by volume. A 25ml standard measure of clear spirit (gin, vodka, white rum) contains 200kJ; dark rum, whisky and brandy contain 250kJ. Dark spirits have far higher concentrations of congeners, biologically active toxic substances produced during fermentation.

Wine

What does it do for me?

▶▶ **Research into the health claims** for wine relate mainly to dark grape skins as a potent source of procyanidins, polyphenols beneficial for heart health. Grape skin is also a source of resveratrol, which may offer some protection against cancer, heart disease and vascular dementia. Non-drinkers need not miss out as grape juice contains resveratrol, too.

▶▶ **Red wines are healthiest** as the dark grape skins are left in the fermenting juices. The most potent effects are found in flavoursome wines such as Madiran (from the tannat grape), Malbec and Cabernet Sauvignon. (*See also* page 118).

▶▶ **Rosé wines** are made mostly with dark grapes, with skins fermented for a shorter time than red, so the wine has some of the same health pluses.

▶▶ **White wines** may be made from white or red grapes. While they may not be so beneficial to heart health, they may improve lung function, thanks possibly to high levels of flavonoids that mop up toxins in the blood.

8 Restaurant food & takeaways

We eat out more than ever in restaurants, wine bars and cafés, while street food stalls and takeaways are booming. Yet what's on offer is often less than healthy – high in saturated fats, salt, sugar and kilojoules. Take control of what you eat and you'll enjoy the experience even more – savouring different foods and knowing that you're getting the best nutrients, too.

Eating out – the healthy way

The smart approach starts with being able to spot which dishes are both delicious and good for you. So whether you're in a luxurious restaurant, grabbing a takeaway, or anything in between – consider what's on offer; sometimes doing a bit of research in advance can help. This does not mean discarding all 'naughty-but-nice' ingredients – just keep them for treats and balance what you eat overall.

Six tips for ...

... making better food choices

1 **Select a restaurant with a varied menu** to give yourself plenty of options for finding something that's healthy and suits your food mood.
2 **Choose by cooking method:** in general go for foods that are steamed, boiled, braised, simmered, stir-fried, grilled, baked or sautéed. Avoid deep-fried or 'crispy' foods.
3 **Opt for brightly coloured foods**. Most high-energy foods are brown, beige, white or pale yellow.
4 **When you order, stick with your choice** – don't be tempted to change when you hear what other people have chosen.
5 **Add extra plain vegetables** and/or salad to any main course.
6 **Don't hesitate to ask questions** about dishes termed 'healthy options' – ask 'Why they are called this?' You are the customer, after all.

How much can I eat?

Is the second big consideration. In some food establishments, 'more is better' seems to be the prevailing wisdom – massive portions are presented as a mark of good value. For the diner, the temptation is to cram in as much food as you can. The healthiest policy is to eat slightly less than you wish to (remembering that your brain takes up to 20 minutes to register fullness), and not a bite more.

Seven tips to ...

... avoid over-eating

1 **Make your restaurant reservation beforehand** – this should cut your waiting time and minimise hunger build-up.
2 **Have a piece of fruit** – an apple, say – an hour or so before you go out. This plugs the hunger gap, so you don't arrive at the restaurant ravenous and ready to eat everything in sight.

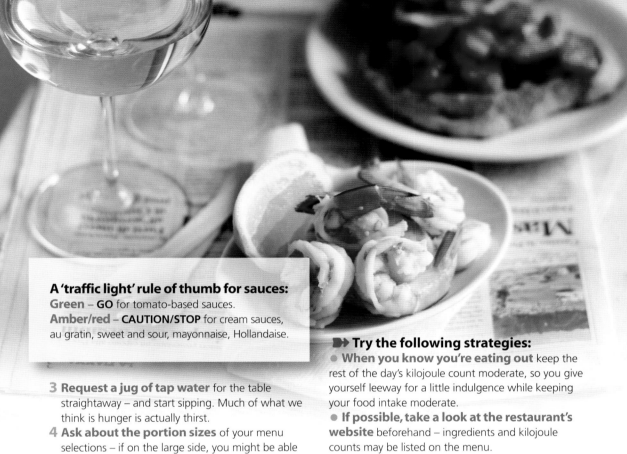

A 'traffic light' rule of thumb for sauces:
Green – **GO** for tomato-based sauces.
Amber/red – **CAUTION/STOP** for cream sauces, au gratin, sweet and sour, mayonnaise, Hollandaise.

3 **Request a jug of tap water** for the table straightaway – and start sipping. Much of what we think is hunger is actually thirst.

4 **Ask about the portion sizes** of your menu selections – if on the large side, you might be able to share, or request a smaller portion.

5 **When ordering a variety of dishes**, get advice from the waiter on how many to go for.

6 **Don't even think about dessert** until you've finished your main course – by which time you may decide to give it a miss.

7 **Don't go on eating if you're no longer hungry** – it's never compulsory to clear your plate.

Take control of eating out

■▶ **You could keep tabs on every kilojoule** (official recommendation: about 8000kJ for an average woman; 10,000kJ for a man) but eating a balanced meal is just as important. Start from the Healthy-Eating Plate on page 120. There's a lot of flexibility. Remember you're in the driving seat – just enjoy it.

■▶ **Try the following strategies:**

● **When you know you're eating out** keep the rest of the day's kilojoule count moderate, so you give yourself leeway for a little indulgence while keeping your food intake moderate.

● **If possible, take a look at the restaurant's website** beforehand – ingredients and kilojoule counts may be listed on the menu.

● **Get to know the components** of different cuisines, so you can recognise which are healthy choices and which are not.

● **Whatever you order**, make sure you get plenty of vegetables.

● **Ignore the freebie** (or otherwise) bread, rolls, pappadums, cornchips and rice crackers.

● **Ask for** dressings and sauces to be served separately on the side.

● **Stick to moderate portions**.

● **Eat low-energy food first** – start with the vegetables.

● **Eat mindfully:** to enjoy the food more fully, put your knife and fork down between mouthfuls and take time to savour the textures and flavours.

● **Say no to sugary drinks with food**. Have kilojoule-free water, or a small glass of wine which will probably have fewer kilojoules and help your digestion.

Best of world cuisines

With so much to enjoy, here's how to combine healthy eating and great tastes.

Chinese

A good Chinese diet balances yin foods (wet and moist) with yang (dry and crisp). Chinese cooking makes good use of steaming and stir-frying, two quick cooking methods that maximise flavour and nutrition. But beware the high salt content of soy sauce or anything labelled 'battered' or 'crispy', which equals deep-fried.

Good menu choices

▶▶ **Try these:** soups (crab or chicken and corn, hot and sour vegetable, wonton); steamed dumplings, vegetables and fish; chop suey and stir-fried main dishes; Szechuan prawns; sizzling dishes.

▶▶ **Healthy accompaniments:** plain steamed rice; stir-fried vegetables.

▶▶ **Dessert:** almond jelly with fruit.

Watch out for

▶▶ **Deep-fried nibbles** such as prawn crackers, spring rolls (deep-fried) and prawn toasts; sweet and sour pork balls (battered, deep-fried) or egg fried rice.

What should I drink?

▶▶ **Drinks with a difference**
● **Chinese wines**, distilled from rice, millet, other grains, herbs and flowers, are higher in alcohol than grape wine. Popular Yellow Wine tastes a little like sherry and is best served warm.
● **Green tea** is a good way to round off a Chinese meal. It has many reputed health benefits, too: its medicinal use dates back almost 5,000 years.

French

French cuisine is rich in regional diversity and displays deep respect for market-fresh, seasonal produce and classic techniques. It can include plenty of fats and butter, but also many healthy options.

Good menu choices

▶▶ **Try these:** salade niçoise; ratatouille; seared scallops; grilled sole; mussels; coq au vin (chicken in red wine); chicken chasseur; tournedos Bordelaise (steak in reduced shallot and red-wine sauce); veal marengo (veal stew with mushrooms and tomatoes); bouillabaisse (fish stew); fish Provençal with tomatoes and herbs.

▶▶ **Healthy accompaniments:** salads; sautéed spinach with garlic and lemon; olive and tomato compote.

Watch out for

▶▶ **Dishes high in fat, such as foie gras;** duck à l'orange; mille feuille; and frites (practically irresistible with steak – so try sharing).

What should I drink?

▶▶ **A French meal without wine** is almost unthinkable:
● **Don't turn down dishes cooked in wine:** when the wine is cooked, the alcohol (and lots of kilojoules) burn away, leaving just the flavour.
● **Enjoy a good red:** there is evidence that cardiovascular benefits stem from the procyanidin flavonoid content of red wine. Other foods rich in procyanidins include grape juice, cranberry juice, apple, cocoa and various teas.

The Mediterranean diet is high in fruit, vegetables, grains and legumes, with moderate amounts of fish, meat and dairy, lots of herbs for flavour and olive oil as the main source of fat. It is a pattern of food proportions, rather than a set list of foods or recipes. This gives infinite scope for invention using locally sourced produce and variation to suit individual tastes.

Greek

Many traditional Greek dishes follow the Mediterranean diet pattern, which can help to reduce heart disease and cancer risk. But not all foods served in Greek restaurants are healthy – additional ingredients vary greatly from restaurant to restaurant.

Good menu choices

▶▶ **Try these:** dolmades (stuffed grape leaves); Greek salad; grilled octopus in olive oil, garlic and oregano; tabbouleh salad (parsley, mint, tomatoes and burghul); beetroot salad with oranges, red onion and rocket.

▶▶ **Kleftiko**, the national dish, was reputedly created by 15th-century Greek freedom fighters; the name means 'stolen'. To cook stolen lamb in a way that could not be seen or smelled, they baked it in earthenware vessels buried underground, with no added fat. Today, kleftiko is made by tightly wrapping lamb in foil and baking until the meat falls off the bone.

▶▶ **Healthy accompaniments:** hummus (a 2-tablespoon serving should be about 200kJ, but recipes vary); grilled vegetables dressed with olive oil.

▶▶ **Dessert:** Greek yogurt with honey, or a small piece of Turkish (Greek) delight.

Watch out for

▶▶ **Moussaka**, a popular dish of minced lamb, fried eggplant and tomatoes can be healthy, but some versions approach 50g of fat per serving; baklava (also Middle Eastern), a rich traditional sweet made with layers of filo pastry, butter, chopped nuts and honey.

Indian

What we think of as Indian food draws mainly on meat-eating culinary traditions, such as Mughal and Kashmiri cuisines, that make up just a small part of the many regional styles of cooking found in the subcontinent. More than a third of people in India are vegetarian, and many more eat meat only occasionally. Indian food as it's found in the West can be high in saturated fat and kilojoules, but there are plenty of delicious, healthy choices on the menu.

Good menu choices

▶▶ **Try these:** dishes with tomato-based sauces such as tandoori and madras; rogan josh; onion-based dishes such as dopiaza; vegetable dishes such as aloo gobi (a potato-cauliflower curry) or saag (spinach); lentil dahls.

▶▶ **Healthy accompaniments:** plain boiled rice; wholemeal chapati; naan bread; lassi.

▶▶ **Dessert:** try low-fat rice kheer or a small piece of burfi.

Watch out for

▶▶ **Buttery and creamy curries** such as korma, passanda, masala with pilau rice; parathas (fried bread); bhajis, pakoras and anything fried, such as samosas (pastry puffs).

The aromatic spices of Indian food, such as turmeric, ginger, red chillies, garam masala (a mix of cumin, coriander, cardamom, black pepper, cinnamon), may do more than give distinctive flavours to a curry. Researchers are finding they may help to protect against neurodegenerative diseases, such as dementia.

Italian

Italian cuisine is acknowledged to be among the finest, simplest and healthiest in the world. Olive oil, fresh vegetables and fibre abound in dishes usually made from just a few select ingredients.

Good menu choices

▶▶ **Try these:** soups such as minestrone; salads dressed with olive oil and balsamic vinegar; veal cacciatore; pasta with napoletana sauce; mussels in wine sauce; thin-crust pizza with fresh vegetable toppings.

▶▶ **Healthy accompaniments:** bread sticks; bruschetta (go easy on the oil); mozzarella and tomato salad; pasta sauces based on tomatoes or other vegetables, such as artichokes.

▶▶ **Dessert:** try gelato made from concentrated natural fruit juice rather than cream; or simply a cappuccino.

Watch out for

▶▶ **Antipasto salads** with lots of high-fat items such as sausages, olives, prosciutto; fried appetisers; pasta with creamy-cheesy sauces; garlic bread; cannoli (cream-filled sweet pastries) and cassata.

The modern pizza has gained an unhealthy reputation for being loaded with high-fat cheeses and meats, contributing to obesity and the risk of life-threatening diseases. But pizza can be healthy. Researchers in Milan found that people who ate pizza at least once a week had less chance of developing cancer of the mouth, oesophagus, throat and colon than those who didn't. Their findings reflect the quality of the ingredients used in traditional Italian pizzas, made with thin crusts and small amounts of nutritious, tasty toppings.

Okinawan Japanese, who often live to 100, **practise a simple diet rule called Hara Hachi Bu, which means 'eat until you are eight parts full'.**

Japanese

Traditional Japanese cuisine is super-healthy – not just a diet rich in fruit and vegetables, but prepared healthily – quickly steamed or stir-fried.

Good menu choices

▶▶ **Try these:** miso soup; vegetable-and-tofu stir-fry; sashimi and other seafood; tempeh (soybean cake from fermented beans).

▶▶ **Sushi sounds a healthy option** – and should be – but watch out for high-sodium, mayonnaise, and high-fat sauces. Drizzle a small amount of soy sauce on top, rather than dipping each roll into a bowl of sauce. Or you could try protein-packed sashimi – plain raw fish, with no added rice.

▶▶ **Healthy accompaniments:** bok choy (calcium-rich); seaweed (iodine); shiitake mushrooms (iron, potassium, zinc, copper, folate); steamed vegetables; edamame (soybeans in the pod).

▶▶ **Dessert:** seasonal fruits; sweetened bean paste; green tea to finish the meal.

Watch out for

▶▶ **Anything with the word 'tempura'** – it means the ingredient has been dipped in batter and deep-fried; stick to small portions.

Native Mexican diet patterns are associated with a lower risk of breast cancer. Spanish 'almonga' beans, used in Mexican cuisine, have been found to reduce triglycerides in people with type 2 diabetes.

Mexican

Mexican cuisine combines the vegetarian heritage of Mayan and Aztec cultures with the food of the Spanish who first arrived in the 16th century. These influences form a cuisine filled with colour, flavour and nutrition. Traditional dishes are rich in healthy ingredients such as legumes, vegetables and whole grains, that provide a delicious range of healthy choices.

Good menu choices

▶▶ **Try these:** grilled chicken with capsicums and onions; ceviche (seafood marinated in a broth of lime, lemon and orange, with onions, tomatoes, capsicums and coriander); chicken fajitas; black or pinto bean burritos; enchiladas (baked, so lower in fat than tacos).

▶▶ **Healthy accompaniments:** soft tortillas; black beans; taco salad with all the salsa you want – it's fat-free, low-energy and a good source of lycopene; guacamole (but limit portion size); brown rice.

▶▶ **Dessert:** flan (similar to a crème caramel); almendrado (eggwhites, lime and almond flavouring).

Watch out for

▶▶ **Fatty dishes** such as corn chips and fried tortillas, refried beans (often prepared with lard); cheese burritos; con queso dips; con queso dips, cheesy nachos, chimichangas; chile relleno.

What should I drink?

▶▶ **Drink with a difference:** Mexican horchata, made from almond and rice milk with cinnamon.

Middle Eastern & North African

From Turkey to Morocco, by way of Israel, Lebanon and Egypt, there are many flavours to experience – dishes seasoned with cardamom, coriander, cumin, thyme, marjoram, sumac – and plenty of healthy options.

Good menu choices

▶▶ **Try these:** lamb and goat are the preferred meat across the region – grilled shish kebabs are a good choice; or kofta (balls of ground lamb and onions, skewered and grilled); shish taouk (marinated chicken skewered and grilled over charcoal).

▶▶ **Healthy accompaniments:** loubieh (green beans cooked with tomatoes); eggplant with garlic, tomatoes and capsicums; hummus (watch out for oil-heavy variations); tabbouleh (a salad of burghul, tomatoes and lots of herbs such as coriander, mint and parsley); labneh (thick yogurt with mint); vegetable sticks to dip (rather than pita); fresh or dried fruit such as figs, dates, apricots, plums.

Watch out for

▶▶ **High-energy dishes:** donor kebab; pastilla (Moroccan chicken pie with almonds); baklava (also Greek, a sweet pastry with butter, honey and nuts).

What should I drink?

▶▶ **Drink with a difference:** mint tea is delicious and aids digestion.

'Fast casual' eateries are a growing trend, combining the ambience of a restaurant with the delivery speed of fast food. They provide a budget-priced alternative that generally pays more attention to food quality than a fast-food outlet. The fast casual Chipotle chain offers Mexican food, while Vapiano is a fresh take on Italian. Nando's specialises in Portuguese food, especially peri peri chicken; you pay as you order so avoid waiting around for a bill.

Spanish

Another Mediterranean cuisine, Spanish food revolves around heart-healthy olive oil as its main source of fat, with lots of fresh fruit, vegetables, legumes, nuts, fish and small amounts of meat. It is noted for the tapas tradition in bars – small portions of tasty dishes, which can be anything from a snack to a sustaining meal depending on how many you order.

Good menu choices

▶▶ Try these: gazpacho (chilled, tomato-based, antioxidant-rich soup); paella (an all-in-one dish of rice, vegetables, seafood, chicken and rabbit); tilapia al ajillo (tilapia with garlic); spinach with pine nuts; jamón Serrano – relatively low in fat and salt for ham; tortilla (Spanish omelette of eggs, potatoes, onions, olive oil).

▶▶ Healthy accompaniments: grilled vegetables; Basque beans; green beans.

▶▶ Dessert: try pinchos des frutas (fruit brochettes); tortas de Aceite (oil cake) – a light dessert originally from Andalucia.

Watch out for

▶▶ Manchego – a rich, creamy sheep's milk cheese (salty, buttery, aromatic and piquant – too good to miss, but keep it small); fatty chorizo and fried foods.

What should I drink?

▶▶ Drink with a difference: batido de fresas – a delicious strawberry milkshake made with yogurt.

Thai

The generous use of herbs, roots and spices is what gives Thai food such freshness and may bring special health benefits, too. Lemongrass is said to help digestion, for example, while galangal, a close cousin of ginger, is used in Ayurvedic medicine and thought to have anti-inflammatory properties helping to relieve muscle and joint pain. Few cuisines boast such a bumper pack of free-radical-fighting antioxidants, but some dishes also contain high levels of fats and sodium so should be avoided.

Good menu choices

▶▶ Try these: tom yum (clear soup with prawns, coriander, lemongrass, ginger) – as with all Thai soups, can be high in sodium; gai pad mamuang him ma pahn (cashew chicken) – the cashews bring healthy fats and protein, but watch portion size for kilojoules; Thai salads; steamed or stir-fried dishes with chicken, fish or vegetables; steamed seafood dishes such as fish or mussels; satay (grilled chicken or meat skewers) – but go easy on the sauces.

▶▶ Healthy accompaniments: summer rolls (soft rice paper around steamed filling); papaya salad (grated unripe fruit in a tangy chilli-lime dressing); steamed rice.

▶▶ Dessert: mango sorbet; mango sticky rice pudding.

Watch out for

▶▶ Thai red and green curries (high in saturated fat from coconut milk); egg fried rice; fish cakes; spring rolls; prawn crackers; sweet and sour dishes.

What should I drink?

▶▶ Drink with a difference: iced tea – served sweet to counteract the hot cuisine.

Eat Well Live Long

Consultant nutritionists
Suzie Ferrie Advanced Accredited Practising Dietitian
Kathy Lewis BCApSc MSc MBA R.Nutr MCIM FRSA, MIHPE

Food writers
Elizabeth Adlam, Sara Altshul, Joanna Blythman, Rose Shepherd

Nutritionist writers
Ursula Arens BSc (Hons) Dip.M
Nicole Berberian BSc (Hons) MSc PG Dip RNutr RD
Sarah Bernard BSc (Hons) ARCS MSc RNutr
Dr Carol Sadler RNutr

Project editor Samantha Kent
Cover designer Melanie Young
Indexer Diane Harriman
Senior production controller Martin Milat

READER'S DIGEST GENERAL BOOKS

Editorial Director Lynn Lewis
Managing Editor Rosemary McDonald
Design Manager Donna Heldon

Eat Well Live Long is published by
Reader's Digest (Australia) Pty Limited
80 Bay Street, Ultimo, NSW, 2007
www.readersdigest.com.au; www.readersdigest.co.nz;
www.rdasia.com;

First published in 2013 in the United Kingdom for The Reader's
Digest Association Inc., under the supervision of Pegasus Regional
Limited. *Eat Well Live Long* is owned and under licence from
The Reader's Digest Association, Inc.

This edition first published 2014

Copyright © Reader's Digest (Australia) Pty Limited 2014
Copyright © Reader's Digest Association Far East Limited 2014
Philippines Copyright © Reader's Digest Association Far East
Limited 2014

All rights reserved. No part of this book may be reproduced, stored
in a retrieval system, or transmitted in any form or by any means,
electronic, electrostatic, magnetic tape, mechanical, photocopying,
recording or otherwise, without permission in writing from the
publishers.

® Reader's Digest and The Digest are registered trademarks of
The Reader's Digest Association, Inc.

National Library of Australia Cataloguing-in-Publication entry
Title: Eat well live long.
ISBN: 978-1-922085-30-6 (hardback)
Notes: Includes index.
Subjects: Nutrition. Diet. Food.
Other Authors/Contributors: Reader's Digest (Australia)
Dewey Number: 613.2

Prepress by Colourpedia, Sydney
Printed and bound by Leo Paper Products, China

We are interested in receiving your comments on the content of
this book. Write to: The Editor, General Books Editorial, Reader's
Digest (Australia) Pty Limited, GPO Box 4353, Sydney, NSW 2001,
or email us at: bookeditors.au@readersdigest.com

Illustrations for *Eat Well Live Long* were supplied by the following
agencies & the following abbreviations are also used:
t = top; c = centre; b = bottom; l = left; r = right

Apple image (Expert Opinion, repeats throughout): Thinkstock;
Thumbs up & down image (True or False, repeats throughout):
Thinkstock/iStockphoto; Newspaper image (Food News, repeats
throughout): iStockphoto

Front cover Shutterstock tl & bl
Back cover Shutterstock bl, bc & br, background
Spine Shutterstock t & b

Getty Images 2–3, 8–9, 10–11, 12, 14, 17, 18, 21, 25 t,
30–31, 33, 43, 49 r, 52, 60, 65, 76, 82–83, 89, 91, 94, 96, 111,
114, 118, 130–1, 133, 134–5, 147, 148, 154, 155, 161 t & b,
162, 163, 164–5, 165 br, 167, 168, 174 b, 175, 176, 199 b,
206, 207, 214, 219, 225, 227, 233, 236, 243, 245, 246, 277

Getty/StockFood 4–5, 41, 71, 84, 95, 99, 106–7, 113, 141,
149, 153, 157, 159, 165 c, 177, 181, 182, 183, 184, 185 l,
187, 189 b, 191, 194, 202, 205, 220–1, 222–3, 226, 229, 230,
234–5, 237, 240–1, 244, 247, 248, 249, 250, 252, 253, 256,
257, 258, 259, 262, 263, 265, 266, 271, 273, 275, 276, 279,
281, 286, 290–1, 293, 294–5, 301, 302, 303, 304–5

Thinkstock iStockphoto 6–7, 13, 15, 19, 23, 26–27, 35, 39,
42, 44 bl & br, 48 cr & r, 49 l & c, 50, 55 l & r, 56, 57, 61, 63,
66, 70, 74 b, 86, 92, 93, 101, 102, 103, 104, 105, 110, 112,
116, 117 both, 119 t, 120 cl, 120 b (all), 122–3, 124–5, 126
l, 145, 146 t, 151, 156, 160, 164, 165 tr, 166, 170–1, 172 t,
173, 174 t, 185 br, 186, 189 t, 192, 193, 199 t, 203, 209, 210,
212, 213, 218, 232, 254, 264, 266–7, 268, 269, 283, 284–5,
288 tl, 292–3, 295, PhotoObjects.net 16; Hemera 26 tr, bl &
br; 28 t & cr; 28–29; 87 all; Photodisc 37; Wavebreak Media
65; BananaStock 68; Stockbyte 77, 80–81, 115, 142, 169, 197;
Lifesize 100; Top Photo Group 137; Digital Vision 152 r; Dorling
Kindersley 196; F1online 208; Fuse 211 t; Purestock 215;
Photos.com 286–7; Wavebreak Media 288–9; Goodshoot 306–7

iStockphoto 20, 22, 59, 72, 75, 78, 85, 109, 170, 171, 178–9,
200, 270–1

Shutterstock 25 b, 34, 36, 44 tr, 45 l, 46, 48 l, 48 cl, 51, 54,
67, 79, 88, 90, 119 b, 120 tl, 126 r, 128–9, 144 both, 146 b,
152, 172 b, 188, 195, 198, 201, 204, 211 b, 216, 251, 255,
260, 267, 272, 282

The information in this book should not be substituted for,
or used to alter, medical treatment without your doctor's
advice. Readers are recommended to consult a qualified
medical specialist for individual advice. The writers,
researchers, editors and publishers of this work cannot
be held liable for any errors and omissions, or actions that
may be taken as a consequence of information contained
within this work.

To order additional copies of *Eat Well Live Long*, please contact us at:
www.readersdigest.com.au or phone 1300 300 030 (Australia)
www.readersdigest.co.nz or phone 0800 400 060 (New Zealand)
or email us at customerservice@readersdigest.com.au

Concept code: US 6514/IC
Product code: 041-5329